Transplant Immunology

Transplant Immunology

EDITED BY

Xian Chang Li, MD, PhD

Professor of Immunology/Surgery, Weill Cornell Medical College,
Cornell University, New York, NY
Director, Immunobiology and Transplant Science, Houston Methodist Hospital,
Texas Medical Center, Houston, TX, USA

and

Anthony M. Jevnikar, MSc, MD, FRCP(C)

Professor of Medicine, Surgery, Microbiology & Immunology
Western University, Director Transplantation Nephrology
Director Matthew Mailing Centre for Translational Transplant Studies
London Health Sciences Centre, London, ON, Canada

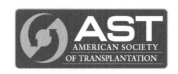

WILEY Blackwell

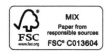
MIX
Paper from
responsible sources
FSC® C013604
www.fsc.org

Contents

Contributors

Andrew B. Adams, MD
Department of Surgery, Emory Transplant Center, Emory University School of Medicine, Atlanta, USA

Maria-Luisa Alegre, MD, PhD
Department of Medicine, Section of Rheumatology, Gwen Knapp Center for Lupus and Immunology Research, The University of Chicago, Chicago, USA

Agnes M. Azimzadeh, PhD
Department of Surgery, Microbiology and Immunology, University of Maryland School of Medicine, Baltimore, USA

William M. Baldwin III, MD, PhD
Department of Immunology, Cleveland Clinic Lerner College of Medicine, Department of Pathology, Case Western Reserve University School of Medicine, Cleveland, USA

Jonathan S. Bromberg, MD, PhD
Department of Surgery, Microbiology and Immunology, University of Maryland School of Medicine, Baltimore, USA

J. Michael Cecka, PhD
UCLA Immunogenetics Center, Department of Pathology and Laboratory Medicine, David Geffen School of Medicine at UCLA, Los Angeles, USA

Anil Chandraker, MD, FASN, FRCP
Transplant Research Center, Renal Division, Brigham and Women's Hospital, Harvard Medical School, Boston, USA

Sung Choi, MD
Blood and Marrow Transplantation Program, Department of Internal Medicine, Division of Hematology/Oncology, University of Michigan Comprehensive Cancer Center, Ann Arbor, USA

Anita S. Chong, PhD
Department of Surgery, Section of Transplantation, The University of Chicago, Chicago, USA

Yaozhong Ding, PhD
Department of Surgery, Microbiology and Immunology, University of Maryland School of Medicine, Baltimore, USA

Gunilla Einecke, MD
Department of Nephrology, Hannover Medical School, Hannover, Germany

Robert L. Fairchild, PhD
Department of Immunology, Cleveland Clinic Lerner College of Medicine, Department of Pathology, Case Western Reserve University School of Medicine, Cleveland, USA

Philip F. Halloran, MD, PhD
Alberta Transplant Applied Genomics Centre, Department of Medicine, Division of Nephrology and Transplant Immunology, University of Alberta, Edmonton, Canada

Choli Hartono, MD
Department of Medicine, Weill Cornell Medical College, New York, USA

Timm Heinbokel, MD
Division of Transplant Surgery and Transplant Surgery Research Laboratory, Brigham and Women's Hospital, Harvard Medical School, Boston, USA

Yiming Huang, PhD
Institute for Cellular Therapeutics, University of Louisville, Louisville, and Duke University, Raleigh, USA

Suzanne T. Ildstad, MD
Institute for Cellular Therapeutics, Jewish Hospital Distinguished Professor of Transplantation, Distinguished University Scholar, Department of Surgery, Physiology, Immunology, University of Louisville, Louisville and Duke University, Raleigh, USA

Haofeng Ji, MD
Dumont-UCLA Transplantation Center, Division of Liver and Pancreas Transplantation, Department of Surgery, David Geffen School of Medicine at UCLA, Los Angeles, USA

Bibo Ke, PhD
Dumont-UCLA Transplantation Center, Division of Liver and Pancreas Transplantation, Department of Surgery, David Geffen School of Medicine at UCLA, Los Angeles, USA

Allan D. Kirk, MD, PhD
Department of Surgery, Emory Transplant Center, Emory University School of Medicine, Atlanta and Department of Surgery, Duke University School of Medicine, Durham, USA

William H. Kitchens, MD
Department of Surgery, Emory Transplant Center, Emory University School of Medicine, Atlanta, USA

Chatchai Kreepala, MD
Alberta Transplant Applied Genomics Centre, Department of Medicine,
Division of Nephrology and Transplant Immunology, University of Alberta,
Edmonton, Canada

Jerzy W. Kupiec-Weglinski, MD, PhD
Dumont-UCLA Transplantation Center, Division of Liver and Pancreas
Transplantation, Department of Surgery, David Geffen School of Medicine
at UCLA, Los Angeles, USA

Fadi G. Lakkis, MD
Thomas E. Starzl Transplantation Institute, Departments of Surgery, Immunology, and
Medicine, University of Pittsburgh, Pittsburgh, USA

Jason R. Lees, PhD
Department of Surgery, Microbiology and Immunology, University of Maryland School
of Medicine, Baltimore, USA

Guangxiang Liu, MD
Division of Transplant Surgery and Transplant Surgery Research Laboratory, Brigham
and Women's Hospital, Harvard Medical School, Boston, USA

Denise J. Lo, MD
Department of Surgery, Emory Transplant Center, Emory University School of Medicine,
Atlanta, USA

Alexandre Loupy, MD
Kidney Transplant Department, Necker Hospital APHP and INSERM UMR 970,
Epidemiology, PARCC Cardiovascular Research Institute, Paris, France

Jonathan S. Maltzman, MD, PhD
Department of Medicine, University of Pennsylvania, Philadelphia, PA, USA

Roslyn B. Mannon, MD
Division of Nephrology, Department of Medicine, University of Alabama at Birmingham,
Birmingham, USA

Thangamani Muthukumar, MD
Department of Medicine, Weill Cornell Medical College, New York, USA

Isam W. Nasr, MD
Thomas E. Starzl Transplantation Institute, Departments of Surgery, Immunology, and
Medicine, University of Pittsburgh, Pittsburgh, USA

Kenneth A. Newell, MD, PhD
Department of Surgery, Emory Transplant Center, Emory University School of Medicine,
Atlanta, USA

Rupert Oberhuber, MD
Division of Transplant Surgery and Transplant Surgery Research Laboratory, Brigham and Women's Hospital, Harvard Medical School, Boston, USA

Raja Rajalingam, PhD
UCLA Immunogenetics Center, Department of Pathology and Laboratory Medicine, David Geffen School of Medicine at UCLA, Los Angeles, USA

Kadiyala Ravindra, MD
Institute for Cellular Therapeutics, University of Louisville, Louisville, and Duke University, Raleigh, USA

Pavan Reddy, MD
Blood and Marrow Transplantation Program, Department of Internal Medicine, Division of Hematology/Oncology, University of Michigan Comprehensive Cancer Center, Ann Arbor, USA

Elaine F. Reed, PhD
UCLA Immunogenetics Center, Department of Pathology and Laboratory Medicine, David Geffen School of Medicine at UCLA, Los Angeles, USA

Leonardo V. Riella, MD, PhD
Transplant Research Center, Renal Division, Brigham and Women's Hospital, Harvard Medical School, Boston, USA

David M. Rothstein, MD
Department of Medicine, Surgery and Immunology, Starzl Transplant Institute, University of Pittsburgh, Pittsburgh, USA

Joana Sellarés, MD
Alberta Transplant Applied Genomics Centre, Department of Medicine, Division of Nephrology and Transplant Immunology, University of Alberta, Edmonton, Canada

Haval Shirwan, PhD
Institute for Cellular Therapeutics, University of Louisville, Louisville, and Duke University, Raleigh, USA

Charles A. Su, MD
Department of Immunology, Cleveland Clinic Lerner College of Medicine, Department of Pathology, Case Western Reserve University School of Medicine, Cleveland, USA

Manikkam Suthanthiran, MD
Department of Medicine, Weill Cornell Medical College, New York, USA

Angus Thomson, PhD
Department of Medicine, Surgery and Immunology, Starzl Transplant Institute, University of Pittsburgh, Pittsburgh, USA

Stefan G. Tullius, MD, PhD
Division of Transplant Surgery and Transplant Surgery Research Laboratory, Brigham and Women's Hospital, Harvard Medical School, Boston, USA

Yoichiro Uchida, MD, PhD
Dumont-UCLA Transplantation Center, Division of Liver and Pancreas Transplantation, Department of Surgery, David Geffen School of Medicine at UCLA, Los Angeles, USA

Tonya J. Webb, PhD
Department of Microbiology and Immunology, Marlene and Stewart Greenebaum Cancer Center, University of Maryland School of Medicine, Baltimore, USA

Qiang Zeng, MD
Thomas E. Starzl Transplantation Institute, Departments of Surgery, Immunology, and Medicine, University of Pittsburgh, Pittsburgh, USA

Yuan Zhai, PhD
Dumont-UCLA Transplantation Center, Division of Liver and Pancreas Transplantation, Department of Surgery, David Geffen School of Medicine at UCLA, Los Angeles, USA

Qiuheng Zhang, PhD
UCLA Immunogenetics Center, Department of Pathology and Laboratory Medicine, David Geffen School of Medicine at UCLA, Los Angeles, USA

Foreword

In hindsight, transplantation has played a major role in advancing basic immunology. Prior to the 1940s, immunology was a relatively small discipline and much of it was centred on the observation that infection resulted in specific immunity, which usually prevented a second case of the same disease. Transplantation was studied much later and was established on a scientific basis only in the 1940s and 1950s. Seminal work by Medawar and colleagues showed that the histologic changes as the graft was rejected had the characteristics of a cell-mediated reaction.

In the 1950s, successful transplantation of the kidney as a vascularized organ showed that surgical success could be obtained in grafts between identical twins. In the late 1950s, it was clear that surgeons could transplant kidneys successfully, but kidney transplants between individuals that were genetically disparate failed universally. There was intense interest in the mechanism of graft rejection. Such interest led to remarkable advancements in basic immunology, and spectacular accomplishments were made in the time that followed.

The major histocompatibility complex (MHC) was unravelled in the 1960s by Dausset, Snell, and Benacerraf, which paved the way for tissue typing. This resulted in major improvements in transplant outcomes. The identification of MHC subsequently led to the revelation of how foreign antigens are processed and presented by antigen-presenting cells and how cells use the MHC molecules to communicate with one another (MHC restriction). Importantly, the concept of MHC restriction proves to be a centrepiece in explaining immunity and immune tolerance.

The thymus was discovered as a filter system, admitting to the circulation only lymphocytes that would accept self and eliminating those that could react against the body's own tissues. Further division of lymphocytes into different subsets in the 1970s and 1980s provided tremendous excitement that the immune system could be better understood or manipulated, and transplantation both contributed to and benefited from such endeavours. The overwhelming drive to prevent graft rejection by immune cells led to the development of powerful immunosuppressive drugs. The introduction of cyclosporine A in the late 1980s revolutionized clinical transplantation, and the subsequent advent of FK506, Rapamycin, Cellcept, among others resulted in an explosion in the number of transplants performed and the types of organs transplanted. These drugs, with the initial goal of extending transplant survival, later became quintessential tools with which to study signalling pathways in lymphocytes. This inquiry led to the identification of calcineurin, cycophilin, FKBP, mTOR, and many other signaling molecules that are strategically positioned in lymphocytes for relaying signals from the cell surface to the nucleus. These drugs are instrumental in illuminating how T cells are activated, and therefore greatly enriched our understanding of the immune mechanisms.

In the past 50 years, organ transplantation has certainly come a long way and has enabled its coat-tails to be grabbed by immunologists who have been able to fly and make extraordinary advancements. Going forward, One of the outcomes of transplant success is the shortage of donors; the better the results, the greater the pressure for patients to be treated by organ transplantation. Expanding the donor pool will present a new set of challenges to immunology research. The "Holy Grail" of tolerance embodies the promises of transplantation as a therapeutic modality as well as the challenges in therapeutic reprogramming of the immune system. It can be said that transplantation remains well positioned to make significant impact on the advance of basic immunology in the future.

Sir Roy Calne, MD
Professor of Surgery
University of Cambridge, UK

Preface

There has been an explosion of new information in immunology and it is increasingly difficult to remain current in any one area. We began this project as a means to collate the insights and information most relevant to transplantation, in a form that would be useful to a broad range of readers. Initially, we had aimed it for those working primarily in clinical transplantation and were in need of broad overviews, as evidenced by the large numbers that attend "Transplant Immunology for the Clinician" at international meetings. However, we realized that there was also a need for information on the aspects of transplant immunology for researchers outside of their primary area of interest. Finally, there remains a need for books with fully annotated illustrations that present principles in simple models, for the purpose of education. We hope that we have been able to provide value for all these audiences.

The chapters in this book have been written by key leaders in their respective areas. There have been several revisions even prior to publication to keep the material as up to date as possible in a textbook. The editors sincerely thank all of the authors for their commitment to this book and the hard work required to summarize their extensive knowledge and insights within the confines of a textbook. We believe the authors have done an extraordinary job on their chapters.

There will be an electronic link with this book that will allow for updated material to be added. We realize that at some time in the future, "books" in their traditional form will evolve to allow real-time updating and provide immediate access to a great wealth of more detailed information for those readers that require more depth. The editors hope that this book will form the foundation for future versions that will follow that evolutionary path.

Finally, the editors would like to sincerely thank Wiley for their support of this book and to the American Society of Transplantation, where the origin of this project began.

Dr. Xian Chang Li, MD, PhD
Dr. Anthony M. Jevnikar, MSc, MD, FRCP(C)

About the companion website

This book is accompanied by a companion website:

www.wiley.com/go/li/transplantimmunology

The website includes:

PPTs of all figures from the book for downloading

CHAPTER 1

Tissues and organs of the immune system

Isam W. Nasr, Qiang Zeng, and Fadi G. Lakkis

Thomas E. Starzl Transplantation Institute, Departments of Surgery, Immunology, and Medicine, University of Pittsburgh, Pittsburgh, USA

CHAPTER OVERVIEW

- Lymphoid organs or tissues are specialized anatomic compartments where lymphocytes develop, reside, and function.

- Primary lymphoid tissues are the sites where lymphocytes undergo development, education, and maturation.

- Secondary lymphoid tissues are the main sites where naïve lymphocytes engage foreign antigens to mount a primary immune response.

- Tertiary lymphoid tissues are secondary lymphoid tissue-like structures that are induced at sites of chronic inflammation, and the function of such structures is not fully defined.

- Memory immune responses can occur outside secondary lymphoid tissues. Memory T cells can also be maintained without secondary lymphoid tissues.

- Primary and secondary lymphoid tissues are also necessary for tolerance induction and maintenance.

Introduction

It is the nature of scientists to be perpetually occupied with questions like "where," "how," and "why" things happen the way they do. Immunologists, in particular, are keen on answering the "where" question as it is central to understanding how immune cells are generated, what is required for their maturation, and whether they might mount productive responses against foreign antigens or not. The immune system is a *bona fide* organ system comprising primary and secondary lymphoid tissues (Figure 1.1). Primary lymphoid tissues (the bone marrow and thymus) specialize in generating immune cells from hematopoietic progenitors and transforming immature cells into mature lymphocytes

---

Transplant Immunology, First Edition. Edited by Xian Chang Li and Anthony M. Jevnikar.
© 2016 John Wiley & Sons, Ltd. Published 2016 by John Wiley & Sons, Ltd.
Copyright ® American Society of Transplantation 2016.
Companion website: www.wiley.com/go/li/transplantimmunology

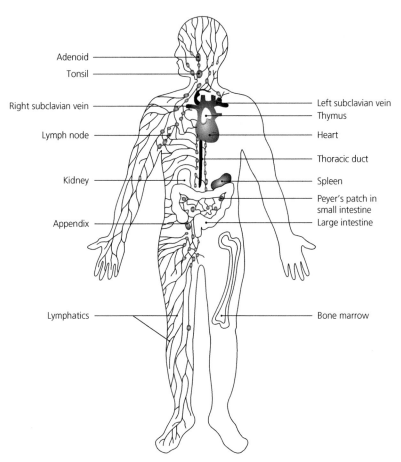

Figure 1.1 Lymphoid tissues of the human body. The primary lymphoid tissues are the bone marrow and thymus. The secondary lymphoid tissues consist of lymph nodes, the spleen, and MALTs. Lymph nodes are arranged in strings along lymphatic vessels where they trap antigens and cells traveling in the lymph. The spleen intercepts antigens and cells circulating in the bloodstream. MALT includes the Peyer's patches, adenoids, tonsils, and appendix. Cells traveling in the lymphatic system re-enter the blood circulation via the thoracic duct. Source: Redrawn from Murphy (2011). Reproduced by permission of Garland Science/Taylor & Francis LLC.

with high specificity to foreign antigens (non-self) but not "self antigens." Secondary lymphoid tissues, namely the spleen, lymph nodes, and mucosa-associated lymphoid tissues (MALTs) on the other hand are organized structures that are strategically located throughout the body to trap foreign antigens and ensure that they are best presented to T and B lymphocytes. The ability of an animal to mount a productive immune response is therefore critically dependent on the presence of the primary and secondary lymphoid tissues as well as the coordinated migration of immune cells into and out of these tissues.

This chapter will provide a comprehensive overview of the anatomy and function of primary and secondary lymphoid tissues and consider their roles in both transplant rejection and tolerance. Tertiary lymphoid tissues, which are secondary lymphoid tissue-like structures that are induced at sites of chronic inflammation, will also be discussed as they are thought to influence allograft outcomes. Controversies and unresolved questions will be highlighted where appropriate to encourage future investigations.

Primary lymphoid tissues

Primary lymphoid tissues are sites where T cells and B cells develop and mature, and mainly include the bone marrow and the thymus in mammals.

Bone marrow

The bone marrow is the site where both red and white blood cells are generated, by a process known as hematopoiesis. The adult human has two types of bone marrow: the red marrow, in which hematopoiesis is actively taking place, and the yellow marrow, consisting mainly of fat cells and lacking hematopoietic activity. At birth, all marrow is red but it is slowly replaced by yellow marrow over time. By adulthood, red marrow is restricted to flat bones (cranium, sternum, vertebrae, pelvis, and scapulae) and the epiphyseal ends of long bones (e.g., the femur and humerus), while the remaining marrow cavities are being occupied by fat cells. The bone marrow also provides a place where subsets of lymphocytes (both T cells and B cells), especially those with memory phenotypes reside.

Structure

Histologically, the red marrow consists of hematopoietic islands; such islands are mixed with fat cells, surrounded by vascular sinusoids, and interspersed throughout a meshwork of trabecular bone (Figure 1.2). The hematopoietic islands are organized into three-dimensional structures that provide optimal microenvironment for hematopoiesis. They contain blood cell precursors at different stages of maturation, stromal reticular cells, endothelial cells, macrophages, osteoblasts, osteoclasts, and the extracellular matrix. Both hematopoietic and nonhematopoietic cells in the islands orchestrate blood cell maturation through cell–cell contacts as well as production of growth factors, cytokines, and chemokines. Mature blood cells enter the circulation by migrating through the discontinuous basement membrane and between the endothelial cells of the vascular sinusoids.

Function

Hematopoietic stem cells (HSCs) are a pluripotent self-renewing cell type in the bone marrow that give rise to progenitor cells. These progenitor cells in turn generate all cells of the megakaryocytic (platelet), erythroid (RBC), myeloid,

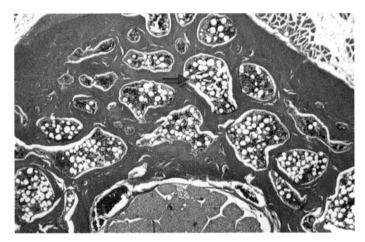

Figure 1.2 Structure of the bone marrow. Example of red bone marrow (vertebra). Arrow points to a hematopoietic tissue island. Note fat cells (white globules) admixed with hematopoietic cells. Trabecular bone fills the space between islands. Source: Reprinted from Travlos (2006). Reproduced by permission of SAGE publications.

and lymphoid lineages (Figure 1.3). Myeloid cells (monocytes, dendritic cells or DCs, neutrophils, basophils, and eosinophils), natural killer (NK) cells, and B lymphocytes develop in the bone marrow, whereas T cell progenitors (pre-thymocytes) migrate to the thymus where they undergo further maturation (see section "Thymus"). The bone marrow also contains mesenchymal stem cells that give rise to nonhematopoietic tissues such as adipocytes, chondrocytes, osteocytes, and myoblasts. Mesenchymal stem cells have attracted considerable interest among transplant immunologists because of their immunosuppressive properties and prolonged survival features when adoptively transferred in select models.

The bone marrow is the site where most stages of B cell maturation occur in mammals. B cell development in the bone marrow proceeds in a stepwise fashion from pro-B cells to pre-B cells, and lastly to immature B cells. During maturation in the bone marrow, B cells rearrange their immunoglobulin genes and express cell-surface IgM (the B cell receptor for antigen). These steps require close interactions with bone marrow stromal cells, which provide critical adhesion molecules, growth factors, chemokines, and cytokines (e.g., Flt3 ligand, thrombopoietin, CXCL12, and IL-7). Finally, autoreactive immature B cells are "weeded out" in the bone marrow through either clonal deletion or receptor editing before they are allowed into the circulation and complete their maturation in secondary lymphoid tissues.

In addition to serving as a primary lymphoid organ, the bone marrow is also a reservoir for mature myeloid and lymphoid cells. The bone marrow contains large numbers of neutrophils and monocytes that are mobilized into the circulation when needed (e.g., after infection). It is also the homing site

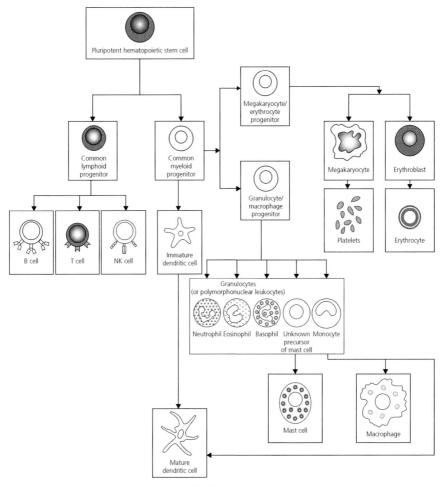

Figure 1.3 Ontogeny of immune cells. Cells of the immune system arise from pluripotent HSCs in the bone marrow. The common lymphoid progenitor gives rise to B cells, T cells, and NK cells. The common myeloid progenitor gives rise to dendritic cells (DCs), monocytes, neutrophils, eosinophils, and basophils.

for mature plasma cells, which are maintained in the bone marrow through the action of IL-6. Plasma cells are the principal source of antibodies in sensitized transplant recipients; therefore, investigators addressing the pathogenesis of antibody (historically referred to as "humoral") rejection are increasingly interested in these bone marrow-resident plasma cells. There is also strong evidence that memory T cells home to or reside in the bone marrow where they can be activated by antigens. Other experiments have suggested that activation of naïve T cells could occur in the bone marrow under certain circumstances, raising the possibility that the bone marrow may additionally serve as a secondary lymphoid tissue (see section "Secondary lymphoid tissues").

Cell trafficking

Cell trafficking is a dynamic process underlying allorecognition and transplantation responses, and remains a potential target in therapeutic strategies. Mature myeloid cells and certain precursor lymphoid cells (pre-thymocytes, immature B cells) migrate out of the bone marrow and enter the circulation. Conversely, mature lymphocytes (e.g., plasma cells) migrate into the bone marrow. The HSCs are also known to exit and re-enter the bone marrow. These trafficking events are primarily regulated by adhesion molecules and guided by chemokines. The integrin VLA-4, for example, maintains the developing B cells in tight contact with stromal cells by binding to VCAM-1. The chemokine CXCL12, which is produced by stromal reticular cells and osteoblasts, is responsible for retaining HSCs as well as myeloid and lymphoid cells in the bone marrow by binding to its receptor CXCR4. Some individuals with "gain of function" mutations in CXCR4 (e.g., WHIM syndrome) have pan-leukopenia because of increased retention of leukocytes in the bone marrow. Conversely, CXCR4 antagonism with the drug plerixafor mobilizes HSCs and myeloid and lymphoid cells from the bone marrow into the circulation. In the mouse, there is abundant evidence that CCR2 and its ligand CCL2 are responsible for monocytes exiting from the bone marrow into circulation.

Role in rejection and tolerance

The role of the bone marrow in organ transplantation has been studied in the context of tolerance induction. Investigators hoping to achieve solid organ allograft acceptance without immunosuppression have used simultaneous bone marrow and solid organ transplantation from the same donor. In this regimen, recipients receive "partial" myeloablative conditioning, followed by infusion of donor HSCs, with the goal being to induce mixed hematopoietic chimerism (both donor and host cells co-exist). Stable mixed chimerism can be attained in small experimental animals. It is more difficult in nonhuman primates (NHPs) and humans, but does result in long-lasting tolerance to allografts as re-emerging donor-specific B cells and T cells in transplant recipients are deleted or become anergic upon encountering donor antigens in the bone marrow and thymus, respectively. One obstacle to the widespread clinical use of the mixed chimerism is the need for toxic myeloablation conditioning prior to HSC infusion, as donor HSC engraftment is dependent on the presence of unoccupied hematopoietic niches or "space" in the recipient's bone marrow. A very small proportion (0.1–1%) of niches are unoccupied under homeostatic conditions, severely limiting the number of exogenous HSCs that could engraft, even if infused in very large numbers. While irradiation and cytotoxic drugs (e.g., cyclophosphamide) have been the mainstay of "freeing up" niches in the recipient, less toxic therapies that target chemokines and chemokine receptors in the bone marrow are currently being investigated. Finally, the bone marrow alone is insufficient for sustaining primary immune responses as seen in mice that lack secondary lymphoid tissues but have an intact bone marrow are severely compromised in their ability to reject a transplanted organ.

Thymus

The thymus is *the* primary lymphoid organ where mature T cells are generated from bone marrow-derived progenitors (pre-thymocytes). The emergence of the thymus in evolution coincides with the emergence of adaptive immunity in jawed fish. In mammals, it is located in the upper anterior thorax above the heart. It owes its name to its lobular shape, which in the eyes of the Greek physician Galen resembled the *thyme* leaf. The thymus was considered to be a nonimmune organ for a long time until seminal work in mice by Jacques F. A. P. Miller and others in the 1960s demonstrated its central role in T lymphocyte development. It was found that removal of the thymus at birth leads to severe immune defects, including the abrogation of skin allograft rejection. Thymectomizing mice that had already reached puberty, on the other hand, had no significant effects on the immune response, indicating that the mature T cell repertoire had completely formed by then. The critical role of the thymus in T cell development in humans was confirmed in individuals with the congenital absence or severe hypoplasia of the thymus (DiGeorge syndrome). These individuals have very few T cells but normal B cell counts. Unlike in mice, removal of the thymus in infants or children does not lead to any obvious immune abnormalities, as T cell development in humans is largely completed prior to birth. Although the human thymus involutes significantly in size after puberty, thymic function persists in adults, especially in those who become lymphopenic secondary to either infection (e.g., HIV) or lymphodepletion (e.g., induction therapy at the time of transplantation).

Structure

Histologically, thymic lobes are made up of two clearly distinguishable areas: the cortex and the medulla and are separated by a highly vascularized corticomedullary border (Figure 1.4). The stroma in both regions consists of a three-dimensional network of thymic epithelial cells (TECs) surrounded by T cells. TECs are known by the acronyms cTECs and mTECs depending on whether they are located in the cortex or medulla, respectively. The cortex is densely populated with immature T cells in various stages of development, while the medulla harbors less tightly packed mature T cells. In addition to T cells, the thymus also contains DCs, macrophages, and B cells. As will be highlighted in the next section, cTECs, mTECs, DCs, and B cells play critical roles in T cell development, selection, and education. The thymic medulla in humans also contains distinct structures known as Hassall's corpuscles that consist of concentric layers of keratinizing epithelium. These structures are a prominent site of T cell apoptosis and of thymic stromal lymphopoeitin (TSLP) production. TSLP is an IL-7-like cytokine believed to activate thymic DC (see section "Function").

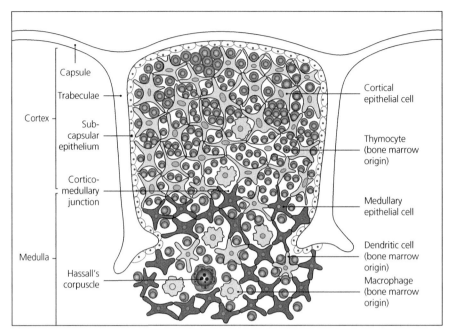

Figure 1.4 Structure of the thymus. The thymus consists of outer (cortical) and central (medullary) regions. Thymocyte maturation and T cell selection occur in both the cortex and medulla, with the outer cortical layer containing mainly proliferating, immature thymocytes and the deeper cortical and medullary areas containing immature T cells undergoing selection. Cortical and medullary epithelial cells, as well as bone-marrow derived DCs and macrophages, participate in the selection process. Source: Redrawn from Murphy (2011). Reproduced by permission of Garland Science/Taylor & Francis LLC.

Function

The thymus is the primary site where T cell maturation and selection occur. The end result of these processes is the generation of a mature T cell repertoire that recognizes myriad foreign peptides in the context of self-MHC (self-restricted) and yet has been successfully purged of autoreactive T cells. Bone marrow-derived T cell progenitors enter the thymus via venules near the corticomedullary junction and begin their maturation in the thymic cortex where they proliferate extensively, acquire classical T cell markers (e.g., the CD4 and CD8 co-receptors), and undergo random rearrangement of T cell receptor (TCR) genes to form mature TCRs. Thymocytes that express functional TCRs then undergo positive and negative selection. Most (>95%) die by "negative selection" because they either fail to sufficiently bind self-MHC and self-peptide complexes, and thus be destined to be poor antigen recognizing cells (leading to immunodeficiency) or bind these complexes too strongly (destined to become potentially autoreactive cells). Only those with proper TCR affinity for self-MHC and peptide complexes are selected to undergo further maturation (positive selection).

T cell selection begins in the cortex but is completed in the medulla, after which mature CD4 and CD8 T cells exit the thymus to enter the blood circulation. Positive selection is mediated by cTECs because they constitutively express both MHC class I and II molecules and can process and present self-peptides. Negative selection is mediated by both cTECs and mTECs for the same reasons mentioned above. Bone marrow-derived DCs are also crucial contributors to both processes. A subset of TECs in the corticomedullary junction is responsible for the production of IL-7, a cytokine critical for T cell survival. Thus, T cells are absent in IL-7 gene knockout mice. Importantly, the expression of a gene called autoimmune regulator (AIRE) allows TECs to present peptides derived from proteins in nonthymic tissues (e.g., insulin). AIRE therefore ensures that autoreactive T cells specific to all possible self-antigens are deleted in the thymus. Humans who harbor AIRE mutations develop autoimmune polyglandular syndrome type I, also known as autoimmune polyendocrinopathy–candidiasis–ectodermal dystrophy (APECED).

In addition to generating mature T cells (mostly with αβ TCRs), the thymus is also indispensable to the production γδ T cells, NKT cells, and natural regulatory T cells (nTreg). γδ T cells originate from the same progenitors as αβ T cells but exit the thymus at an early "double negative" stage (i.e., they lack both CD4 and CD8 expression) and populate epithelial sites such as the gut and skin. NKT cells are NK-like T cells that express an invariant TCR and are positively selected in the thymus by the nonclassical MHC molecule CD1d. Their main function is recognition of glycolipids produced by certain microbes such as mycobacteria. nTreg are CD4+ T cells that express conventional αβ TCR with an intermediate affinity to self-MHC and self-peptide complexes (thus, they are positively selected). They regulate immune responses by suppressing the function of effector T cells. The discovery of thymic-derived nTreg came from elegant observations in mice and humans. Although thymectomy at birth led to severe immunodeficiency in mice, immunologists noted that thymectomy on the third post-natal day paradoxically caused severe autoimmunity. The autoimmunity could be attributed to the absence of nTreg. It was later discovered that the transcription factor Foxp3 is required for the development of Treg and thus loss of function Foxp3 mutations in mice and humans cause fatal autoimmune disease (scurfy in mice and immunodysregulation, polyendocrinopathy, enteropathy, X-linked syndrome, or IPEX in humans).

Cell trafficking

Chemokines play a key role in guiding cell trafficking in the thymus. The entry of progenitor cells from the bone marrow into the thymus is dependent on the chemokines CCL21 and CCL25, which bind the receptors CCR7 and CCR9, respectively. The chemokines CCL21 and CXCL12, the ligand for CXCR4, direct the migration of immature thymocytes during their maturation journey through the thymic cortex and medulla. Disruption of CCL21 expression causes defective deletion of autoreactive T cells. The chemokine that is central to the emigration of mature T cells from the thymus into the blood is CXCL12. CXCL12 repels mature T cells out of the thymus, which contrasts to its function in retaining myeloid and lymphoid cells in the bone marrow (see section "Cell trafficking"). Emigration also requires binding of sphingosine-1-phosphate (S1P), which is present in high concentrations in the blood and lymph, to its receptor $S1PR_1$ on mature T cells. This interaction drives mature T cells to the periphery and alteration of cell trafficking through this pathway in transplantation has been tested in transplantation using the S1P agonist FTY720, which had adverse effects in transplant patients and was not further developed for this indication.

Role in rejection and tolerance

In solid organ transplantation, the thymus is exploited for tolerance induction because it is indispensable to the generation of nTreg and for the negative selection of newly developing T cells (commonly referred to as central tolerance). As mentioned earlier, unless performed at birth, thymectomy does not prevent allograft rejection. However, thymectomy around day 3 after birth eliminates nTreg and prevents graft acceptance in mouse models in which Tregs are needed for tolerance. In the mixed hematopoietic chimerism approach, the process of thymic T cell selection is recapitulated; DCs derived from donor HSC induce the apoptosis of newly developing, donor-reactive T cells in the thymus, leading to central tolerance. The key role of thymus in tolerance has prompted some investigators to co-transplant thymus and kidney or heart (referred to as thymo-kidney, thymo-heart or thymo-islet) grafts from the same donor to MHC-mismatched recipients. The rationale behind this procedure rests on the ability of epithelial cells of the thymic graft to express donor antigens, including donor MHC, and to delete donor-reactive T cells from the recipients, thus leading to donor-specific, central tolerance. Finally, the thymus also plays a role in the maintenance of allograft tolerance in some animal models by either providing a steady source of nTreg or a site for continual negative T cell selection.

Secondary lymphoid tissues

After exiting the thymus and bone marrow, mature naïve T and B cells populate the secondary lymphoid tissues, which include not only compartmentalized or encapsulated tissues such as the lymph nodes, spleen, tonsils, appendix, and Peyer's patches of the small intestine but also other lymphoid structures that are relatively less well delineated. Secondary lymphoid tissues are strategically located throughout the body at sites where antigen and antigen-presenting cells (APCs) are efficiently concentrated. Specifically, lymph nodes drain distinct organs or geographical areas of the body via afferent lymphatic vessels, the spleen traps antigens that enter the blood circulation, and MALTs capture antigens at mucosal surfaces (Figure 1.1). This arrangement maximizes the chance that antigen-specific T and B cells, which exist in very low frequencies (about 1 in 100,000 T cells express the TCR specific for an individual antigen), encounter their cognate antigens. Importantly, the architecture of secondary lymphoid tissues is such that contacts between APCs, T cells, and B cells occur not only in the most effective way but also in the correct sequence to initiate productive responses. T and B cells that have been successfully activated by antigens then leave secondary lymphoid tissues to enter the blood circulation and eventually the tissues to execute their function. Secondary lymphoid tissues are the quintessential sites for initiating primary immune responses.

We will focus on lymph nodes, spleen, and Peyer's patches and discuss their direct relevance to solid organ transplantation. The roles of secondary lymphoid tissues in rejection and tolerance will be discussed collectively at the end of the section.

Lymph nodes

Lymph nodes are encapsulated, bean-shaped structures distributed along the lymphatic system throughout the body. The lymphatic system drains the extracellular fluid from the tissues and returns it to the blood via the thoracic and right lymphatic ducts in the chest. Antigens and migrating APCs are present in the lymphatic fluidand, therefore, lymph nodes are ideally positioned to capture the antigens arriving via the lymph for presentation to T and B cells in the nodes. Lymphocytes enter the lymph nodes through specialized blood vessels known as high endothelial venules (HEVs) that are localized to specific areas within the lymph nodes (see section "Structure" below). Lymph nodes are classified as either peripheral or mucosal, based on subtle differences in the adhesion molecules they express as well as their function (see sections "Function" and "Cell trafficking and lymph nodes"). Peripheral lymph nodes encompass most lymph nodes in the body, while mucosal lymph nodes include the mesenteric, cervical, sacral lymph nodes as well as bronchial lymph nodes, which participate in mucosal immune responses.

Structure

From a histological perspective, lymph nodes are organized structures surrounded by a capsule and sinus (Figure 1.5). Lymph flows from the afferent lymphatics into the subcapsular sinus and exits the lymph node through the efferent lymphatic vessel via the medullary sinus. A conduit system lined by fibroblastic reticular cells and collagen, fibrillin, and laminin layers allows lymph-carrying antigens and APCs to penetrate deep into the parenchyma of the lymph node. Antigens diffuse across sinus and conduit walls and are taken up by APCs that reside within lymph nodes or are picked up by DCs that extend cellular processes (dendrites) into the lymph. Mature APCs carrying antigens that reach lymph nodes from peripheral tissues via lymphatic vessels migrate across the sinus and conduit walls and then localize in T cell areas under the guidance of chemokines (see section "Cell trafficking and lymph nodes").

A point of entry for T and B cells to lymph nodes is the highly specialized HEV. HEV are post-capillary vessels unique to lymph nodes and Peyer's patches. They are lined by tall, cuboidal endothelial cells, which express adhesion molecules and chemokines necessary for the transmigration of T and B cells (see section "Cell trafficking and lymph nodes"). Importantly, T and B cells are not randomly distributed in the lymph node but are highly organized into two anatomic regions in the cortex. B cells are grouped within follicles in the outer cortex, while T cells are more diffusely distributed in the paracortical (or deep cortical) areas underneath the B cell follicles. The areas with T and B cells also contain stromal cells, macrophages, and DCs. A network of follicular dendritic cells (FDCs) located in the B cell follicles is specialized to capture antigens or antigen–antibody complexes. They play an important role in the formation of germinal centers, which are the central part of lymphoid follicles where memory B cells and antibody-producing plasma cells are generated (see section "Function"). FDCs are distinct from other DCs in that they are not derived from bone marrow precursors; they neither express MHC class II molecules nor do they have phagocytic activities. The innermost region of the lymph node consists of medullary cords that protrude into the medullary sinus (Figure 1.5); such medullary cords are rich in macrophages and plasma cells.

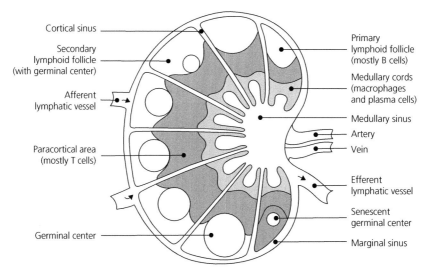

Figure 1.5 Structure of the lymph node. A cross-section of a lymph node reveals the outer cortex where B cell follicles reside and the paracortical (or deeper cortical) areas where the T cell zones are. The medulla (or medullary cords) are rich in plasma cells and macrophages. Lymph-carrying antigens and DCs arrive from peripheral tissues via the afferent lymphatic vessel and empties into the cortical sinus. Activated lymphocytes leave lymph nodes via the efferent lymphatic vessel and eventually enter the bloodstream via the thoracic ducts. Source: Redrawn from Murphy (2011). Reproduced by permission of Garland Science/Taylor & Francis LLC.

Function

Lymph nodes are the principal sites where naïve T and B cells are exposed to antigens to initiate activation and maturation. Mice that lack lymph nodes have abnormalities in their adaptive cellular and antibody immune responses. Lymph nodes are also crucial for the maintenance of naïve and memory T cells, especially those of the CD4+ subpopulation. This is due to the presentation of self-antigens by MHC on lymph node-resident DC, which provides survival signals to T cells. Lymph nodes and the spleen are also the sites where immature B cells that emerge from the bone marrow complete their final maturation during which autoreactive B cells that bind abundant self-antigens are deleted and purged.

The activation of naïve T cells occurs in the cortical zones (T cell zone), whereas B cell priming occurs in the follicles in the outer cortex. Classical imaging studies have established that T and B cell activation in lymph nodes occurs following a sequence of events. Naïve T and B cells enter lymph nodes via HEV and migrate to the T cell zones and B cell follicles, respectively. T cells sample DCs as they journey within the T cell zone. An antigen-specific T cell that encounters its cognate antigen on DCs leads to a protracted contact (or synapse) with the DC, and divides with daughter cells differentiating into effectors. T cells that do not encounter cognate antigen rapidly exit the lymph node via cortical sinuses, eventually returning to the blood via the thoracic duct. Naïve T cells may re-enter other lymph nodes via the lymph. Activated T cells on the other hand are retained for a few days in the lymph node to complete their proliferation and differentiation before exiting. Retention is in part mediated by the membrane lectin CD69 induced on activated T cells. Many follicular T helper cells (referred to as Tfh), however, migrate toward the B cell follicles. B cells activated in the follicles localize to the border between the follicle and the adjacent T cell zone where they are much more likely to interact with helper T cells. This interaction leads to B cell proliferation and differentiation into plasma blasts. Some plasma blasts migrate back to the center of the follicle where they continue to divide and differentiate into memory B cells or antibody-producing plasma cells, forming what is known as germinal centers where immunoglobulin gene rearrangements and affinity maturation occur. Affinity maturation refers to the selection of B cells that produce antibodies with high affinity to antigen. Mature plasma cells arising in germinal centers either migrate to the medullary cords or leave the lymph node altogether. Like T cells, B cells that do not encounter their cognate antigens rapidly exit lymph nodes via the efferent lymphatic vessel and then into the blood.

Cell trafficking and lymph nodes

DC, T cell, and B cell trafficking into, within, and out of lymph nodes is orchestrated by chemokines. DCs express the chemokine receptor CCR7 and migrate from nonlymphoid tissues to lymph nodes in response to the CCR7 ligand CCL19 and CCL21. CCL21 bound to extracellular fibrils in the walls of lymphatic vessels and in the paracortical areas (T cell zones) of the lymph node guides DC migration by a process known as haptokinesis. Naïve T cells and a subset of memory T cells (central memory T cells) also express CCR7; therefore, they co-localize with DCs in the paracortical areas. CCR7 gene knockout mice lack T cell zones and have impaired primary T cell responses. Unlike T cells, naïve B cells express the chemokine receptor CXCR5 and home to follicles in the cortex in response to the chemokine CXCL13. Upon activation by antigens, B cells express CCR7 and migrate toward the periphery of the follicle in response to CCL21 (produced by mature DC) where B cells receive help from activated CD4+ T cells that express CXCR5. Follicular helper T cells (Tfh) also express CXCR5 and reside in B cell follicles in the lymph nodes, spleen, and other secondary lymphoid tissues. Tfh cells participate in B cell activation and germinal center formation. More recently, a subset of regulatory T (Treg) cells known as follicular Treg has been described. These cells inhibit B cell activation and humoral immunity.

The process by which naïve T cells enter lymph nodes via HEV has been well characterized. Initial adhesion of T cells on HEV is mediated by the binding of L-selectin (CD62L) on T cells to the sugar moiety (sulfated sialyl-Lewis^x) of mucin-like molecules (CD34 and GlyCAM-1) on endothelial cells. CD34 and GlyCAM-1 are specific to HEV in peripheral lymph nodes and are referred to as peripheral node addressins (PNAd), while MAdCAM-1 is expressed on endothelial cells in mucosal lymph nodes and Peyer's patches. MAdCAM-1 is the ligand for the integrin $\alpha_4\beta_7$ expressed on gut homing T cells. Firm adhesion and subsequent transendothelial migration of T cells is dependent on the binding of high-affinity LFA-1 on T cells to ICAM-1 on endothelial cells. LFA-1 is a β2 integrin that changes its confirmation from low to high affinity in response to G protein-coupled chemokine receptor signaling. Pertussis toxin, a potent inhibitor of Ga_i, therefore, abolishes T cell entry into lymph nodes. The exit of effector T cells from the lymph node is dependent on sphingosine-1-phospate (S1P), which is also required for the egress of mature T cells from the thymus. The immunosuppressive drug FTY720 is an S1P receptor agonist that causes the retention of activated T cells in secondary lymphoid tissues, presumably by rapid downregulating S1P receptors. Although effective in preventing organ transplant rejection at high doses (but with significant side effects), it is currently approved for the treatment of multiple sclerosis where lower doses appear to be effective and with less side effects.

Spleen

The spleen is a highly vascularized organ that serves several functions. First, it clears aging and abnormal blood cells and platelets in the blood as well as opsonized bacteria and immune complexes. Second, it serves as a site for extramedullary hematopoiesis in conditions where the bone marrow is compromised. Third, it is an organized secondary lymphoid tissue that plays an important role in initiating adaptive immune responses. Unlike lymph nodes, the spleen is not connected to lymphatic vessels but only to the bloodstream. In the absence of the spleen, humans are at higher risk for sepsis caused by encapsulated bacteria such as *Streptococcus pneumoniae*, which are normally opsonized and cleared by the spleen. Splenectomy in experimental animals also leads to certain immunologic defects and has been used clinically in some forms of aggressive solid organ transplant rejection.

Structure

Histologically, the spleen is made up of two areas: the red pulp and white pulp (Figure 1.6). The red pulp consists of large blood-filled venous sinusoids where red blood cells and platelets are removed. The white pulp, on the other hand, carries out the immunologic functions of the spleen. It consists of discrete, organized collections of lymphocytes surrounding arterioles and interspersed among the venous sinusoids of the red pulp. The arterioles of the white pulp branch off from trabecular arteries and are distinct from those that form the red pulp. A cross-section of a white pulp area reveals a central arteriole, a sheath of lymphocytes around the arteriole (also known as the peri-arteriolar lymphoid sheath or PALS), lymphocyte follicles interspersed at intervals along the PALS, and a peri-follicular zone or marginal sinus surrounding the follicles. PALS contain mainly T cells (like the T cell zones of lymph nodes), while the follicles consist primarily of B cells and FDCs. The marginal zone of the follicles is abundant in macrophages, DCs, and a noncirculating population of marginal zone B cells unique to the spleen. The peri-follicular zone (marginal sinus) consists of small blood vessels that fan out from the central arteriole and empty into open blood-filled spaces surrounding the marginal zone of the follicles. The peri-follicular zone is the site of entry of antigens into the white pulp. The central arteriole and the blood spaces of the peri-follicular zone eventually drain into trabecular veins.

Function

Microbes, antigens, and antigen–antibody complexes present in the blood are picked up by macrophages and immature DCs in the marginal zone of the splenic white pulp. Activated DCs migrate to the T cell zones where they prime T cells with internalized and processed antigen. Activated T cells then either leave the spleen via the blood or migrate to the border of the follicles to provide help to B cells. Activated B cells in turn form germinal centers and differentiate into antibody-producing plasma cells and memory B cells. The spleen is also an important site where immature B cells arriving from the bone marrow undergo their final maturation and selection steps.

A distinguishing feature of the spleen is the presence of unique marginal zone macrophage and B cell populations not present in other secondary lymphoid tissues. The marginal zone has an outer ring of marginal zone macrophages and an inner ring of metallophilic macrophages. These macrophages capture a wide variety of pathogens from the blood through specialized surface receptors. Marginal

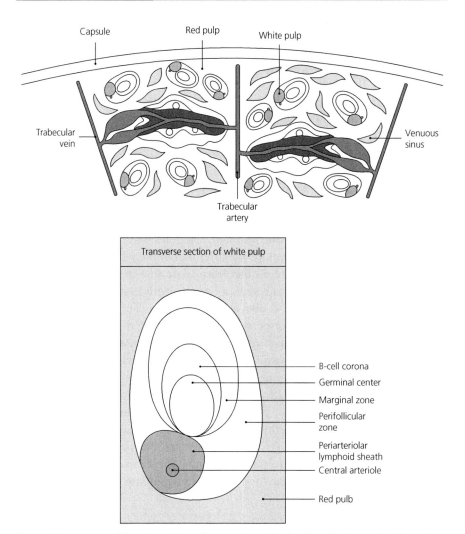

Figure 1.6 Structure of the spleen. The spleen consists of red pulp and white pulp. The red pulp is the site where aging RBCs and platelets are removed. The white pulp is the area in the spleen where lymphocytes are activated. T cells reside in the periarteriolar lymphoid sheaths (PALS) that immediately surround central arterioles while B cells reside in the adjacent follicles (inset). The marginal zone is rich in DCs and macrophages, some unique to the spleen. The spleen has no connections to the lymphatic system. Source: Redrawn from Murphy (2011). Reproduced by permission of Garland Science/Taylor & Francis LLC.

zone B cells are distinct from follicular B cells in that they express high levels of IgM (instead of IgD) and the toll-like receptor (TLR)-9, and have a limited B cell receptor repertoire. They resemble B-1 cells in the peritoneal cavity and likely provide T cell-independent responses to bacterial antigens. The marginal zone, therefore, is often regarded as a defense system strategically positioned to capture pathogens that enter the bloodstream and present them to the adaptive immune cells.

Cell trafficking and the spleen

Unlike lymph nodes, the spleen does not contain HEV and does not have significant PNAd expression. Naïve T cells and B cells enter the splenic white pulp via the marginal sinus and localize to the PALS and follicles in response to the chemokines CCL19/CCL21 and CXCL13, respectively. In contrast to their entry into lymph nodes, the transmigration of lymphocytes into the white pulp is not dependent on G protein-coupled chemokine receptors and the requirement for integrins is not clear. Although ICAM-1, MAdCAM-1, and VCAM-1 are expressed on the endothelial cells lining the marginal sinus, none is absolutely essential for T and B cell entry. The mechanisms and routes of T and B cell egress from the spleen are also not well understood.

Peyer's patches

Peyer's patches are organized lymphoid aggregates present in the intestinal mucosa. They are present in the ileum but are absent in the jejunum and duodenum. Like lymph nodes and the spleen, they consist of B cell follicles and T cell zones (Figure 1.7). The area just underneath the intestinal epithelium is rich in DCs and is known as the subepithelial dome. DCs are attracted there by the chemokines CCL20 and CCL25 (TECK) produced by epithelial cells. The receptors for these chemokines are CCR6 and CCR9, respectively, and are expressed on gut-homing DCs. Peyer's patches do not have afferent lymphatics, so antigen uptake is dependent on specialized epithelial cells called microfold or M cells intercalated between intestinal epithelial cells. M cells lack microvilli and mucus; they are transcytotic, and therefore specialize in transporting antigens (they express receptors for certain pathogens such as Salmonella and HIV) from the gut lumen to Peyer's patches, but are not involved in antigen processing and presentation to T cells. The latter function is carried out by DCs, which acquire antigen directly from the gut lumen via interepithelial dendrites. Naive lymphocytes enter Peyer's patches via HEV that express MAdCAM-1, which binds $\alpha_4\beta_7$ integrin on lymphocytes. Primary immune responses take place in Peyer's patches in a regulated process analogous to what occurs in lymph nodes and the spleen. Newly minted effector cells exit Peyer's patches through efferent lymphatic vessels that drain into the mesenteric lymph nodes. Effector T and B cells eventually reach the circulation via the thoracic duct and re-enter the small intestinal wall via blood vessels. The homing of an effector or memory T cell back to the site where its naïve predecessor was initially primed is an example of "imprinting." In case of the gut, imprinting occurs at the time of naïve T cell activation by DCs in Peyer's patches. Gut DCs induce the expression of $\alpha_4\beta_7$ and CCR9 on effector T cells, mainly through the production of rentinoic acid derived from dietary vitamin A. $\alpha_4\beta_7$ and CCR9 are responsible for the "gut-tropism" of these cells. The $\alpha_4\beta_7$ receptor MAdCAM-1 is expressed on intestinal endothelal cells, while CCR9 ligand CCL25 is secreted by intestinal epithelial cells. It is important to note that not all DC–T cell interactions in the gut induce immune

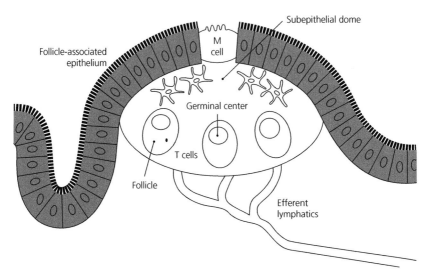

Figure 1.7 Structure of Peyer's patches. Peyer's patches are located in the ileum under the intestinal epithelium. A distinctive feature of Peyer's patches is M cells. They are specialized epithelial cells that transcytose antigens from the gut lumen to the Peyer's patch. The basic architecture of Peyer's patches is similar to that of other secondary lymphoid tissue and is characterized by B cell follicles and more loosely organized T cell zones. Source: Redrawn from Murphy (2011). Reproduced by permission of Garland Science/Taylor & Francis LLC.

responses. In fact, a significant proportion of such interactions are necessary for maintaining tolerance to harmless antigens in the gut, such as those derived from food.

In addition to Peyer's patches, the gut contains a large number of less well-defined DC and lymphocyte aggregates, referred to as "cryptopatches," that are distributed throughout the lamina propria. Cryptopatches are quite plastic; they organize into lymph node-like structures during infection or autoimmunity and participate in the mucosal immune response, but disintegrate back to lose lymphoid aggregates upon resolution of the response. The lamina propria also contains a large number of scattered T and plasma cells. The T cells include effector, memory, and Treg cells, while the lamina propria plasma cells are responsible for IgA production. Another lymphocyte population in the gut residing in the epithelial layer called intra-epithelial lymphocytes (IELs) are virtually all antigen-experienced CD8+ T cells and γδ T cells. They play an important role in host defense against pathogens.

Role of secondary lymphoid tissues in rejection and tolerance

Adaptive immune responses to foreign antigens are mainly initiated within the organized structures of secondary lymphoid tissues. In transplantation immunology, however, controversy has lingered regarding the site where primary alloimmune responses are initiated. While some contend that the alloimmune response follows the same rules as adaptive immunity to nontransplant antigens, others argue that naïve T cells can be activated within the graft itself, as allografts present a unique form of antigenic challenge: they come with their own DCs and more often, their own vasculature, which can also present donor antigens. It was shown that rejection of skin allografts is dependent on the graft having access to host lymphatics whereas the rejection of vascularized allografts is not. The latter observation led to the "peripheral sensitization" concept that donor endothelial cells lining vascularized grafts are capable of directly activating allospecific naïve T cells. This peripheral sensitization hypothesis has been revisited more recently using genetically modified mice that lack secondary lymphoid tissues; for example, *aly/aly* mice that harbor a mutation in the NF-kB-inducing kinase (NIK) or LTβR gene knockout mice that lack the lymphotoxin (LT) receptor central to the ontogeny of lymph nodes and Peyer's patches (see section "Genesis"). The data so far indicate that rejection of vascularized organ allografts by naïve mice is impaired if all secondary lymphoid tissues are absent, with the exception of small intestinal allografts, which provide their own Peyer's patches, and lung allografts in the mouse, which contain bronchus-associated lymphoid tissues (BALTs). Another key exception is the host that harbors alloreactive memory T cells. Unlike naïve T cells, memory T cells home directly to nonlymphoid tissues (e.g., the allograft) and initiate immune responses within the graft. This is particularly important in the field of organ transplantation because the alloreactive T cell repertoire is composed of both naïve and memory T cells. Alloreactive memory T cells are ubiquitous, even in humans who have never been exposed to alloantigens, due to heterogonous immunity (cross-reactivity). Heterogonous immunity refers to the presence of memory T cells specific to microbial antigens that are also alloreactive.

Secondary lymphoid tissues are also important for tolerance induction and maintenance. Transplantation tolerance is an *active* process dependent on the deletion or regulation of mature alloreactive T cells. Both of these phenomena occur predominantly in secondary lymphoid tissues. This is best illustrated by experiments that show that allograft acceptance in mice that lack secondary lymphoid tissues is due to immunologic ignorance and not tolerance. T cells from these mice are not deleted or rendered tolerant because they rapidly precipitate allograft rejection upon transfer to recipients that have intact secondary lymphoid tissues. There is also evidence that Treg maintain tolerance by suppressing immune responses within lymph nodes that drain the transplantation site. In the case of tolerance to gut antigens (e.g., food antigens), Tregs generated in the mesenteric lymph nodes migrate to the *lamina propria* of the intestine where they maintain mucosal tolerance by producing IL-10 and other immune modulatory cytokines.

Tertiary lymphoid tissues

Tertiary lymphoid tissues are organized, ectopic lymphoid aggregates, often developed in nonlymphoid tissues in response to chronic inflammation, or in the case of transplantation, chronic rejection. They are referred to as tertiary lymphoid tissues or tertiary lymphoid organs (TLOs) because they structurally resemble lymph nodes. The process by which they arise is known as lymphoid neogenesis. In humans, TLO have been described in the thyroid gland (Hashimoto's thyroiditis), central nervous system (multiple sclerosis), thymus (myasthenia gravis), joints (rheumatoid arthritis), salivary glands (Sjogren's syndrome), gastric mucosa (*Helicobacter pylori* infection), liver (primary sclerosing cholangitis and chronic hepatitis C), skin (*Borrelia burgdorferi* infection), and in transplanted kidneys, hearts, and lungs. TLO propagate immune responses locally by functioning as "lymph nodes." There is evidence, however, that TLO also participate in immune regulation.

Structure

TLO contain elements of both chronic inflammation and secondary lymphoid tissues, specifically those of peripheral lymph nodes (Figure 1.8). Structural elements reminiscent of lymph node architecture include (a) HEV, (b) discrete T and B cell areas including follicles and germinal centers, (c) DC and FDC networks, and (d) lymphatic channels. As in lymph nodes, HEV in TLO express L-selectin ligands (PNAd) or MAdCAM-1. Chemokines that attract T cells, B cells, and DCs (CCL19, CCL21, and CXCL13) are produced by stromal cells in TLO.

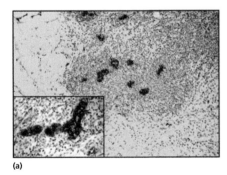 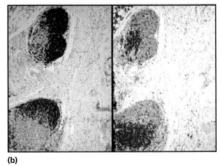

(a)   (b)

Figure 1.8 Tertiary lymphoid tissues in the transplanted heart. Examples of lymph node-like aggregates within the parenchyma of murine cardiac allografts undergoing combined acute and chronic rejection. (a) Lymphoid aggregate rich in high endothelial venules (HEVs) stained positive for peripheral node addressins (PNAds). The insert depicts PNAd+ HEV with stronger staining evident on the luminal side of the endothelium (arrows). (b) Lymphoid aggregates demonstrating distinct compartmentalization of B cells (left panel, CD220+ cells) and T cells (right panel, CD3+ cells). Source: Baddoura et al. (2005). Reproduced by permission of John Wiley & Sons Ltd.

TLO also contain cellular elements of chronic inflammation and are not always organized, including in some instances of scattered HEV surrounded by lymphocyte aggregates. TLO are plastic; they form, dissolve, and reform as inflammation fluctuates. Therefore, TLO are considered as an end-product of inflammation.

Genesis

Generation of TLO is a well-defined process that recapitulates the ontogeny of secondary lymphoid tissues (lymphoid organogenesis). Key to both lymphoid neogenesis and lymphoid organogenesis is the tumor necrosis factor (TNF) family of inflammatory cytokines, namely the lymphotoxins (LT). Lymphotoxins include the secreted cytokine $LT\alpha_3$ and the membrane-bound cytokine $LT\alpha_2\beta_1$. $LT\alpha_3$, which signals through TNFR1 p55, and $LT\alpha_2\beta_1$, which signals through LTβR, is essential for the development of secondary and tertiary lymphoid tissues. LTα or LTβR gene knockout mice lack lymph nodes and Peyer's patches and have a disorganized splenic white pulp. Inactivation of the NIK enzyme downstream of LTβR, either due to a naturally occurring mutation (*aly*) or to a genetically engineered NIK gene knockout, leads to the same secondary lymphoid tissue defects. Mice that lack the LTβ gene on the other hand are devoid of peripheral lymph nodes but retain mucosal (mesenteric, sacral, and cervial) lymph nodes, indicating that $LT\alpha_3$ is sufficient for the genesis of the latter, while $LT\alpha_2\beta_1$ is required for the former. The fusion protein LTβR-Ig is a potent, immunosuppressive agent, which disrupts lymph node and splenic white pulp architecture by interrupting the binding of $LT\alpha_2\beta_1$ to its receptor. This implies that lymphotoxins are important not only for lymphoid organogenesis but also for the maintenance of secondary lymphoid tissues in the adult animal.

During chronic inflammation, lymphoid neogenesis is initiated by bone marrow-derived lymphoid-tissue inducer (LT_i) cells that express $LT\alpha_2\beta_1$ as well as the chemokine receptor CXCR5. Engagement of LTβR on tissue stromal cells by $LT\alpha_2\beta_1$ on LT_i cell leads to the production of secondary lymphoid tissue chemokines (CXCL13 and CCL21, among others). These attract more LT_i cells as well as T, B, and DCs, eventually leading to the formation of tertiary lymphoid structures. The transcription factor RORγt responsible for the development of LT_i is also critical for the development of the Th17 T cell subset. Recent data demonstrated that Th17-mediated autoimmune disorders (e.g., autoimmune allergic encephalitis in mice) are characterized by TLO formation in the affected tissues, suggesting that Th17 cells also initiate lymphoid neogenesis.

Function

Studies in humans and mouse models of autoimmunity have shown that TLO are responsible for T cell and B cell activation and antibody production at the sites where they form; for example, in joints affected by rheumatoid arthritis, the central nervous system in multiple sclerosis, or the pancreas of nonobese diabetic (NOD) mice. These studies provided direct evidence that B cells undergo antigen-driven proliferation and somatic hypermutation within TLO, leading to the generation of plasma cells that produce high-affinity autoantibodies. The autoantibodies are specific to antigens abundant in the tissue where the TLO are located and often display the phenomenon of epitope spreading. Although direct evidence of T cell activation within TLO is lacking, elegant studies in mice have shown that TLO are sufficient for sustaining T cell-mediated autoimmune diabetes and for mounting antitumor and antiviral T cell responses. Therefore, TLO are beneficial to the host in the setting of tumors or infection but are deleterious in autoimmunity.

Role in rejection and tolerance

Either fully formed TLO or PNAd+ HEV, lymphocyte clusters, and lymphatic channels reminiscent of lymph node architecture have been documented in chronically rejected human and mouse heart and kidney allografts (Figure 1.8). PNAd+ blood vessels, in the absence of lymphocyte clusters, have also been reported in allografts undergoing acute rejection. In lung transplantation, lymphoid neogenesis occurs under the epithelial lining of the airways. These structures are referred to as inducible BALTs (iBALTs) and have been also described after infection with the influenza virus. What function do TLO then serve in transplantation? Most studies point to a pathogenic role for TLO. However, TLO are also observed in allografts accepted long term in mice and humans, suggesting a role in tolerance or immune regulation. Thus, the exact role of TLO in transplantation requires further testing.

Summary

The lymphoid organs and tissues are complex structures that support generation, function, homeostasis, and regulation of lymphocytes. The primary lymphoid organs are sites where T cells and B cells develop and mature. A mature repertoire of lymphocytes consists of cells that are selected and educated to respond to foreign antigens, including alloantigens. Secondary lymphoid organs provide places for mature lymphocytes to reside and also as ideal sites for their activation and functional differentiation. Although T cells and B cells are developed in separate primary sites, they interact extensively at secondary sites to mount productive responses to antigens. Importantly, proper regulation of the immune system and additionally the immune responses to antigens require both primary and secondary lymphoid tissues. The exact role of tertiary lymphoid tissues in the overall immune responses remains incompletely defined. Clearly, immune responses that lead to rejection or even tolerance requires the interaction of multiplicity of cells and precisely choreographed interactions within exquisitely engineered anatomic structures. Strategies to exploit these interactions within lymphoid structures continue to hold promise for the induction of transplant tolerance.

References

Baddoura FK, Nasr IW, Wrobel B, Li Q, Ruddle NH, Lakkis FG. Lymphoid neogenesis in murine cardiac allografts undergoing chronic rejection. Am J Transplant 5(3): 510–516, 2005.

Murphy, K (2011). *Janeway's Immunobiology*, 8th edition, Garland Science, New York.

Travlos GS. Normal structure, function, and histology of the bone marrow. Toxicol Pathol 34: 548, 2006.

Further reading

Aloisi F, Pujol-Borrell R. Lymphoid neogenesis in chronic inflammatory disease. Nat Rev Immunol 6:205–217, 2006.

Anderson MS, Venanzi ES, Klein L, Chen Z, Berzins SP, Turley SJ, et al. Projection of an immunological self shadow within the thymus by the AIRE protein. Science 298:1395–1401, 2002.

Bhattacharya D, Rossi DJ, Bryder D, Weissman IL. Purified heamtopoietic stem cell engraftment of rare niches corrects severe lymphoid deficiencies without host conditioning. J Exp Med 203:73–85, 2005.

Chalasani G, Dai Z, Konieczny BT, Baddoura FK, Lakkis FG. Recall and propagation of allospecific memory T cells independent of secondary lymphoid tissues. Proc Natl Acad Sci U S A 99:6175–6180, 2002.

Drayton DL, Ying X, Lee J, Lesslauer W, Ruddle NH. Ectopic LTab directs lymphoid organ neogenesis with concomitant expression of peripheral node addressin and a HEV-restricted sulfotransferase. J Exp Med 197:1153–1163, 2003.

Gelman AE, Li W, Richardson SB, Zinselmeyer BH, Lai J, Okazaki M, et al. Cuttine edge: acute lung allograft rejection is independent of secondary lymphoid organs. J Immunol 182:3969–3973, 2009.

Itoh M, Takahashi T, Sakaguchi N, Kuniyasu Y, Shimizu J, Otsuka F, et al. Thymus and autoimmunity: production of CD25+CD4+ naturally anergic and suppressive T cells as a key function of the thymus in maintaining immunologic self-tolerance. J Immunol 162:5317–5326, 1999.

Karrer U, Athage A, Odermatt B, Roberts CWM, Korsmeyer SJ, Miyawaki S, et al. On the key role of secondary lymphoid organs in antiviral immune responses studied in alymphoplastic (*aly/aly*) and spleenless (*Hox11-/*) mutant mice. J Exp Med 185:2157–2170, 1997.

Kawai T, Cosimi AB, Spitzer TR, Tolkoff-Rubin N, Suthanthiran M, Saidman SL, et al. HLA-mismatched renal transplantation without maintenance immunosuppression. N Engl J Med 358:353–361, 2008.

Lakkis FG. Where is the alloimmune response initiated? Am J Transplant 3:241–242, 2003.

Lakkis FG, Arakelov A, Konieczny BT, Inoue Y. Immunologic ignorance of vascularized organ transplants in the absence of secondary lymphoid tissues. Nat Med 6:686–688, 2000.

Mazo IB, Honczarenko M, Leung H, Cavanagh LL, Bonasio R, Weninger W, et al. Bone marrow is a major reservoir and site of recruitment for central memory CD8+ T cells. Immunity 22:259–270, 2005.

Mercier FE, Ragu C, Scadden DT. The bone marrow at the crossroad of blood and immunity. Nat Rev Immunol 12:49–60, 2012.

Miller JFAP. The golden anniversary of the thymus. Nat Rev Immunol 11:489–495, 2011.

Mora JR, Bono MR, Manjunath M, Weninger W, Cavanagh LL, Rosemblatt M, von Andrian, UH Selective imprinting of gut-homing T cells by Peyer's patch dendritic cells. Nature 424:88–93, 2003.

Nasr IW, Reel M, Oberbarnscheidt MH, Mounzer RH, Baddoura FK, Ruddle NH, et al. Tertiary lymphoid tissues generate effector and memory T cells that lead to allograft rejection. Am J Transplant 7:1071–1079, 2007.

Ruddle NH, Akirav EM. Secondary lymphoid organs: responding to genetic and environmental cues in ontogeny and the immune response. J Immunol 183:2205–2212, 2009.

Serbina NV, Pamer EG. Monocyte emigration from bone marrow during bacterial infection requires signals mediated by chemokine receptor CCR2. Nat Immunol 7:311–317, 2006.

Thaunat O, Patey N, Morelon E, Michel J-B, Nicoletti A. Lymphoid neogenesis in chronic rejection: the murderer in the house. Curr Opin Immunol 18:576–579, 2006.

Yamada K, Shimizu A, Ierino FL, Utsugi R, Barth RN, Esnola N, et al. Thymic transplantation in miniature swine: development and function of the "thymokidney". Transplantation 68:1684–1692, 1999.

Zinkernagel RM, Ehl S, Aichele P, Oehen S, Kundig T, Hengartner H. Antigen localisation regulates immune responses in a dose- and time-dependent fashion: a geographical view of immune reactivity. Immunol Rev 156:199–209, 1997.

CHAPTER 2

Cells of the immune system

Jason R. Lees[1], Agnes M. Azimzadeh[1], Yaozhong Ding[1], Tonya J. Webb[2], and Jonathan S. Bromberg[1]

[1] Department of Surgery, Microbiology and Immunology, University of Maryland School of Medicine, Baltimore, USA
[2] Department of Microbiology and Immunology, Marlene and Stewart Greenebaum Cancer Center, University of Maryland School of Medicine, Baltimore, USA

CHAPTER OVERVIEW

- The immune system consists of innate and adaptive immune cells, and both cell types are involved in the allograft response.

- T cells are critical effector cells of graft rejection; various T cell subsets have been identified, including T cells that inhibit immune responses.

- B cells produce antibodies and are involved in antibody-mediated rejection; the definition of pathogenic versus regulatory B (Breg) cells is still unclear.

- Recent knowledge about NK and NKT cell subsets is likely to bring new insights regarding graft rejection and acceptance.

- Immune regulation is critical but complex, involving multiple cell types and regulatory mechanisms.

Introduction

Cells of the immune system consist of innate immune cells and adaptive immune cells. Innate immune cells include dendritic cells (DCs), monocytes, macrophages, and natural killer (NK) cells as well as other myeloid and lymphoid cells. As a front line defense to "danger," they rapidly exert their effector functions. Adaptive immune cells are primarily composed of two types of lymphocytes, T cells and B cells, which clonally express a large repertoire of antigenic receptors. Naïve T and B cells encounter antigens in specialized lymphoid organs and undergo proliferation and maturation before exerting their effector functions.

Experimental studies in genetically modified mice lacking T and B cells have demonstrated the critical role of adaptive immune cells in allograft rejection.

Transplant Immunology, First Edition. Edited by Xian Chang Li and Anthony M. Jevnikar.
Companion website: www.wiley.com/go/li/transplantimmunology

T cells mediate acute cellular rejection, usually within a week after organ transplantation. Accordingly, most therapeutic strategies in the clinic target T cell activation or function. However, these T cell-directed therapies do not protect against the insidious and largely uncontrolled chronic and antibody-mediated rejection. In addition, T cell inhibition does not prevent hyperacute or acute rejection in patients previously sensitized to donor alloantigens. In this context, B cells have been recently recognized as important mediators of graft rejection, in addition to antibody production as plasma cells. However, subsets of B cells also mediate regulatory functions of alloimmune responses. In order to better prevent pathogenic B cell responses while sparing their regulatory capacity, there is a clear need to improve our understanding of phenotypes of B cells that mediate these diverse functions, the effect of immunosuppressive therapies on B cells, and how B cell responses evolve over time after transplantation.

In this chapter, we will discuss key features of innate and adaptive immune cells in the allograft response, and how they interact with and regulate each other in tolerance induction. We also discuss the emerging role of innate immune cells in rejecting or protecting solid organ transplants, as well as the challenges and opportunities in targeting these cells to further improve transplant outcomes in the clinic.

Innate immune cells

Dendritic cells (DCs)
DCs are a rare cell type in the immune system, with distinct stages of development, activation, and maturation. This heterogeneous population of cells forms a cellular network that is involved in immune surveillance, antigen capture and antigen presentation, and capable of inducing both immunity and immune tolerance.

Dendritic cell origin and differentiation
DCs are generated from bone marrow hematopoietic stem cells. During hematopoiesis, multipotent CD34$^+$ stem cells give rise to common myeloid progenitors (CMPs) and common lymphoid progenitors (CLPs). This divergence occurs early during hematopoiesis and leads to the generation of megakaryocytes, erythrocytes, monocytes, macrophages, and granulocytes from CMP, while T cells, B cells, and NK cells originate from CLP (Figure 2.1). However, recent studies have shown that purified CLP or CMP injected into irradiated mice differentiate into DCs. Therefore, DCs may arise from both the myeloid and lymphoid ontogenic pathways. Furthermore, many individual tissues can generate local tissue resident DCs from a reservoir of immediate DCs precursors, rather than depending on a continuous flux of DCs from the bone marrow.

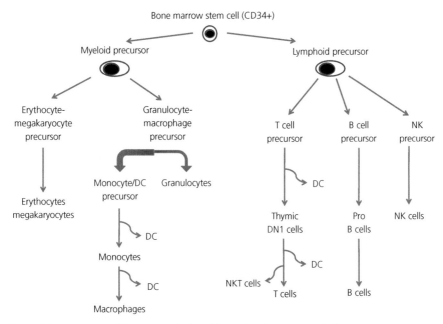

Figure 2.1 Ontogeny of hematopoietic cells. During hematopoiesis, bone marrow stem cells give rise to common myeloid progenitors (CMPs) and common lymphoid progenitors (CLPs). Megakaryocytes, erythrocytes, monocytes, macrophages, and granulocytes originate from CMP, while T cells, and B cells and natural killer cells originate from CLP.

Phenotypes and classification of DCs

DCs can be broadly classified into three major categories. Pre-dendritic cells are cells without the characteristic dendritic appearance and antigen presenting function, but have the capacity to develop into DCs upon stimulation. Examples in this category include blood plasmacytoid DCs and monocytes. A second category is composed of conventional DC (cDC), which already have a dendritic appearance and exhibit DCs functions. cDC themselves comprise two subsets: migratory DCs and lymphoid-resident DCs. Migratory DCs constitute the classical DCs subset involved in immune surveillance, that is transporting antigens from the peripheral tissues to lymph nodes. In contrast, lymphoid DCs are restricted to particular lymphoid organs and are specialized in the presentation of self-antigens (e.g., thymic DCs). A last category of DCs includes cells that are not normally present in the steady state, but are induced as a consequence of inflammation. Inflammatory mediators such as tumor necrosis factor (TNFα) and inducible nitric-oxide synthase (iNOS) produced during inflammation have the potential to induce inflammatory DCs. DCs derived from inflammatory $CCR2^+$ monocytes are a prototypic example of an inflammation-induced DCs type.

Phenotypically, DCs are characterized by their expression of major histocompatibility complex (MHC) class II, but lack other lineage-specific markers such as CD3, CD19, CD16, NK1.1, and CD14 that identify T cells, B cells, NK cells, and monocytes, respectively. In the circulation, DCs have been traditionally described as lineage negative (Lin$^-$) with expression of blood DCs markers. In humans, mDC are defined as Lin$^-$/MHCII$^+$/CD11c$^+$ CD123$^-$ (IL-3R) BDCA-1$^+$ and pDC as Lin$^-$ MHCII$^+$ CD11c$^-$ CD123$^+$ BDCA-2$^+$ and Ig-like transcript 7$^+$. The nomenclature of blood DCs has been reviewed recently for both mouse and human systems, with new human subset definitions based on markers BDCA-1 (CD1c), BDCA-2 (CD303), and BDCA-3 (CD141).

In mice, most DCs express CD11c. Two main subsets have been defined primarily based on their differential expression of CD11b and B220, which appear to functionally correspond to myeloid (conventional) and plasmacytoid DCs: myeloid DCs are B220$^-$ CD11c^{hi} CD11b$^+$ NK1.1$^-$, whereas pDC are B220$^+$ CD11c^{lo} CD11b$^-$ Gr-1$^+$. Other mouse pDC markers include the murine pDC Ag-1, BM stromal cell Ag (BST)-2/CD317, Siglec-H, and the chemokine receptor CCR9. In mouse spleen, DCs express high levels of MHC class I and class II proteins, CD11c, and the mannose-receptor-like protein DEC-205, as well as adhesion (CD11a, CD54) and costimulatory (CD40, CD80, CD86) molecules. In addition, a subset of splenic DCs also expresses the lymphocyte antigen CD8, as a αα homodimer.

Dendritic cell function

DCs play key roles in the immune responses, including responses leading to transplant tissue rejection or acceptance. The main function of DCs is to process antigens and present them to T cells and B cells. As such, DCs function as antigen-presenting cells (APCs) and provide a key link between innate and adaptive immunity. While other cell types (macrophages, B cells) can present antigens to T cells, DCs are by far the most potent APCs, as they efficiently activate both naïve and memory T cells. Thus, DCs play a crucial role in the initiation of immune responses and as such, represent an attractive target for manipulation of immune responses in transplantation.

The process of antigen presentation can occur via one of three pathways. In the major histocompatibility complex (MHC) class I pathway, endogenous (intracellular) antigens are presented by MHC class I molecules. Antigens generated within a cell (for example, donor MHC or viral proteins in an infected cell) are degraded into small peptides within DCs by a specialized enzyme complex, the proteasome. The MHC class I/peptide complex on the surface of DCs is able to present antigens to CD8$^+$ T cells expressing the corresponding TCR. In contrast, in the class II pathway, exogenous (extracellular) antigens are presented by MHC class II molecules. External molecules (e.g., soluble donor MHC molecules or bacteria) are engulfed by APCs through endocytosis. The antigenic peptides are then uploaded onto MHC class II molecules and the resulting complex is expressed on the cell surface available for recognition by CD4$^+$ T cells. Finally, the "cross-presentation" pathway permits the transfer of extracellular antigens into the class I pathway. Dead cells (injured graft cells or infected cells) or cell

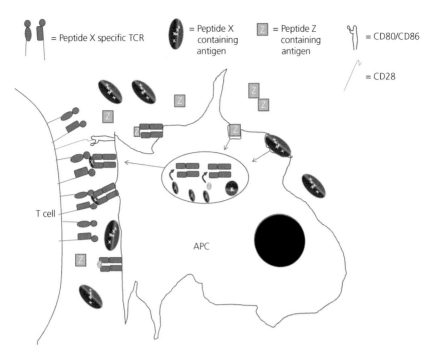

Figure 2.2 T cell recognition of antigen. APCs capture, process, and present antigenic peptides in the context of self-MHC molecules. Following uptake, antigenic epitopes are produced allowing selective activation of T cells expressing specific TCR. Robust T cell activation requires both antigen/MHC complex and costimulatory molecules such as CD80 and CD86 on APCs.

debris (exosomes, small vesicles released by various cells) are engulfed by endocytosis. The antigenic peptides formed can be inserted into MHC class I molecules and the complex expressed on the cell surface (Figure 2.2).

The ability of DCs to take up and process antigens is not the same in all DCs subsets, a point that is relevant to DCs manipulation in transplantation. For cDC, the phagocytic activity is linked to the degree of cell maturation. Immature DCs are able to efficiently engulf and process antigens. Pro-inflammatory signals from the environment (CD40L, TLR, IFN, TNF) induce DCs to mature, resulting in the upregulation of critical costimulatory molecules (CD80, CD86). Mature DCs are more efficient at antigen presentation, but less efficient in phagocytosis. During DCs maturation, there are changes in the expression of chemokine receptors, which induce DCs migration to lymphoid organs, where they can stimulate T and B cells. pDC are well known for their ability to respond to viral nucleic acids via Toll-like receptors (TLR7 and TLR9). While several signals (IL-3Rc, CD40, OX40L, IFN) can promote the maturation of pDC, the recognition of nucleic acids by endosomal TLR7 and TLR9 is the key signal that results in an initial burst of Type I IFNs, due to high levels of IRF7 in pDC. This property thus provides a mechanism by which viral infections can promote or amplify graft rejection mechanisms. Interestingly, the activation of pDC by self-nucleic acids was recently demonstrated with tissue injury as well as autoimmunity, suggesting that graft injury (triggered by ischemia-reperfusion injury or rejection) may promote pDC activation, thereby amplifying immune responses via IFN expression. DCs control many adaptive responses via the release of soluble factors. DCs are potent producers of IL-12 and IL-23, cytokines that drive Th1 and Th17 phenotypes, respectively. Moreover, interactions with T and B cells lead to reciprocal activation of both cell types via upregulation of costimulatory molecules and their ligands (e.g., CD28/B7, CD40/CD40L, OX40/OX40L for T cells; APRIL/BAFF for B cells), again amplifying immune responses.

Importantly, and relevant to therapeutic strategies in clinical transplantation, dendritic cells can not only activate T cells but also tolerize T cells. Interestingly, the decision between immunity and tolerance appears to depend largely on the environment in which the immune response is elicited. Pro-inflammatory signals with inflammation (i.e., TLR, TNF, and IFN) induce DCs maturation and thus enhance adaptive immune responses. In contrast, antigen presentation in the absence of inflammation generally leads to unresponsiveness or tolerance. Such a response would appear to minimize autoimmune reactions to self-antigens presented in the absence of infection (i.e., "danger"). Several mechanisms appear to be involved in the induction of tolerance by DCs. In the thymus, DCs are crucial to the induction of central tolerance, while under steady-state conditions in the periphery, DCs are also thought to play an important role in the induction of peripheral tolerance. T cell clones may be tolerized to self-antigens presented in draining lymph nodes by mechanisms of deletion or anergy. Finally, DCs mediate the induction of regulatory T cells (Tregs), which can suppress immune responses via different molecular pathways, including (i) the production of suppressive factors (IL-10, transforming growth factor [TGFβ]), (ii) expression of metabolism rate-limiting enzymes such as indoleamine-deoxygenase (IDO), and (iii) expression of coinhibitory molecules like PD-L1.

Effect of immunosuppressive drugs on DCs

Although most current therapeutic drugs in transplantation target T cells, these same immunosuppressive therapies can have effects on DCs. Cyclosporine A (CsA) failed to interfere with the differentiation of monocyte-derived DCs *in vitro* and its effect on DCs maturation remains controversial. However, inhibitory effects of CsA on antigen presentation and cytokine production have been reported. Similar results were found with tacrolimus, another widely used calcineurin inhibitor (CNI). In contrast, rapamycin, a mammalian target of rapamycin (mTOR) inhibitor, had no effect on DCs differentiation but induced DCs apoptosis in a time- and dose-dependent manner. The inhibitory role of rapamycin in several DCs functions (e.g., IL-12 production) has been clearly demonstrated. Glucocorticoids have extensive effects on DCs; they inhibit DCs differentiation and maturation, and also alter their function by enhancing endocytosis, decreasing the production of IL-1, IL-6, IL-12, and TNF, and enhancing IL-10 expression. Interestingly, aspirin exhibits some but not all of the effects of glucocorticoids. Desoxyspergualin (DSG), which has been tested in clinical transplantation, inhibits DCs maturation via inhibition of NF-κB nuclear translocation. Finally, mycophenolic acid and mycophenolate mofetil (MMF) have been shown to impair the maturation and function of DCs, resulting in reduced allo-stimulating capacity.

Natural killer cells

NK cells were identified in the 1970s, and are classified as lymphocytes based on a number of parameters. NK cells are components of innate immunity and important in early antiviral immune responses, as well as tumor immune surveillance. NK cells were originally described as "natural killers" because of their ability to directly induce the death of tumor cells and virally infected cells in the absence of specific priming. This is in contrast to adaptive CD8$^+$ T cells, which require antigen priming for their killing function.

In humans, NK cells are characterized by the absence of the T cell receptor complex (CD3, TCR) and the expression of CD56. Based on levels of CD56 expression, human NK cells can be defined as CD56^{dim} or CD56^{bright}. The majority of circulating NK cells are CD56^{dim} and also express CD16, while the remaining approximately 10% are CD56^{bright}CD16$^{neg/low}$. The CD56^{dim} NK population is considered to be classical killer cells. In mice, NK cells can be identified by the expression of NK1.1 (in certain strains), DX5, or asialo GM1. NK cells also produce inflammatory cytokines, most notably IFN-γ, TNF-α), and immunosuppressive cytokines, such as interleukin IL-10. Finally, NK cells secrete many chemokines and express multiple chemokine receptors, adhesion receptors, and cytokine receptors (Figure 2.3).

NK cells express an array of receptors that can either stimulate (activating receptors) or diminish (inhibitory receptors) their activities. In addition, cytokine receptors that belong to the common gamma chain (γc), such as IL-15R, IL-2R, and IL-21R, are critical for NK cell development and function. TLRs and cytokine receptors that are linked to the adaptor protein MyD88 are also necessary for NK cell maturation and function, specifically IL-1R in humans and the IL-18R in mouse.

NK activation and signaling

NK cells function by producing cytokines or directly lysing target cells. NK cells also detect antibody-coated cells through the FcγRIIIA (CD16) cell surface receptor to exert antibody-dependent cell-mediated cytotoxicity (ADCC). CD16 is coupled to the CD3ζ and FcRγ signal transduction cascades containing cytoplasmic "Immunoreceptor Tyrosine-based Activation Motifs" (ITAMs). The natural killer receptors (NKp46, NKp44, and NKp30) are also activating receptors linked to

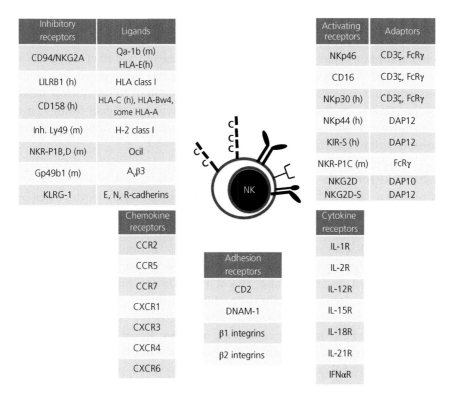

Inhibitory receptors	Ligands
CD94/NKG2A	Qa-1b (m) HLA-E(h)
LILRB1 (h)	HLA class I
CD158 (h)	HLA-C (h), HLA-Bw4, some HLA-A
Inh. Ly49 (m)	H-2 class I
NKR-P1B,D (m)	Ocil
Gp49b1 (m)	A_vβ3
KLRG-1	E, N, R-cadherins

Activating receptors	Adaptors
NKp46	CD3ζ, FcRγ
CD16	CD3ζ, FcRγ
NKp30 (h)	CD3ζ, FcRγ
NKp44 (h)	DAP12
KIR-S (h)	DAP12
NKR-P1C (m)	FcRγ
NKG2D	DAP10
NKG2D-S	DAP12

Chemokine receptors
CCR2
CCR5
CCR7
CXCR1
CXCR3
CXCR4
CXCR6

Adhesion receptors
CD2
DNAM-1
β1 integrins
β2 integrins

Cytokine receptors
IL-1R
IL-2R
IL-12R
IL-15R
IL-18R
IL-21R
IFNαR

Figure 2.3 NK cell receptors, adaptors, and ligands. NK cells express multiple receptors on the cell surface that are divided into activating, inhibitory, adhesion, cytokine and chemotactic receptors. NK cells express inhibitory receptors specific for self-MHC class I and some non-MHC ligands. Adaptor molecules that mediate downstream signaling cascades are also depicted. NK receptors shown in the figure are conserved in both species, unless indicated (h, human; m, mouse).

the ITAM-bearing CD3ζ, FcRγ, or DAP12 molecules. A characteristic of many NK cell activating receptors is their ability to detect self-molecules induced during cellular stress, such as B7-H6 (a ligand for NKp30), which is expressed on many tumor cells. In addition, NKG2D on NK cells interacts with various ligands (MIC-A, MIC-B, ULBP in human, and Rae-1, H60, MULT-1 in mice) that are expressed at low levels in most tissues, but are upregulated following the induction of cellular distress (Figure 2.3). In fact, the expression of MIC-A and MIC-B on renal and pancreatic allografts is correlated with rejection. Conversely, shedding of the NKG2D ligands into the serum will block NKG2D-mediated NK cell activation by receptor internalization and degradation. Consistent with this, cardiac transplant patients with favorable graft function have been found to have elevated levels of soluble MIC-A.

The "missing self" hypothesis

Unlike T or B cells, which depend on specific antigen receptor recognition of the MHC/antigen complex, NK cells respond to the absence of MHC class I which enhances their cytotoxic activities. This is referred to as the "missing self" hypothesis, a situation that can occur during virus infections, cellular transformation, and cancer. The recognition of "missing self" is mediated by a variety of MHC class I specific inhibitory receptors that include killer immunoglobulin-like receptors (KIRs) in humans, lectin-like Ly49 molecules in mice, and CD94/NKG2A heterodimers (in both humans and mice). These MHC class I binding receptors belong to the large family of inhibitory receptors that mediate their function by signaling through cytoplasmic "Immunoreceptor Tyrosine-based Inhibitory Motifs" (ITIMs). Consequently, NK cells selectively kill stressed cells, which have downregulated MHC class I molecules and/or highly express stress-induced activating ligands, such as those for NKG2D, and at the same time ignore healthy cells that express high levels of self-MHC class I molecules.

NK cells and solid organ transplant

Initial studies showed that NK cells were not involved in rejection of solid organ transplants because the depletion of NK cells did not alter the kinetics of rejection. However, NK cells are known to mediate rejection of MHC-mismatch hematopoietic stem cells. It has been shown that NK cells become activated by stress ligands expressed on allografts, which leads to the production of inflammatory cytokines that enhance T cell responses to the allograft. This was specifically demonstrated for cardiac allograft vasculopathy (CAV). It has been shown that advanced CAV lesions develop in cardiac allografts transplanted from parental to unmanipulated F1 hybrid mice, a transplant model that lacks specific antidonor T cell reactivity but retains antidonor NK cell responses. Thus, NK cells activated by the mismatched MHC class I molecules on donor endothelium result in alloreactive T cell stimulation, leading to the pathogenesis of CAV. Similar responses occur in kidney transplants, as NK cells can injure tubular epithelial cells (TECs) through direct interaction of NKG2D on NK cells with the Rae-1 ligand on TEC. Recently it was shown that kidney transplants from parental to F1 hybrid mice lacking T and B cells (Rag null mice) result in chronic kidney injury, which can be abrogated by antibody depletion of NK cells. In other models, however, NK cells promote transplant tolerance by killing donor-derived APCs, thus reducing priming of host alloreactive T cells.

Macrophages and monocytes

Monocytes are derived from bone marrow stem cells and constitute between 3 and 8% of the leukocytes in the blood. They traffic into tissues and differentiate into tissue resident macrophages. There are two major monocyte subsets in the mouse. Grl$^+$/Ly-6C ^{high} monocytes can differentiate into many types of macrophages as well as DCs subtypes. This subtype is important for host defense and inflammatory responses. Grl$^-$/Ly-6C ^{low} monocytes mostly differentiate into macrophages, including alveolar macrophages, and may play a role in tissue repair. The majority of human monocytes express high levels of CD14 and are negative for Fcγ receptor type III (CD16). However, about 8% of all monocytes co-express CD14 and CD16. The CD14+CD16+ population exhibits a pro-inflammatory phenotype, with features of tissue macrophages; they rapidly expand during acute and chronic inflammatory diseases, with increased phagocytosis capacity and higher levels of IL-1 and MHC class II molecules. Thus, monitoring the pro-inflammatory CD14+CD16+ subset may be of interest in patients under immunosuppressive and/or anti-inflammatory therapy. Monocytes and their macrophages as well as DCs progeny exert three main functions in immune responses: (i) phagocytosis, (ii) antigen presentation, and (iii) cytokine production.

Macrophage activation

Activated macrophages can be polarized into M1 (classically activated macrophages) or M2 (alternatively activated macrophages) phenotype. Two key signals are required for the activation of M1 macrophages, namely, IFNγ and TLRs, which recognize pathogen or cellular damage-associated molecular patterns (PAMP, cDAMP). After activation, macrophages take up microbes, process and present antigen in the context of MHC molecules, produce IL-12 to initiate Th1 development, and express both NO through inducible nitric oxide (iNOS) and TNF-α to exert cytotoxicity. In addition to recognizing PAMP, TLRs also recognize endogenous cellular products from damaged cells or cDAMP, suggesting an early involvement of macrophages in allograft rejection. Alternatively, M2 macrophages can be activated in IL-4 and/or IL-13 rich environments, producing little NO, and thus having limited cytotoxic activities. Such M2 macrophages play a role in tissue repair and fibrosis and thus affect long-term allograft survival. Macrophages can also be activated by engagement of cell surface FcγR and signaling through TLRs and CD40 to produce IL-10 and have anti-inflammatory capacities. Macrophages, like many other cells of the immune system, show a recurring theme of "context specific" capacity to either promote or attenuate inflammation and injury.

Macrophages in transplant rejection

Infiltration by macrophages is observed in acute rejection, and studies using human biopsies show that they comprise 38–60% of the cellular infiltrate. Macrophages may use their phagocytic abilities to process and present alloantigens to T cells and initiate rejection. Macrophages can also influence graft rejection by producing potent pro-inflammatory cytokines such as IL-1, IL-12, IL-18, TNF-α, and IFN-γ. They also directly act as effector cells to cause tissue damage by producing reactive nitrogen and oxygen species. In fact, elevated NO in serum correlates with the kinetics of allograft rejection. Depleting macrophages by administration of liposomal clodronate reduced rejection responses, as nitric oxide was reduced by more than 90%. This confirms an important role of macrophages in acute rejection and perhaps as a therapeutic target in clinical transplantation.

Macrophage accumulation has been shown to both predate and accompany chronic rejection leading to end-stage transplant failure. In a miniature swine model, persistence of macrophage infiltrates following resolution of acute rejection was predictive of chronic rejection. Similarly in a rat model, significantly increased macrophage infiltration in addition to T cells correlated with progressive chronic rejection, indicating a role for macrophages in the development and progression of chronic graft injury. Administration of a macrophage inhibitor or an angiotensin II type 1 receptor antagonist to inhibit chemoattraction of macrophages resulted in the suppression of chronic rejection in a rat model. In humans with chronic transplant arteriopathy, macrophages have been detected in arteries. In fact, the ratio of macrophages/monocytes versus T lymphocytes was significantly increased in chronic kidney rejection, further supporting the involvement of macrophages in chronic rejection. Despite their observations, little is known about the precise mechanisms by which macrophages contribute to chronic rejection, apart from broadly stimulating tissue inflammation.

Adaptive immune cells

T cells
Pathways of T cell activation in transplantation
Mature T cells in the periphery demonstrate a strong potential for cross-reactivity with non-self allogeneic MHC proteins, due to an intrinsic ability of the T cell receptor to engage MHC molecules. Particularly relevant to transplantation is that extremely high numbers of mature T cells exist, which are directly cross-reactive with donor MHC. This results in somewhat more robust T cell responses to alloantigens than those observed during immunity to pathogens. As a reference, the frequency of T cells that can directly respond to allogeneic MHC on a transplant is estimated to be as high as 1–10% of the total T cell pool. The remarkable number of T cells capable of recognizing alloantigens is the result of selective T cell maturation in recipients and unique antigen presentation pathways that take place following transplantation. T cells specific to alloantigens can be activated in three different pathways, which have been broadly termed indirect, direct, and semi-direct presentation (Figure 2.4).

Indirect presentation is the default and robust antigen recognition pathway used by T cells to recognize exogenous antigens such as viruses. APCs traffic through grafted tissue and take up, process, and display donor antigens in the context of recipient MHC molecules. A key feature of this type of presentation is the requirement of recipient MHC molecules for T cell activation, and thus will activate alloreactive T cells similar to those activated by exogenous nominal

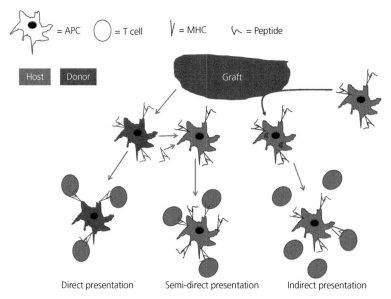

Direct presentation   Semi-direct presentation   Indirect presentation

Figure 2.4 Pathways of antigen presentation in transplantation. There are three pathways of antigen presentation in transplantation. Recipient T cells recognize donor antigens complexed to recipient MHC on recipient APC (indirect presentation), donor antigens complexed with donor MHC on donor APC (direct presentation), or donor antigens complexed with donor MHC on recipient APC (semidirect presentation).

antigens. Direct presentation involves donor APCs presenting alloantigen peptides in the context of donor MHC to recipient T cells and is unique to transplantation as donor APC, rather than recipient APC, participate. Many T cells will display reactivity to the entire donor MHC/donor peptide complexes, accounting for the large T cell precursor frequencies in transplantation. Direct presentation appears to be a major pathway for the induction of acute rejection of allografts. Semidirect presentation is similar to the direct presentation pathway in that donor alloantigenic peptides in the context of donor MHC molecules together activate recipient T cells, but it differs in that recipient APC participate in antigen presentation. This occurs with a unique transfer of donor cell membrane components, including MHC/peptide complexes, to recipient APCs, either through cell–cell contact or by the uptake of donor exosomes that fuse with recipient APC cell membranes. Recipient APCs then present the donor MHC/peptide complex to recipient T cells.

T cell effector function

Effector T cells are a heterogeneous cell population. Mature T cells are capable of recognizing specific peptides in the context of either MHC class I (CD8+ T cells) or MHC class II (CD4+ T cells), which generates different effector populations. Both CD8+ and CD4+ effector cells are capable of expressing a variety of trafficking and effector molecules, allowing tropism for specific tissues and differential capacities to respond to secondary stimulations. The major recognized effector subsets are described in the following text.

CD8+ T cells are a critical component of alloimmune responses as they can recognize ubiquitously expressed MHC class I/peptide complexes and induce cytolysis of cells bearing their cognate antigens. Thus, in their active form, they are also called cytotoxic (or previously "killer") T cells, which contribute greatly to graft destruction. Killing of target cells is carried out by exocytosis of preformed toxic granules or through ligation of death receptors on target cells. The ability of CD8 T cells as well as other cells using perforin-Granzyme B to efficiently induce target cell death is modified by the target cells' ability to resist death by the expression of endogenous Granzyme B inhibitors (SPI-6 in mouse or PI-9 in humans). Accelerated allograft rejection was recently demonstrated in a mouse transplant model in which the transplanted kidney lacked SPI-6. The alternate pathway for CD8-mediated donor cell lysis occurs following ligation of TNF-α superfamily members with death domain containing receptors on donor cells. Activated CD8+ T cells express Fas ligand (CD178) that triggers caspase-dependent lysis in target cells expressing a trimerized ligand Fas (CD95). Currently, there are several members in the death receptor family known to be involved in graft rejection, including Fas (CD95), the tumor necrosis α receptor TNFR1 (CD120a), and the TRAIL receptors DR4 and DR5 (Figure 2.5).

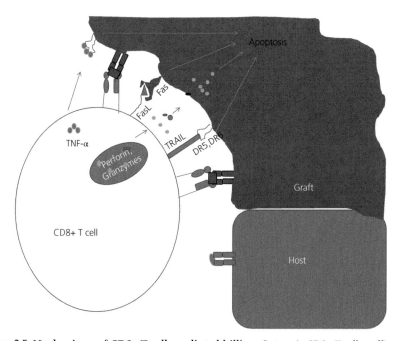

Figure 2.5 Mechanisms of CD8+ T cell-mediated killing. Cytotoxic CD8+ T cells traffic to the site of rejection and are in close contact with target cells. The cytotoxic CD8+ T cells then kill target cells through release of pre-formed cytotoxic granules containing perforin and granzymes or through engagement of death receptors (Fas, DR5, DR6) on target cells via expression of ligands for such death receptors (FasL, TRAIL). Cytokines produced by cytotoxic T cells, such as TNF-α, are also capable of binding to receptors on graft tissue and inducing cell death.

CD4 T cell help is vital to productive CD8+ T cell responses and to the production of high-affinity antigraft antibodies by B cells. Overall, CD4+ T cells have great capacity to further differentiate into functionally different subsets, exemplified by the expression of unique cytokine profiles. However, the precise role(s) of individual effector subsets in different transplantation settings remains incompletely defined, which limits the specific targeting strategies for clinical transplantation.

CD4+ T cell subsets

It has long been recognized that CD4+ T cells often exhibit different cytokine production patterns that are associated with diverse pathologic states. Initially, CD4+ T cells that produce IFNγ or IL-4 were termed T helper 1 subset (Th1) and T helper 2 subset (Th2), respectively. Now, CD4+ T cell subsets have been expanded to include Th9, Th17, Th22, T follicular helper cells or Tfh, and inducible T regulatory cells (iTregs). Such diverse CD4+ T cell subsets develop in response to specific cytokine milieu in which T cells are activated, primarily through the induction of key subset specific transcription factors.

Th1 cells are induced in response to IL-12 during T cell activation, resulting in an increased expression of the transcription factor T-bet, a key transcription factor now shown to be critical to the development of Th1 responses. Th1 cells produce the signature cytokine IFN-γ, as well as IL-2 and TNF-α. These effector cytokines allow Th1 cells to target intracellular pathogens and also mediate significant tissue damage. Th1 cells are known to be deleterious to transplants and are strongly associated with cellular rejection in many transplant models.

Th2 cells are induced by IL-4, resulting in the expression of the transcription factor STAT6 and GATA-3, which are required for development of Th2 responses. In addition to the signature cytokine IL-4, Th2 cells also produce IL-5 and IL-13. Th2 cells typically mediate immune responses to parasites and allergens. While Th2 cells may be less damaging or even beneficial in some transplant settings because of their ability to inhibit other cell types, including Th1 cells, they may directly mediate graft rejection in other models; they also participate in the production of antidonor antibodies through promoting B cell activation and Ig class switching.

Th17 cells are cells capable of producing diverse cytokines, including IL-17A, IL-17F, IL-21, and IL-22. These cells are generated following exposure to TGF-β in the context of inflammatory cytokines such as IL-1 and IL-6. The expression of the transcription factor RORγt is required for Th17 induction. In addition, IL-23 clearly plays a role in driving Th17 responses. Th17 cells induce tissue infiltration of inflammatory cells and are thought to play a role in autoimmune responses and immune responses to fungal pathogens. Th17 cells have been shown to be involved in chronic allograft rejection in both animal models and humans.

Recent studies demonstrate cytokine profiles associated with IL-9 production (Th9), IL-22 production in the absence of IL-17 production (Th22), and high

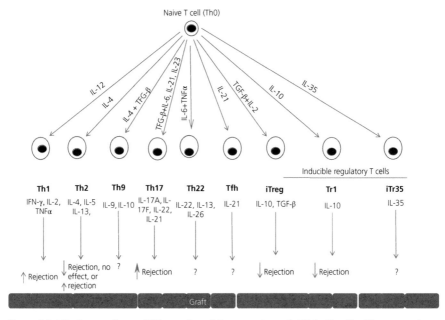

Figure 2.6 T helper subsets differentiated from activated CD4+ T cells. The currently recognized CD4+ T cell subsets and the cytokine milieu known to drive differentiation of individual subsets are shown here. The relative contribution of each subset to graft rejection is highlighted.

levels of IL-21 production associated with expression of the transcription factor Bcl-6 (Tfh). While the role(s) for Th9 and Th22 cells in clinical allograft rejection is currently unknown, there is an emerging appreciation for the role of Tfh cells. Tfh cells are characterized as CXCR5+Bcl6+PD1+) CD4+ T cells that provide B cell help and is needed for antibody-affinity maturation. Thus, Tfh cells may be involved in the production of high-affinity antigraft antibodies, which induce humoral allograft rejection (Figure 2.6).

T cell regulation

T cell responses are tightly controlled, and multiple layers of "checks and balances" are required to fine-tune the immune responses in terms of tempo, duration, and intensity. The activity of Tregs has been shown to be essential to the formation of immune tolerance and thus has long been viewed as the key to long-term successful transplantation strategies without chronic immunosuppression.

T Regulatory cells that express the transcription factor FoxP3 have been extensively studied. These regulatory cells are collectively called Tregs and can be divided into two subsets. Cells that express FoxP3 during thymic development are called natural Tregs (nTregs), while mature T cells that acquire FoxP3 expression extra-thymically, typically following exposure to antigens and immunoregulatory cytokines, are termed induced Tregs (iTregs). Tregs suppress T effector cells by a variety of mechanisms, including production of (i) immunoregulatory agents such as adenosine, TGF-β, and IL-10, (ii) tryptophan metabolism via indoleamine deoxygenase (IDO), (iii) direct cell–cell transfer of inhibitory levels of cAMP, and (iv) competition for common costimulatory signals (signal 2) or downregulation of costimulatory molecule expression on APCs. In addition to Foxp3+ Tregs, several other types of T cells are involved in the control of immune responses. CD8+CD28- T cells (referred to as T suppressor cells) have been shown to inhibit immune responses directly by suppressing T effector cells, and indirectly by preventing DCs activation. Subsets of γδ T cells have also been linked to the regulation of immunity in tissue inflammation and graft rejection.

Drugs used in clinical transplantation can alter Treg subsets. mTOR inhibitors such as rapamycin can promote the expansion of Tregs while inhibiting the expansion of activated T effector cells. Glucocorticoids have also been suggested to enhance the accumulation of FoxP3+ Tregs following transplantation. This increase in Tregs may reflect a previously unrecognized component of the immunosuppressive effect of these currently used drugs. In contrast, CNIs, such as tacrolimus and cyclosporin, appear to have a negative effect on Tregs in transplant models. Indeed, in many models, tolerance induction can be blocked by CNI. Combination therapies or altered timing might be required to minimize these negative effects on regulatory cells and potentially augment the immunosuppressive capacity of CNI drugs.

T cell memory

A hallmark of adaptive immunity is the ability to generate "memory cells" that can mount rapid secondary responses to the same antigens encountered in the primary response. Memory T cells are of particular concern in transplantation, as their heightened responses to lower levels of antigens without a stringent requirement for costimulation increases the chance that these cells will cross-react with one or more directly presented donor antigens, resulting in earlier and stronger rejection responses that are more difficult to reverse. This is compounded by the relative resistance of memory cells to conventional immunosuppression drugs and the increased numbers of memory cells due to heterologous immunity or homeostatic proliferation following lymphocyte depletion strategies that are used as induction therapies in transplant patients.

B cells
B cell development, subsets, and function

Similar to T cells, B cells arise from hematopoietic progenitor cells in the bone marrow. The development of B cells is outlined in Figure 2.7. The expression of immunoglobulin (IgM) on the cell surface that functions as a B cell receptor (BCR) defines the immature B cell stage. Immature B cells are subjected to a negative selection process via one of three mechanisms: deletion, anergy, or receptor editing. Selected B cells express delta chains and membrane IgD and

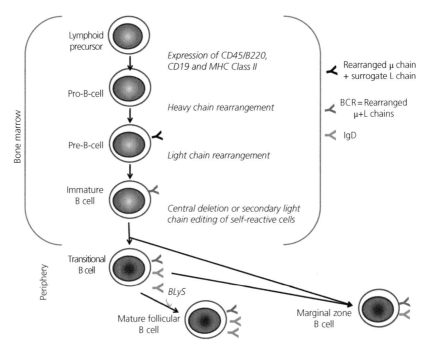

Figure 2.7 Schematic diagram of B cell development. Early pro-B cells are derived from lymphoid progenitor cells in the bone marrow. This step is defined by the recombination of genes encoding the Ig heavy chain and expression of CD45/B220, CD19, MHC class II. The cells then become large pre-B cells, and express a rearranged heavy chain and surrogate light chain. Expression of both heavy and light chains on the cell surface defines immature B cells. B cells leave the bone marrow at this stage, but they usually undergo clonal selection to delete self-reactive clones in the bone marrow before they reach the periphery. Mature B cells express membrane IgD.

become mature B cells. While the majority of conventional B cells are generated this way in the bone marrow, functional B cells can also be derived from hematopoietic stem cells in the fetal liver.

There are at least three major subsets of mature B cells in the periphery, namely, B1, B2, and marginal zone (MZ) B cells. B1 cells are subdivided into B1a and B1b subsets based on CD5 expression and are mostly located in the peritoneal and pleural cavities. B2 cells are "conventional" B cells and are predominantly located in follicles of secondary lymphoid organs. MZ B cells segregate anatomically into the marginal zone of the spleen, which also contains DCs and macrophages. While MZ B cells are noncirculating in mice, cells with a similar phenotype are found in the blood in humans. Such differences again highlight the limitations of animal models in transplantation.

B1 B cells spontaneously secrete IgM and IgG3 antibodies. These natural low-affinity antibodies bind to various carbohydrate moieties expressed by bacteria and also display certain self-reactivity. MZ B cells are well positioned to trap systemic blood-borne antigens. Both B1 and MZ B cells can rapidly produce

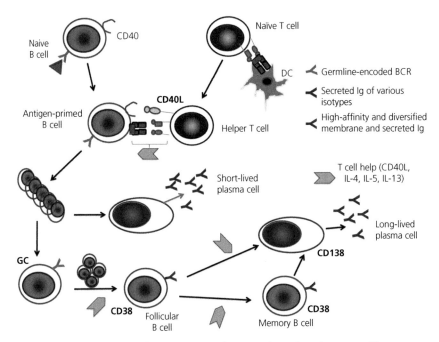

Figure 2.8 Key steps in B cell activation and generation of antigen-specific memory B cells. The antigen-specific B cell captures antigen via its BCR, and with the help of T_{FH} cells, antigen-primed B cells expand in secondary lymphoid organs; they either enter the germinal center (GC) pathway or give rise to short-lived (half-life of 3–5 days) plasma cells (PCs). During this process, activated B cells undergo antibody isotype class-switching, and in the GC, B cells also undergo somatic diversification of their antibody variable region genes, followed by selection of high-affinity clones. The generation of high-affinity memory B cells, including long-lived plasma cells and antigen specific memory B cells requires cognate interactions with GC T_{FH} cells.

antibodies to bacterial cell wall components and to various antigens with multivalent epitopes in a T cell-independent manner. B2 B cells express a diverse BCR repertoire and mediate T cell-dependent humoral immunity. Upon antigen encounter and with help from Tfh, B2 B cells differentiate into antibody-producing plasma cells and long-lived memory B cells (Figure 2.8).

Role of B cells in transplantation

The general belief is that B cells play a pathogenic role in transplant rejection, though emerging evidence suggests that certain B cells exhibit immunoregulatory functions. Thus, therapeutic strategies are hampered by lack of specificity in targeting harmful but not helpful, B cell populations. The presence of antidonor antibody (*alloantibody*) in transplant patients is associated with antibody-mediated rejection as well as the development of chronic rejection. Thus, activation of B cells and the induction of "humoral responses" against allografts are generally associated with poor transplant outcomes (Figure 2.9). In addition, B cells may also participate in the *priming* of CD4+ T cells by virtue of their antigen presentation

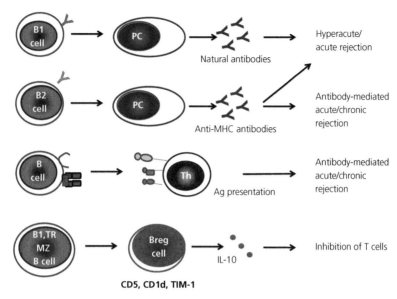

Figure 2.9 Role of B cells in transplant rejection. B cells are antibody-producing cells. Pre-existing antibodies (natural ABO antibodies or anti-HLA antibodies in transplant patients) mediate hyper-acute or acute graft rejection. Production of alloantibodies post-transplantation leads to antibody-mediated acute and chronic graft injury. B cells also amplify indirect donor antigen presentation to CD4+ T cells. Regulatory B cells (Bregs) have a protective effect by suppressing T cell responses.

capacity. As B cells can directly bind to soluble antigens via their BCR, recipient B cells can pick up soluble antigens released by the graft and present them to naïve or memory CD4+ T cells, thereby amplifying or sustaining T cell responses.

Recent studies suggest that B cells can also inhibit immune responses by acting as regulatory cells. It was shown that a subset of "small" B cells can mediate the induction of tolerance to soluble protein antigens by acting as tolerogenic APCs. Recent clinical data have also identified a strong B cell signature in kidney transplant patients with stable graft survival and were not on any immunosuppressive drugs. These findings are consistent with the recent recognition of Breg) under various tolerizing conditions. Several Breg phenotypes have been described, including but not restricted to the marginal zone (MZ) population or to a CD1d^{hi}CD5+ subset. Functionally, Bregs are characterized by the production of high levels of IL-10. Indeed, the T cell Ig domain and mucin protein-1 (TIM-1) molecule was recently identified as a marker for Breg. TIM-1 is expressed by >70% of the IL-10+ B cells and TIM-1 ligation on B cells induced B cells with regulatory activity. B cells may have other functions in transplantation. The formation of intra-graft B cell clusters reminiscent of ectopic germinal centers identified in autoimmune diseases has been reported in humans and mice. The phenotype and role of B cells in these tertiary lymphoid organs is unclear, but a role in chronic rejection has been suggested.

Targeting B cells in transplantation

Approximately 30% of patients on the waiting list for kidney transplant are classified as "sensitized"; they have high levels of preformed antidonor HLA antibodies before transplantation. In keeping with the critical role of B cells as crucial mediators of antibody production, preemptive B cell depletion using a monoclonal antibody against CD20 (rituximab) decrease *de novo* alloantibody production and attenuate chronic rejection of islet and cardiac allografts in monkeys, a finding that has now been extended to clinical trials. Furthermore, B cell depletion combined with intravenous immunoglobulin (IVIG) has been used to "desensitize" patients with high levels of alloantibody. The proteasome inhibitor Bortezomib used to treat myeloma cancer patients was shown to induce apoptosis of antibody-producing plasma cells and has been used as a strategy to desensitize transplant patients. However, its use is associated with side effects, which has limited greater use. New therapies are also emerging to control B cell survival, activation, or differentiation, and those therapies are currently in clinical trials for the treatment of systemic lupus erythematosus and other autoimmune diseases. For example, TACI-Ig (Atacicept or Etanercept) is a soluble receptor that binds to BLyS and APRIL, which are TNF family cytokines that promote B-cell survival, and neutralizes their functions. Belimumab (Benlysta) is a monoclonal antibody that specifically recognizes and inhibits the biologic activity of B-Lymphocyte stimulator (BLyS). Additional reagents targeting various surface receptors on B cells or growth factors are also under clinical development.

As differentiation of B cells into memory and antibody-producing plasma cells is dependent on the help they receive from Tfh cells, targeting costimulation pathways required for Tfh induction is an alternative strategy to modulate B cell responses. Targeting costimulatory molecules, including CD28, CD154, and ICOS, can drastically improve transplant survival in various models; such costimulatory pathways may also affect Tfh cells, thereby, indirectly modulating antidonor antibody responses.

Natural killer T (NKT) cells

NKT cells express both a restricted TCR repertoire and the traditional NK cell marker, NK1.1. However, NKT cells are distinct from NK cells and conventional T cells in multiple aspects (Figure 2.10). NKT cells recognize lipid antigens in the context of CD1 molecules, unlike classical T cells, which recognize peptide antigens presented by MHC molecules. The majority of NKT cells express an invariant TCR, which is Vα14Jα18 in mice and Vα24Jα18 in humans, respectively, and they pair with the Vβ chain of limited diversity. These are referred to as canonical or invariant NKT (*i*NKT) cells. In contrast to conventional $\alpha\beta$ T cells, which are selected by MHC-peptide complexes presented by thymic epithelial cells, NKT cells are selected by CD1d-lipid antigen complexes presented on the

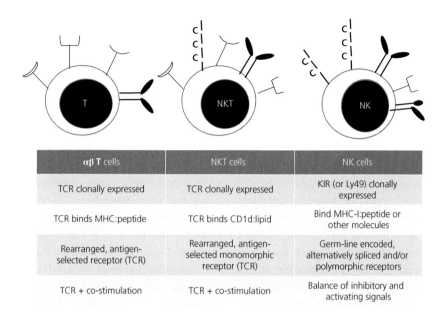

αβ T cells	NKT cells	NK cells
TCR clonally expressed	TCR clonally expressed	KIR (or Ly49) clonally expressed
TCR binds MHC:peptide	TCR binds CD1d:lipid	Bind MHC-I:peptide or other molecules
Rearranged, antigen-selected receptor (TCR)	Rearranged, antigen-selected monomorphic receptor (TCR)	Germ-line encoded, alternatively spliced and/or polymorphic receptors
TCR + co-stimulation	TCR + co-stimulation	Balance of inhibitory and activating signals

Figure 2.10 Comparison of NKT, T, and NK cells. NKT cells display molecules characteristic of both NK and T cells. Unlike classical T cells, NKT cells are activated by lipid antigens presented by CD1d molecules. Similar to NK cells, NKT cells express germline encoded inhibitory and activating receptors. Thus, NKT cells function to bridge the innate and adaptive immune responses.

surface of cortical thymocytes. One hallmark of NKT cells is their ability to produce large amounts of Th1 and Th2 cytokines within hours after activation. NKT cells constitutively express mRNA encoding IFN-γ and IL-4, which allows them to rapidly exert their effector functions. Functionally, NKT cells interact with NK cells, neutrophils, macrophages, DCs, B cells, and T cells.

NKT cells and transplant response

Although some data suggest that NKT cells play a role in the immune response to transplants, it is not clear whether NKT cells can directly recognize alloantigens in the context of CD1d molecules or if they are activated during transplantation by the cytokine milieu generated from immune activation. NKT cells may promote transplant rejection or tolerance, depending on their response to these antigens.

In an islet transplant model, NKT cells have been reported to promote graft loss of intraportal transplanted islets. Moreover, it was shown that wild-type diabetic mice required 400 syngenetic islets, while NKT-deficient mice needed only 100 islets to achieve euglycemia, demonstrating a detrimental role for NKT cells in transplant rejection. In other models, NKT cells are required for the induction of tolerance to cardiac allografts, rat xenografts, and corneal transplants. The mechanism(s) by which NKT cells prolong graft survival are largely unknown, but production of immunoregulatory cytokines, including IL-10 or IFN-γ, has been suggested.

Summary

As most therapeutic strategies in the clinic target T cells to prevent acute cellular rejection, this chapter highlights the complexity of cell types in transplant rejection. Existing therapeutics appear to be effective in preventing rejection mediated by some cell types, but less so in rejection by other cell types. Nonetheless, it is obvious that different strategies may be required to limit organ injury by immune and nonimmune mechanisms before transplant and to induce donor-specific tolerance after transplant. It is clear now that the T cell-centric strategy alone is not sufficient for the induction of indefinite transplant survival. By contrasting what is known about the biology of immune cells derived from various models with existing studies in clinical transplantation, we may be able to develop a deeper understanding of the mechanisms of transplant rejection and identify potential new therapeutic targets. It is also likely that future improvement in transplant outcomes will depend on new drugs and biologics to target various pathways of both the innate and adaptive arms of the immune system.

Further reading

Clatworthy MR. Targeting B cells and antibody in transplantation. Am J Transplant 2011;11(7):1359–1367.

Cua DJ, Tato CM. Innate IL-17-producing cells: the sentinels of the immune system. Nat Rev Immunol 2010;10(7):479–489.

Ezzelarab M, Thomson AW. Tolerogenic dendritic cells and their role in transplantation. Semin Immunol 2011;23(4):252–263.

Ford ML, Larsen CP. Overcoming the memory barrier in tolerance induction: molecular mimicry and functional heterogeneity among pathogen-specific T-cell populations. Curr Opin Organ Transplant 2010;15(4):405–410.

Garcia MR, Ledgerwood L, Yang Y, Xu J, Lal G, Burrell B et al. Monocytic suppressive cells mediate cardiovascular transplantation tolerance in mice. J Clin Invest 2010;120(7):2486–2496.

Geissmann F, Manz MG, Jung S, Sieweke MH, Merad M, Ley K. Development of monocytes, macrophages, and dendritic cells. Science 2010;327(5966):656–661.

Halloran PF. T cell-mediated rejection of kidney transplants: a personal viewpoint. Am J Transplant 2010;10(5):1126–1134.

Idoyaga J, Steinman RM. SnapShot: dendritic cells. Cell 2011;146(4):660–660 e662.

Jordan SC, Kahwaji J, Toyoda M, Vo A. B-cell immunotherapeutics: emerging roles in solid organ transplantation. Curr Opin Organ Transplant 2011;16(4):416–424.

Kim CH, Butcher EC, Johnston B. Distinct subsets of human Valpha24-invariant NKT cells: cytokine responses and chemokine receptor expression. Trends Immunol 2002;23(11): 516–519.

Liu K, Nussenzweig MC. Origin and development of dendritic cells. Immunol Rev 2010; 234(1):45–54.

Lu LF, Lind EF, Gondek DC, Bennett KA, Gleeson MW, Pino-Lagos K et al. Mast cells are essential intermediaries in regulatory T-cell tolerance. Nature 2006;442(7106):997–1002.

Mantovani A, Cassatella MA, Costantini C, Jaillon S. Neutrophils in the activation and regulation of innate and adaptive immunity. Nat Rev Immunol 2011;11(8):519–531.

Murphy SP, Porrett PM, Turka LA. Innate immunity in transplant tolerance and rejection. Immunol Rev 2011;241(1):39–48.

Orr MT, Lanier LL. Natural killer cell education and tolerance. Cell 2010;142(6):847–856.

Parsons RF, Vivek K, Redfield RR, 3rd, Migone TS, Cancro MP, Naji A et al. B-lymphocyte homeostasis and BLyS-directed immunotherapy in transplantation. Transplant Rev (Orlando) 2010;24(4):207–221.

Stegall MD, Dean PG, Gloor J. Mechanisms of alloantibody production in sensitized renal allograft recipients. Am J Transplant 2009;9(5):998–1005.

Vivier E, Raulet DH, Moretta A, Caligiuri MA, Zitvogel L, Lanier LL et al. Innate or adaptive immunity? The example of natural killer cells. Science 2011;331(6013):44–49.

Wieckiewicz J, Goto R, Wood KJ. T regulatory cells and the control of alloimmunity: from characterisation to clinical application. Curr Opin Immunol 2010;22(5):662–668.

Zhu J, Paul WE. Heterogeneity and plasticity of T helper cells. Cell Res 2010;20(1):4–12.

CHAPTER 3

Soluble mediators in the immune system

Charles A. Su, William M. Baldwin III, and Robert L. Fairchild

Department of Immunology, Cleveland Clinic Lerner College of Medicine,
Department of Pathology, Case Western Reserve University School of Medicine, Cleveland, USA

CHAPTER OVERVIEW

- Cytokines mediate communication among cells in the immune system.
- Acute phase cytokines are produced immediately after injury and mediate the intensity of inflammation.
- Cytokines of the common γ_c chain family primarily mediate lymphocyte homeostasis, survival, and effector differentiation.
- Cytokines produced by antigen-presenting cells direct the differentiation of T lymphocytes to acquire specific functions during immune responses.
- Cytokines are also involved in suppression of immune responses that favor allograft survival.

Introduction

Proper immune cell function requires that they receive and respond to signals within their environment. These signals are transduced to the nucleus to evoke the expression of genes that regulate cell movement, positioning, and/or expression of specific functions. Such signals are essential for directing cell behavior and function in response to injury. Delivery of signals can be mediated during cell–cell contact or by soluble molecules. This chapter will focus on families of cytokines that play key roles in initiating, maintaining, and/or resolving tissue inflammation, as well as in the function of the immune system, emphasizing their roles in the response to an allograft.

Transplant Immunology, First Edition. Edited by Xian Chang Li and Anthony M. Jevnikar.
© 2016 John Wiley & Sons, Ltd. Published 2016 by John Wiley & Sons, Ltd.
Copyright ® American Society of Transplantation 2016.
Companion website: www.wiley.com/go/li/transplantimmunology

Cytokines

Cytokines are small, soluble proteins produced by almost all cells that mediate cellular communication. Cytokines are involved in morphogenesis; the development of lymphoid architecture; the generation of leukocytes and other cells in the bone marrow; the induction, amplification, and resolution of inflammation; and as effector and regulatory molecules during immune responses. Cell-to-cell communication by cytokines is transmitted through receptors specific for particular cytokines on the target cell. Different groups of cytokines transmit signals to target cells through different signal transduction mechanisms that begin with cytokine binding to the receptor and end with the induction of transcription factors to promote gene expression (Figure 3.1). Obviously, the different stages of transplantation, from ischemia-reperfusion injury (IRI) to acute and chronic forms of injury leading to allograft failure, and even the induction and maintenance of tolerance to the allograft involve the activities of specific cytokines. Here we will briefly summarize the properties of specific cytokines and their receptors and comment briefly on the roles of key cytokines known to play roles in allograft injury and protection.

Acute phase cytokines (i.e., IL-1β, IL-6, and TNFα) are produced immediately following reperfusion of organ grafts. This production is stimulated in part by the oxygen radicals generated by tissue-resident macrophages and endothelial cells that have converted to a glycolytic form of respiration during ischemia and the sudden provision of oxygenated blood during reperfusion. The acute phase cytokines stimulate a number of downstream inflammatory processes that contribute to graft injury. In response to allografts, donor antigen-reactive T cells in recipient lymphoid organs are activated and differentiate to distinct functional phenotypes during which the common γ_c cytokines are critically involved. The trafficking of donor antigen-primed T cells to the allograft and their activation results in cytokine-mediated injury to the graft tissue. IFN-γ is by far the most frequently observed cytokine produced by donor antigen-primed T cells during the rejection response. In some animal models, donor antigen-specific T cells have been shown to differentiate into IL-17-producing cells, which result in a distinct pathology in rejecting graft tissue. The development of T cell responses to tissue-specific antigens may be skewed to IL-17 production, particularly during the rejection of lung allografts. Finally, it is also important to understand the consequences of TGFβ signaling during the priming of donor antigen-reactive T cells as well as in the development of chronic graft injury. Details regarding the production of these cytokines and their impact on acute and chronic allograft injury are discussed here.

Acute phase cytokines

The acute phase cytokines IL-1, IL-6, and TNFα are typically produced during the initiation of inflammatory processes. These cytokines have pleiotropic downstream effects including the activation of endothelial cells with mobilization of

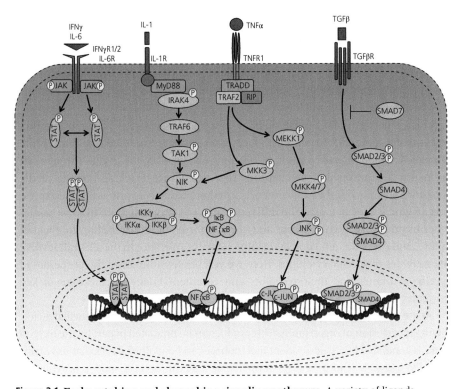

Figure 3.1 Early cytokine and chemokine signaling pathways. A variety of ligands including cytokines such as IL-6 and IFN-γ propagate their signals through the JAK/STAT pathway. JAK activation occurs upon ligand-mediated receptor multimerization when two JAKs are brought into close proximity, allowing trans-phosphorylation. The activated JAKs subsequently phosphorylate STATs, which dimerize and enter the nucleus where they bind specific regulatory sequences to activate or repress transcription of target genes. Pro-inflammatory cytokines such as IL-1 signal through pathways that converge on the activation of NF-κB. MyD88 functions as an adaptor between receptors of the TLR or IL-1R families and downstream signaling kinases. Phosphorylated IκB releases NF-κB dimers from the cytoplasmic NF-κB-IκB complex, allowing them to translocate to the nucleus to mediate gene transcription. TNF-α acts by binding to its trimeric receptors, TNFR1 (p55) and TNFR2 (p75). Ligand binding results in the recruitment of signal transducers that activate either the NF-κB or the MAPK pathways. Two MAPK kinases (MAPKKs), MKK4 and MKK7, phosphorylate and activate JNK, which translocates to the nucleus and activates transcription factors such as c-Jun. TGF-β-triggered signals are transduced by proteins belonging to the Smad family. The type I receptor recognizes and phosphorylates Smad2 and Smad3, which associates with Smad4, forming complexes that participate in DNA binding and recruitment of transcription factors. Smad7 inhibits Smad2 and Smad3 phosphorylation.

Weibel–Palade bodies to the luminal surface and expression of von Willebrand factor and P-selectin, induction of ICAM-1 and ICAM-2 and the production of chemoattractants that direct leukocytes into the tissue inflammation site. TNFα and IL-1β also induce the liver to produce acute phase proteins, including serum amyloid A, C-reactive protein, and importantly, complement C3.

The IL-1 family cytokines

IL-1β

Although IL-1α and IL-1β are structurally related, they are distinct cytokines that play key roles in tissue inflammation. Monocytes and macrophages that have been stimulated through Toll-like receptors (TLRs) or by TNFα are the primary sources of IL-1α and IL-1β. However, IL-1α and IL-1β are produced by almost all cells during inflammatory stress. Following translation, IL-1α is mostly retained in the cytosol of the producing cells. In contrast, IL-1β is produced as a pro-form that has no biological activity until it is processed by TLR-activated caspase 1 within the organized inflammasome, and then is released from the producing cell. A critical pro-inflammatory function of IL-1β is the stimulation of the liver to produce acute phase proteins, including C-reactive protein and serum amyloid protein. IL-1β also stimulates the production of chemokines, including IL-8 and CXCL1, which are key neutrophil chemoattractants. IL-1β can also regulate the development of different cell populations from hematopoietic precursor cells in the bone marrow. During adaptive immune responses to bacteria and fungi, IL-1β promotes the differentiation of CD4+ T cells to IL-17-producing Th17 cells.

IL-1α and IL-1β signal through binding to the IL-1 type 1 receptor, a member of the Toll-IL-1 receptor superfamily. Similar to most TLRs, binding of IL-1β to the IL-1R1 transduces signals through the MyD88 adaptor molecule and IL-1 receptor-associated kinases (IRAKs) to induce IKK-mediated phosphorylation of IκB. This phosphorylation provokes the release of NF-κB from IκB and the translocation of NF-κB to the nucleus permits binding to the promoters of target genes encoding pro-inflammatory mediators. The IL-1 type 2 receptor binds both IL-1α and IL-1β but acts as a "decoy" receptor incapable of transducing signals upon binding. It is important to note a soluble form of an IL-1 receptor, IL-1Rα can bind IL-1β to act as an antagonist for IL-1β binding and blocks binding to the functional IL-1R1 receptor. Production of IL-1Rα is also induced during tissue inflammation and the intensity of inflammation is likely to be, at least in part, a balance between the production of IL-1Rα and IL-1β. In support of this, infants with loss of function mutations in IL-1Rα, quickly develop auto-inflammatory manifestations including skin pustule eruptions, high serum levels of C-reactive protein, neutrophilia, and bone abnormalities.

IL-6

The IL-6-related cytokines includes leukemia inhibitory factor (LIF), oncostatin M, and IL-6. These cytokines are small-molecular-weight proteins with a four α-helix bundle structure. They also share a requirement for binding to the gp130 receptor subunit to transduce signals into receptor-expressing target cells. IL-6 mediates a broad range of functions on a diverse target cell population as it is involved in promoting inflammation, the development of T cells to specific functional phenotypes, alters lymphocyte survival by inducing expression of the anti-apoptotic molecule Bcl-2, and promotes the differentiation of B lymphocytes to antibody-producing plasma cells. Although gp130 is expressed on almost all cells, IL-6-mediated signaling requires initial binding of the cytokine to a subunit chain of the receptor, IL-6Rα that is produced by hepatocytes and leukocytes. IL-6/IL-6Rα dimers then form complexes with two of the receptor chains, having the intracellular signaling domains. These complexes activate JAK-mediated phosphorylation of STAT3 and translocation of STAT3 dimers into the nucleus to bind promoter elements of responsive genes and induce gene transcription.

IL-6 transcripts are observed during the reperfusion of grafts and during acute rejection of heart and kidney allografts in rodent models as well as in clinical kidney transplants. In mouse models, transplant of IL-6 deficient cardiac or kidney allografts results in a threefold prolongation of allograft survival that correlates with increased Treg activity. Antibody neutralization of IL-6 abrogates CD4 T cell-mediated rejection of complete MHC mismatched heart allografts and when combined with CTLA-4Ig results in allograft survival beyond 60 days.

IL-6 plays a critical role in the development of graft hypertrophy and fibrosis during chronic injury of cardiac allografts. This is consistent with *in vitro* studies indicating the ability of IL-6 to enhance cardiac fibroblast expression of collagen mRNA and proliferation. IL-6 enhances the pro-fibrotic TGFβ signaling to cells by increasing TGFβ receptor trafficking to nonlipid rafts within the plasma membrane. Recent studies demonstrate synergism of IL-6 and TGFβ1 in chronic rejection in cardiac allografts by the induction of connective tissue growth factor (CTGF), which appears to be the key factor mediating the fibrosis that develops during the chronic injury.

TNFα

TNFα in its active form is a 17 kD cytokine produced primarily by monocytes and macrophages that has a key role in tissue inflammation; TNFα induces the expression of many components of inflammation. TNFα induces IL-6, multiple chemokines, cyclo-oxygenase 2 (COX2), inducible nitric oxide synthase (iNOS), adhesion molecules, and activates endothelial cell to translocate Weibel-Palade bodies containing P-selectin and von Willebrand factor, to the cell surface. The key role of TNFα in sepsis and endotoxic shock, rheumatoid arthritis, Crohn's disease, and psoriasis is highlighted by the ability of neutralizing antibodies or engineered soluble TNFα receptors to attenuate inflammation and tissue pathology in these diseases.

TNFα is produced as a 26 kD precursor protein that is expressed on the cell membrane and cleaved by TNFα-converting enzyme (TACE/ADAM17) to a secreted form that then organizes into non-covalently associated trimers. The effect of TNFα trimers is transduced by two different receptors: TNFR1 and TNFR2. The intracellular domains of the two receptors differ, suggesting different intracellular pathways and functions of the two receptors. Importantly, TNFR1 activates caspase 8-mediated apoptosis, while TNFR2 mediates the activation of NF-κB leading to transcription of many of the downstream inflammatory components. The balance between TNFR-1 and TNFR-2 signaling may determine whether cell death or cell survival occurs. Recently, it has been shown that TNFα exposure in cells with caspase-8 inhibition results in an intense form of programmed necrosis, termed "necroptosis."

TNFα is a key mediator of many inflammatory events. TNFα is produced within minutes to hours of reperfusion of vascularized iso- and allografts. Neutralization of TNFα at this time results in marked decreases in TNFα production as well as IL-1β, but not IL-6. Interstitial dendritic cell emigration from inflammatory tissue sites is promoted by TNFα. TNFα also upregulates MHC class I and class II molecule expression on the dendritic cell surface, implicating TNFα as a promoter of donor antigen-reactive T cell priming.

Many studies have documented a beneficial effect of anti-TNFα antibodies in delaying the rejection of organ allografts in animal models. A recent study indicated that administration of a single dose of anti-TNFα monoclonal antibody (mAb) at the time of allograft reperfusion attenuated post-transplant inflammation including the production of neutrophil and macrophage chemoattractants and the infiltration of these leukocytes and endogenous memory CD8+ T cells into the allograft post-transplant. TNFα mAb treatment also inhibited the priming of donor-reactive T cells and extended complete MHC-mismatched heart allograft survival. In rat models, administration of TNFα neutralizing antibody with low-dose cyclosporine A extended heart allograft survival and in combination with CD4-depleting antibodies resulted in the long-term survival of 60% of MHC-mismatched small bowel transplants, thus documenting the beneficial effect of TNFα neutralization in transplant settings.

IL-18

Similar to IL-1, IL-18 is transcribed as a biologically inactive precursor that is processed by caspase 1 cleavage to generate the active cytokine. The IL-18 receptor is a heterodimer expressed by T cells, NK cells, and macrophages. Typical of IL-1R family signaling pathways, IL-18 binding induces recruitment of MyD88 to activate IRAK-1 and then phosphorylation of IκB to provoke release of NF-κB and its translocation to the nucleus to induce pro-inflammatory cytokine gene expression. IL-18 induces T cell and NK cell production of IFN-γ, and this production is amplified in the presence of IL-12.

IL-18 expression is upregulated during reperfusion of ischemic kidneys in mouse models and genetic deletion of IL-18 or of caspase-1 (and IL-18 processing) attenuates this injury. In patients with acute tubular necrosis and in recipients of cadaveric renal grafts experiencing delayed graft function after transplant, high levels of IL-18 protein are detected in the urine and may constitute a biomarker of proximal tubular injury. IL-18 expression is also upregulated during acute rejection of renal allografts in a rat model, although renal allografts are rejected at similar times in wild-type and IL-18$^{-/-}$ mice. IL-37 is a newly described IL-1 family member, which inhibits IL-18-dependent pro-inflammatory cytokine production. Interestingly, a mouse homolog of IL-37 has not been reported, but human IL-37 has been shown to be active on mouse cells. Recently it has been demonstrated that kidney and other epithelial cells express IL-37, possibly representing an endogenous control mechanism to reduce inflammation during ischemia-reperfusion injury. IL-1, IL-18 and its family members, continue to have appeal as potential targets in limiting inflammation in transplantation.

The common γ_c family of cytokines

Cytokines that bind to multiunit receptors that include the common γ_c chain (CD132) constitute a large family, also with diverse functions. These cytokines include IL-2, IL-4, IL-7, IL-9, IL-15, and IL-21, and are arranged in a four α-helix bundle configuration. The receptors for the cytokines in this group consist of a private α chain, which defines cytokine specificity, and a shared β chain or the common γ_c chain that permits the transduction of signals from cytokine binding to the surface receptor to JAK-STAT-mediated intracellular signaling pathways (Figure 3.2).

IL-2
IL-2 is a central target of current immunosuppression using calcineurin inhibitors (CNI) as well as IL-2 receptor targeting by antibody (anti-CD25). It is produced primarily by activated CD4$^+$ T cells, but can be produced by CD8$^+$ T cells

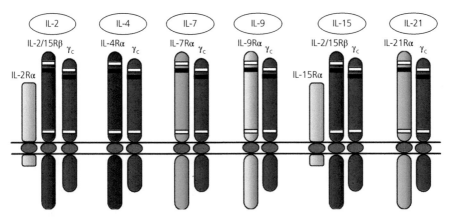

Figure 3.2 The common γ_c cytokines. The receptors for γ_c family cytokines are multimeric cell surface structures. The receptors for IL-2 and IL-15 are trimers, consisting of a private α chain and the shared IL-2Rβ chain and the common γ_c chain. The receptors for IL-4, IL-7, IL-9, and IL-21 are dimers, composed of a distinct α chain, which defines the cytokine specificity, and the common γ_c chain.

as well. IL-2 is rapidly produced during TCR engagement of cognate peptide/MHC complex and is the cytokine primarily responsible for clonal expansion during the activation of the peptide/MHC-specific T cells. Although IL-2 can increase susceptibility to apoptosis and activation-induced cell death through Fas (CD95) by cell-cycle-dependent downregulation of anti-apoptosis proteins (c-FLIP), its major effect appears to be on cell proliferation rather than tolerance induction.

The IL-2 receptor is composed of 3 subunits: the α (CD25), β (CD122), and the common γ_c chain. The β chain and the γ_c are constitutively expressed on the T cell surface and confer low-affinity binding of IL-2. During T cell receptor engagement of peptide/MHC complexes, signals transduced through CD3 and through CD28-mediated costimulation induce the expression of the IL-2 receptor α chain, CD25, which in complex with the β chain and γ_c provides for high-affinity IL-2 binding. CD4$^+$ T cells that express the transcription factor FoxP3 (Tregs) constitutively express CD25, thereby allowing Tregs to have a competitive advantage in being able to bind IL-2 under static conditions. Tregs require IL-2 signaling for their survival and expansion, but can be maintained with low levels.

CD4 T cells are the major source of IL-2 during the initiation of alloreactive T cell responses. IL-2 can promote the clonal expansion of alloreactive CD4$^+$ and CD8$^+$ T cells in recipients of allografts, which can be attenuated by treating the recipients with anti-CD25 mAb. In clinical transplantation, this strategy is commonly used as induction therapy. Although there might be theoretical concerns that treatment with anti-CD25 mAb might interfere with the graft prolonging effects of Treg cells, this has not been the case in clinical practice. Indeed induction with anti-CD25 mAb has been observed to be very effective in improving allograft outcomes, particularly when the graft is from a living donor.

IL-7

IL-7 serves functions as a key "rheostat" for T cell development in the thymus as well as regulating peripheral T cell numbers and their homeostasis. Stromal cells in the bone marrow and skin and intestinal epithelial cells are the major sources of IL-7, while dendritic cells and macrophages are secondary sources of IL-7. The IL-7 receptor is a heterodimer expressed on thymocytes, naïve T cells, as well as on B cells. It consists of an α chain (CD127) paired with the common γ_c chain (CD132). During T cell responses to foreign peptide/MHC complexes, IL-7Rα chain expression on reactive T cells is downregulated and IL-7 is not used to drive the clonal proliferation of the T cells. Interestingly, regulatory T cells express low levels of IL-7Rα chain, which may reflect continuous or frequent TCR-mediated stimulation from self-peptide/MHC complexes in the periphery.

IL-7 is produced by epithelial cells in the thymus and provides key survival and differentiation signals for developing T cells. IL-7 maintains the survival of peripheral T cells by inducing homeostatic cycling and the expression of anti-apoptotic molecules such as Bcl-2 and Mcl-1. Memory T cells also express the IL-7Rα chain and signaling through the receptor maintains their survival. Under lymphopenic conditions such as those generated following the administration of lymphocyte-depleting antibodies or during the course of an HIV infection, stromal cells increase IL-7 production inducing homeostatic proliferation of the remaining T cells or T cells introduced into the lymphopenic environment until homeostatic numbers of T cells are achieved. Importantly, this homeostatic proliferation results in the transition of the proliferating T cells to a memory phenotype.

During acute and chronic antibody-mediated rejection of renal grafts, increases in alloreactive T cells expressing high levels of CD127 are observed in the peripheral blood and in the graft. Furthermore, homeostatic proliferation and conversion of proliferating T cells from a naïve to a memory phenotype may be particularly important with regards to the use of lymphocyte-depleting strategies used to condition higher risk allograft recipients. As proof of principle, depletion of T cells in cardiac allograft recipients results in the generation of alloreactive memory T cells that are resistant to tolerance induction using costimulatory blockade strategies that otherwise induce tolerance. The potential clinical use of anti-CD127 antibodies to target memory cells in patients that have been conditioned with lympho-depleting regimens is currently being considered.

IL-9

IL-9 was originally identified as a T cell-derived growth factor for other T cells, primarily by those also producing IL-4, IL-5, and IL-13. Recent studies have identified specific populations of T cells that produce IL-9 but not IL-4 or IFN-γ. IL-9-producing CD4$^+$ T cells have been termed Th9 cells and are best induced *in vitro* by a combination of TGFβ and IL-4. IL-9 binds to a receptor composed of the IL-9 receptor α chain and the common γ$_c$ chain.

IL-9 also promotes the expansion and recruitment of mast cells to peripheral tissues and stimulates mast cell production of pro-inflammatory (e.g. IL-1β, IL-6, and IL-13) as well as anti-inflammatory (e.g. TGFβ and IL-10) cytokines. In some transplant models, the induction and maintenance of tolerance to skin allografts requires Treg production of IL-9. However, the tolerogenic effect of this mechanism is conditional. Mast cell degranulation readily breaks transplant tolerance and triggers the rejection of an otherwise tolerant graft.

IL-15

IL-15 is a growth and survival factor for T cells, especially CD8$^+$ T cells and NK cells through binding to a receptor consisting of the IL-15Rα chain, the IL-2Rβ chain (CD122), and the γ$_c$ chain. Macrophages, monocytes, and dendritic cells are the primary producers of IL-15, particularly during acute phase cytokine mediated inflammation. As well, IL-15 can be produced by renal tubular epithelial cells and other parenchymal cells. Unlike the IL-2 receptor, the IL-15Rα chain alone has a high affinity for IL-15. Thus, IL-15 can be bound by the IL-15Rα chain expressed on dendritic cells or macrophages, and this IL-15/IL-15Rα complex is "trans-presented" to responding cells to provoke T cell proliferation and survival.

IL-15 transcripts are detected in clinical renal grafts during acute rejection episodes. A mutant IL-15/Fc construct designed to be an antagonist for IL-15 binding to its receptor has been generated by Strom et al. and tested for its ability to promote long-term survival of islet and heart allografts in mouse models. In a complete MHC-mismatched model, recipient treatment with the usion protein resulted in a modest prolongation in survival of 60% of islet grafts and in long-term survival of 40% of the allografts, but was more efficacious in promoting allograft survival when combined with CTLA-4Ig. Recipient treatment with the construct in addition to a suboptimal dose of anti-CD154 mAb conferred long-term survival of complete MHC-mismatched heart allografts and tolerance to subsequent challenge with a heart donor skin allograft in 50% of the treated recipients. A similar strategy applied to nonhuman primate recipients indicated that short-term treatment with an antagonist IL-15/Fc construct in combination with an agonist IL-2/Fc construct and sirolumus extended survival of islet and heart allografts. Together, these studies demonstrate an important role for IL-15 in allograft rejection, and supports further studies.

The IL-12 family of cytokines

Structurally, cytokines of the IL-12 family are heterodimeric molecules consisting of two chains; the subunits of the cytokine chains, as well as their receptor chains are shared among family members. This provides a structural basis for functional diversity and redundancy of these cytokines. The IL-12 family of cytokines plays key roles in directing the differentiation of CD4+ T cells to specific functional phenotypes. While the role of IL-12 in the rejection of allografts has been well documented in mouse models, the role of other family members is less clear and requires further investigations.

IL-12

IL-12 is a heterodimer consisting of 35 (p35) and 40 (p40) kD subunits. Each subunit is encoded on different chromosomes and the expression of each is differentially regulated. When produced in excess, the p40 chains can form homodimers and in mice these homodimers antagonize binding of the p35–p40 heterodimer to its specific receptor. Many cells produce the p35 subunit, but the p40 subunit and the functional IL-12 heterodimer is produced mainly by dendritic cells, monocytes, and macrophages, as well as neutrophils following activation via TLR binding.

The IL-12 receptor is similarly composed of two subunits, a β1 and a β2 chain, and the expression and association of both are required for high-affinity binding to IL-12. The β2 chain transduces signals into receptor-bearing cells through the activation of JAK2 and STAT4, and, upon phosphorylation, STAT4 translocates into the nucleus to provoke gene expression. IL-12 binding to the receptor also induces the expression of T-bet, a key transcription factor that upregulates expression of IL-12R β2 expression on CD4 T cells and directs CD4 T cell development to IFN-γ-producing Th1 cells that are critical for responses to intracellular pathogens. IL-12 also stimulates the growth and activation of NK cells to produce IFN-γ. Studies have indicated that the production of IL-12 within inflammatory tissue sites provokes infiltrating memory CD8 T cells to proliferate and express effector function including TNF-α and IFN-γ production as well as perforin/granzyme B mediated cytolysis.

In mouse models, neutralization of IL-12 or genetic deletion of IL-12 p40 in complete MHC-mismatched heart allograft recipients did not inhibit the development of donor-reactive T cells producing IFN-γ or the rejection of the allografts. However, neutralization of IL-12 in recipients depleted of CD8 T cells did lead to significant prolongation in allograft survival, implicating IFN-γ-producing donor-reactive CD8 T cells that are independent of IL-12 as the effector T cells capable of mediating acute rejection in previous studies.

IL-23

IL-23 is a disulfide-linked heterodimer composed of a 19 kD chain and the IL-12 p40 chain. The functional IL-23 heterodimer is produced by activated dendritic cells and macrophages, primarily originating from the intestinal tract, the skin, and the lungs. IL-23 production by these cells is stimulated through engagement of TLR2, NOD2, and C-type lectins, such as dectin-1 and β-glucan curdlan from fungi. The receptor for IL-23 shares the IL-12β1 subunit, which is associated with a second chain, IL-23R, conferring specificity for the p19 chain of the cytokine and induction of gene transcription through the activation of the JAK/STAT transduction pathway. The products of this stimulation can enhance CD4 T cell differentiation to an IL-17-producing phenotype (i.e., Th17) and stabilize the differentiated T cells to maintain the Th17 phenotype.

IL-27

IL-27 is a heterodimer composed of a 28 kD chain and the Epstein Barr virus-induced gene 3 (EBI3) chain. Dendritic cells and macrophages are the major sources of IL-27, but it is also produced by endothelial cells following stimulation with TLR ligands. The production of the p28 and EBI3 chains are induced by TLR ligands as well as by engagement of CD40. IL-27 binds to a heterodimer receptor composed of the IL-27Rα chain and the gp130 chain shared by receptors for IL-6 and OSM. The α chain confers specificity for the IL-27 heterodimer and the gp130 transduces signals upon cytokine binding through the activation of JAKs to phosphorylate STAT1. This STAT1 activation induces the expression of T-bet, which drives IFN-γ production, CXCR3 expression, and other cellular processes involved in the differentiation of CD4 T cells to Th1 cells during immune responses. IL-27 also inhibits the differentiation of CD4 T cells to Th2 and Th17 cells by inhibiting the expression of GATA-3 and RORγt, key transcription factors required for the differentiation to Th2 and Th17 cells, respectively. Paradoxically to its pro-inflammatory properties, IL-27 also has anti-inflammatory effects that are involved in downmodulation of immune responses. These effects are due in part to IL-27 inhibiting IL-2 production and stimulating T cell production of IL-10.

The role of IL-27 in transplant models is not well understood. In a rat model, IL-27 p28 and EBI3 mRNA were expressed in long-term surviving cardiac allografts in recipients subjected to tolerance inducing strategies at higher levels than in cardiac allografts undergoing chronic rejection. The implication of this finding in transplant survival remains to be studied.

Adaptive immunity cytokines

IFN-γ

IFN-γ is a pleiotropic cytokine that induces many pro-inflammatory effects; most cells express the receptor and thus respond to IFN-γ production. The IFN-γ receptor is composed of two chains, IFN-γR1 which primarily functions in binding the cytokine and IFN-γR2 that transduces the JAK1/JAK2-STAT2 mediated signals to promote expression of genes involved in inflammation, phagocytosis and bacterial killing, and the initiation and maintenance of adaptive immune responses.

IFN-γ is produced primarily by NK cells and CD4 or CD8 T cells during antigen priming. For CD4 T cells this requires the production of IL-12 and/or IL-27 by the antigen-presenting cell and the activation of transcription factors including T-bet, that direct development to an IFN-γ-producing Th1 phenotype. CD8 T cells do not require stimulation with IL-12 to develop into IFN-γ-producing cells, but use either T-bet or another transcription factor eomesodermin to direct IFN-γ production. These transcription factors are required for the activation of several genes involved in IFN-γ-mediated inflammation including the chemokine receptor CXCR3, which binds to the IFN-γ-induced chemokines CXCL9/Mig, CXCL10/IP-10 and CXCL11/I-TAC. These chemokines direct recruitment of IFN-γ-producing CD4 Th1 and CD8 T cells to inflammatory sites.

The pro-inflammatory effects of IFN-γ are numerous. Importantly, IFN-γ is critical for the elimination of intracellular parasites as it stimulates the production and assembly of the NAPDH oxidase complex needed for the digestion of parasites and to stimulate lysozomal-phagosome fusion to generate the phagolysosomes where digestion occurs. IFN-γ also stimulates the production and assembly of proteins involved in peptide transport into the endoplasmic reticulum where it is bound by class I MHC molecules prior to their delivery to the cell surface and upregulates the expression of both class I and class II MHC molecules on cells. Interestingly, IFN-γ can induce the expression of MHC class II molecules that constitutively do not express class II, including renal tubular epithelial cells. Thus, cellular rejection with IFN-γ expressing cells may result in the enhanced expression of MHC, that can then be targeted by both class I and class II directed alloantibody.

IFN-γ transcripts and protein are typically observed during acute injury of renal, cardiac, and pancreatic islet transplants and anti-IFN-γ antibody has been shown to prolong the survival of allografts. Furthermore, the enumeration of donor antigen-specific CD4 and CD8 T cells producing IFN-γ in ELISPOT assays is a frequently used approach to assess the presence and levels of donor-reactive T cells in recipients both in experimental and clinical studies.

In addition to its pro-inflammatory functions, IFN-γ exhibits immunoregulatory functions. The absence of IFN γ in genetic depletion models impairs the development of tolerance. In the absence of IFN-γ signaling, many T cell responses are of higher magnitude and longer duration indicating a function for IFN-γ in the homeostasis of adaptive immune responses. One of the mechanisms underlying this homeostatic function is the ability of IFN-γ to upregulate Fas expression on activated T cells, promoting activation-induced cell death. This leads to a reduction in effector T cell numbers to favor transplant survival.

IL-17

IL-17 is actually a family of six cytokines and is part of a complex system. IL-17A through IL-17F are secreted as homodimers linked by disulfide bonds. IL-17A and IL-17F are produced by CD4 and CD8 T cells and bind to a dimeric receptor, IL-17RA, and IL-17RC. Epithelial cells, endothelial cells, and leukocytes express IL-17RA and IL-17RC and respond to IL-17 produced by antigen-primed T cells. Signals are transduced from the IL-17RA chain through the adaptor molecule Act1 leading to NF-κB activation and cytokine gene transcription. Binding of IL-17 to this receptor stimulates the production of many pro-inflammatory cytokines. Stimulation of endothelial and epithelial cells with IL-17 induces production of IL-6 and IL-8, resulting in intense neutrophil infiltration, as observed in IL-17 mediated immune responses in the intestine, central nervous system, and skin. In addition, IL-17 is a key cytokine in responses to extracellular bacterial and fungal infections, and also in the development and exacerbation of many autoimmune diseases including multiple sclerosis, rheumatoid arthritis, psoriasis, and Crohn's disease.

The role of IL-17 in these immune-based conditions has raised questions about a potential role in acute and/or chronic injury in allografts. Indeed, IL-17 transcripts have been observed in allografts shortly after reperfusion and during acute rejection episodes in heart allografts in mouse models as well as in clinical renal grafts. However, BALB/c (H-2^d) heart allografts are rejected at similar times by wild-type C57BL/6 (H-2^b) and B6.IL-17$^{-/-}$ recipients, suggesting that IL-17 plays a limited role in acute rejection of these allografts. In contrast, FVB (H-2^q) heart allografts have a substantial prolongation in survival in B6.IL-17$^{-/-}$ recipients and about 40% survive past day 60, post-transplant. This prolongation is associated with an increase in Treg cell numbers in the allografts. MHC class II MHC-disparate H-2^{bm12} heart grafts develop severe vasculopathy and failure in transgenic C57BL/6 recipients that lack expression of T-bet and this rejection is inhibited by neutralizing anti-IL-17 antibody. In another mouse model, donor-reactive CD8 T cells producing IL-17 mediate acute rejection of BALB/c heart allografts in B6.T-bet$^{-/-}$ recipients conditioned with anti-CD154mAb and this rejection was obviated by treatment with neutralizing anti-IL-17 antibody. Overall, these results indicate that IL-17 is present during acute injury of heart allografts in mouse models. However, IL-17 does not appear to be required for progression to allograft failure except under circumstances where the recipient immune system is compromised by lack of T-bet, and therefore, represents a compromised host Th1 response.

In human lung transplant patients, seminal studies by Burlingham and Wilkes showed the appearance of IL-17-producing CD4 T cells reactive to collagen V and that the strength of this IL-17-dependent response was associated with the incidence and severity of bronchiolitis obliterans. In a minor histocompatiblity mismatched orthotopic lung model in mice, development of bronchiolitis obliterans was associated with splenic mRNA and serum protein levels of IL-17, and neutralizing anti-IL-17 antibody inhibited the development of the fibrotic pathology in the allografts. In another model of lung fibrosis, intra-bronchial administration of anti-MHC class ImAb into native lungs led to the production of autoantibodies to collagen V and K-α1 tubulin antibodies promoting lung fibrosis; however, this antibody response and lung pathology was attenuated by treatment with anti-IL-17 antibody.

Immunoregulatory cytokines

TGF-β

The transforming growth factors belong to a "superfamily" of cytokines. There are three TGF-β isoforms in mammals with TGF-β1 being the major isoform active within the immune system. TGF-β is synthesized as a latent precursor that cannot bind to its receptor unless processed to form dimers that are then capable of binding to its receptor. TGF-β dimers bind to a tetrameric receptor complex composed of paired chains, TGFβRI and TGFβRII, to initiate transduction of intracellular signals to the nucleus. This binding activates phosphorylation of SMAD proteins that translocate to the nucleus and bind to the promoters of target genes to modulate transcription.

TGF-**β** is a key regulator of adaptive immune responses and the prevention of autoimmune disease. Genetic deletion of TGF-**β** or TGF**β**RII results in accelerated T cell proliferation and activation, which results in a lethal autoimmune condition in mice. TGF-**β** directly inhibits the proliferation of T cells as well as their functional differentiation to cytolytic and Th1 cells. TGF-**β** also inhibits the activation and differentiation of B lymphocytes including the inhibition of heavy and light chain production, with the exception that the differentiation of B cells to IgA-producing cells is promoted by TGF-**β**. As another mechanism of TGF-**β**-mediated immune regulation, TGF-**β** provides critical signals for the development of CD4$^+$FoxP3$^+$ regulatory T cells and their homeostasis through stabilization of FoxP3. Furthermore, these Tregs mediate immune regulation and inhibit autoimmune disease through the production of TGF-**β** in some models. In nonimmune effects, TGFβ is profoundly capable of inducing fibrosis through both the direct effects on matrix formation as well as the effects on remodeling enzymes. This is of significance in renal transplantation as CNI therapy induces the expression of TGFβ from parenchymal cells.

TGF-**β** being such a potent immune regulatory cytokine has provoked many studies attempting to increase TGF-**β** production and inhibit alloimmune responses to promote allograft survival. Systemic infusion of an adenoviral vector expressing human TGF-β1 allowed successful transplantation of syngeneic islets under the kidney capsule of diabetic NOD mice, with more than 80% of grafts surviving longer than 50 days versus rejection by day 18 in recipients not treated with the construct. Also in a mouse model, complete MHC-mismatched heart allografts perfused with liposomes carrying human TGF-β1 or an adenoviral vector expressing the TGF-β1, resulted in prolonging allograft survival in CD8-depleted recipients. More than 50% of the allografts survived longer than 60 days in treated group versus rejection at day 8 in nontreated recipients. However, the allografts surviving long term developed interstitial fibrosis and neointimal vasculopathy that were absent in isografts treated with the TGF-β vectors. As noted, TGF-β has been associated with the development of fibrosis and arteriopathies in many different organs and the predominance of fibrosis effect over immunosuppression *per se*, has hampered its use therapeutically.

An alternate strategy for TGF-β has been in expanding Treg cell populations. TGF-β1 has been used to expand Tregs that are then infused into autoimmune or allograft recipients. Cell culture in the presence of rapamycin and TGF-β has been shown to induce functionally potent CD4$^+$CD25$^+$FoxP3$^+$ Tregs from human naïve CD4 T cells that were effective in inhibiting graft-versus-host disease when co-transferred with human T cells in an SCID mouse model. These strategies are currently transitioning from the preclinical models to human patients.

IL-10

IL-10 is a homodimer. The major activity of IL-10 is the attenuation of inflammation through binding to receptors on mononuclear cells. Its effects on antigen-presenting cells (i.e., monocytes/macrophages, dendritic cells) include the downregulation of MHC and costimulatory molecules as well as attenuation of pro-inflammatory cytokines, namely, IL-1β, TNF-α, and IL-12p40. IL-10 inhibits T cell proliferation and expression of IL-2, IFN-γ, and GM-CSF. In contrast, IL-10 promotes the proliferation and survival of B cells and Ig class switching.

IL-10 mediates these effects by binding to a tetrameric receptor composed of two IL-10R1 and two IL-10R2 chains. IL-10 first binds to the dual IL-10R1 chains, which through conformational changes, allows the recruitment of two IL-10R2 chains into a single complex. Formation of this tetrameric complex activates JAK1 and Tyk2 to phosphorylate STAT3. Translocation of the phosphorylated STAT-3 dimer into the nucleus then induces the expression of target genes including IL-10, TNF-α, and IL-12p40, as well as the transcription repressor suppressor of cytokine signaling 3 (SOCS3), which inhibits JAK and STAT function in IL-10 target cells.

The major sources of IL-10 are monocytes/macrophages and some populations of CD4+FoxP3+ regulatory cells. Although dendritic cells, B cells, and NK cells can also produce IL-10, they are considered relatively minor sources during inflammatory processes. Recently, a novel population of CD4 T cells (Tr1) isolated from several SCID patients that had received HLA-mismatched bone marrow and became tolerant to the donor HLA antigens were shown to be immunosuppressive and donor HLA-specific, and produce high amounts of IL-10, similarly to what have also been identified in mice. In addition, a population of influenza virus antigen-primed CD8 T cells producing high amounts of IL-10 has been identified in a mouse influenza infection model; neutralization of IL-10 resulted in increased inflammation and lethal injury in the infected lung.

IL-10 has been recognized for some time as key regulators of inflammation, and loss of IL-10 in genetic mutations leads to autoimmunity in mice, and diffuse intestinal inflammation that has features similar to Crohn's colitis. The immune inhibitory functions of IL-10 have raised considerable interest in transplant research to potentially induce tolerance and long-term allograft survival. Studies infusing a gene encoding viral IL-10 into allografts using an adenoviral vector showed modest prolongation of cardiac allograft survival in a mouse model. In addition, transduction of complete MHC-mismatched cardiac allografts with retroviral vectors encoding IL-10 delayed T cell graft infiltration and increased survival times of heart allografts from 12 to 39 days in a mouse model and from 7 to 14 days in a rat model. Given such results, IL-10 may not work as a sole agent and likely will have to be paired with other approaches to produce long-term engraftment.

In summary, the soluble mediators involved in inflammation and immune responses represent a diverse and incredibly complex biologic response network. While they are clearly present in transplant responses and are thus of potential utility in diagnostics, their diversity and complexity provides a substantial challenge to their use in therapeutics. As well, many of the observations regarding utility have been made in small animal models, and translation to human studies will require careful selection. Despite these challenges, the targeting of small molecules has already shown great clinical effect such as the reduction of rejection by attenuating IL-2 and other T cell growth factors by current drugs. The targeting of other cytokines and chemokines may similarly prove to be beneficial in clinical transplantation.

Further reading

Adachi, O., T. Kawai, K. Takeda, M. Matsumoto, H. Tsutsui, M. Sakagami, K. Nakanishi, and S. Akira. 1998. Targeted disruption of the MyD88 gene results in loss of IL-1- and IL-18-mediated function. Immunity 9:143–150.

Akira, S., K. Takeda, and T. Kaisho. 2001. Toll-like receptors: critical proteins linking innate and acquired immunity. Nat Immunol 2:675–680.

Auffray, C., M. H. Sieweke, and F. Geissmann. 2009. Blood monocytes: development, heterogeneity, and relationship with dendritic cells. Annu Rev Immunol 27:669–692.

Charo, I. F., and R. M. Ransohoff. 2006. The many roles of chemokines and chemokine receptors in inflammation. N Engl J Med 354:610–621.

Devarajan, P. 2006. Update on mechanisms of ischemic acute kidney injury. J Am Soc Nephrol 17:1503–1520.

Dinarello, C. A. 2009. Immunological and inflammatory functions of the interleukin-1 family. Annu Rev Immunol 27:519–550.

Groom, J. R., J. Richmond, T. T. Murooka, E. W. Sorensen, J. H. Sung, K. Bankert, U. H. von Andrian, J. J. Moon, T. R. Mempel, and A. D. Luster. 2012. CXCR3 chemokine receptor-ligand interactions in the lymph node optimize CD4+ T helper 1 cell differentiation. Immunity 37:1091–1103.

Hildalgo, L. G., and P. F. Halloran. 2002. Role of IFN-gamma in allograft rejection. Crit Rev Immunol 22:317–349.

Katstelein, R. A., C. A. Hunter, and D. J. Cua. 2007. Discovery anad biology of IL-23 and IL-27: related but functionally distinct regulators of inflammation. Annu Rev Immunol 25:221–242.

Kee, B. L., R. R. Rivera, and C. Murre. 2001. Id3 inhibits B lymphocyte progenitor growth and survival in response to TGFb. Nat Immunol 2:242–247.

Korn, T., E. Bettelli, M. Oukka, and V. K. Kuchroo. 2009. IL-17 and Th17 cells. Annu Rev Immunol 27:485–517.

Li, M. O., Y. Y. Wan, S. Sanjabi, A.-K. L. Robertson, and R. A. Flavell. 2006. Transforming growth factor-b regulation of immune responses. Annu Rev Immunol 24:99–146.

Liao, W., J.-X. Lin, and W. J. Leonard. 2013. Interleukin-2 at the crossroads of effector responses, tolerance, and immunotherapy. Immunity 38:13–25.

Ma, A., R. Koka, and P. Burkett. 2006. Diverse functions of IL-2, IL-15, and IL-7 in lymphoid homeostasis. Annu Rev Immunol 24:657–679.

Mosser, D. H., and X. Zhang. 2008. Interleukin-10: new perspectives on an old cytokine. Immunol Rev 226:205–218.

Plantanias, L. C. 2005. Mechanisms of type-I- and type-II-infterferon-mediated signalling. Nat Rev Immunol 5:375–386.

Pratt, J. R., S. A. Basheer, and S. H. Sacks. 2002. Local synthesis of complement component C3 regulates acute renal transplant rejection. Nat Med 8:582–587.

Raue, H.-P., C. Beadling, J. Haun, and M. K. Slifka. 2013. Cytokine-mediated programmed proliferation of virus-specific CD8+ memory T cells. Immunity 38:131–139.

Rot, A., and U. H. von Andrian. 2004. Chemokines in innate and adaptive host defense: basic chemokinese grammar for immune cells. Annu Rev Immunol 22:891–928.

Townsend, J. M., G. P. Fallon, J. D. Matthews, P. Smith, E. H. Jolin, and N. A. McKenzie. 2000. IL-9-deficient mice establish fundamental roles for IL-9 in pulmonary mastocytosis and goblet cell hyperplasia but not T cell development. Immunity 13:573–583.

CHAPTER 4

Costimulatory molecules

Maria-Luisa Alegre[1] and Anita S. Chong[2]

[1] Department of Medicine, Section of Rheumatology, Gwen Knapp Center for Lupus and Immunology Research, The University of Chicago, Chicago, USA

[2] Department of Surgery, Section of Transplantation, The University of Chicago, Chicago, USA

CHAPTER OVERVIEW

- Structurally, costimulatory molecules are divided into three major families: the immunoglobulin (Ig) family, the tumor necrosis factor receptor (TNFR) family, and the T cell immunoglobulin mucin (TIM) family.
- Costimulation can be stimulatory or inhibitory to T cell activation.
- Costimulatory signals are critical to productive immunity and immune tolerance.
- Costimulatory molecules are promising therapeutic targets in tolerance induction.

Introduction

It has long been recognized that at least two signals are required to fully activate lymphocytes. In T cells, the first signal is delivered by the T cell receptor (TCR) upon engagement of cognate antigen, while the second signal is provided upon ligation of costimulatory receptors on T cells by their ligands on neighboring APCs. Ligation of the TCR without costimulatory signals often induces T cell anergy or apoptosis, thus placing costimulatory molecules as key determinants of T cell fate. Naïve T cells express few costimulatory receptors (e.g., CD28 and CD27) but upregulate many others following activation, several of which are retained following differentiation into effector and memory cells. While some costimulatory molecules support T cell activation, others can terminate an ongoing immune response by inhibiting TCR signaling. The interest in costimulatory molecules in transplantation stems from the assumption that blockade of positive costimulatory signals or agonistic trigger of negative ones should specifically inactivate those T cells that are actively recognizing antigen (i.e., alloreactive T cells in transplantation) while

---

Transplant Immunology, First Edition. Edited by Xian Chang Li and Anthony M. Jevnikar.
© 2016 John Wiley & Sons, Ltd. Published 2016 by John Wiley & Sons, Ltd.
Copyright ® American Society of Transplantation 2016.
Companion website: www.wiley.com/go/li/transplantimmunology

leaving T cells of other specificities intact. Such an approach should promote donor-specific unresponsiveness or even tolerance. Several families of costimulatory molecules have been described, including the immunoglobulin superfamily, the TNFR superfamily, and the immunoglobulin mucin family. The individual members of these families, their role in alloimmuneresponses, and therapeutic targeting in transplant survival will be discussed in this section.

Costimulatory molecules

The classic T cell activation involves stimulation via the TCR and costimulatory receptors by APCs bearing cognate antigen and costimulatory ligands in secondary lymphoid structures (Figure 4.1) (Li et al., 2009). However, there are many

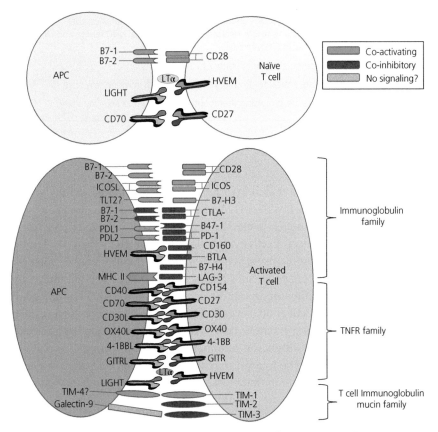

Figure 4.1 Costimulatory and coinhibitory family members. Naïve T cells express CD28, CD27, and HVEM, although only the role of CD28 in naïve T cells is well understood. Activated T cells express a variety of immunoglobulin, TNFR, and TIM family members. Costimulatory receptors and activating ligands are depicted in green, while coinhibitory receptors are in red, and molecules not thought to signal are in gray.

exceptions to these rules. For instance, not all receptors (capable of signaling) are on T cells, with ligands on APCs. The costimulatory receptor CD40 is mainly expressed on APCs rather than T cells, while its ligand, CD154, is expressed on activated T cells rather than APCs. Signaling via CD40 enables upregulation of MHC molecules and costimulatory ligands on APCs, which in turn enhance their capacity to activate T cells. Moreover, some costimulatory ligands can transmit signals through the acytoplasmic tail, such that they function as receptors in the cells expressing them. For example, B7-1 (CD80), the ligand for CD28, can act as a coinhibitory receptor on T cells when ligated by PDL-1. Adding yet another level of complexity, some ligands are known to have several receptors and some receptors to have several ligands, with sometimes opposing effects. Furthermore, T cell activation may occur in secondary lymphoid organs as well as in tissues including the transplanted organ itself. Finally, nonhematopoietic cells such as epithelial and endothelial parenchymal cells can express a limited repertoire of costimulatory ligands as well as MHC molecules, especially under inflammatory conditions. Thus, costimulatory signals delivered to T cells may be provided not only by professional APCs but also by many parenchymal cell types in the vicinity of the T cells. Over all, their contribution to allograft responses is highly complex, and this has hampered rapid translation to clinical transplantation.

Immunoglobulin (Ig) superfamily

The Ig superfamily refers to the members of the CD28/B7 family. This family includes CD28 and ICOS; their ligands B7-1 (CD80), B7-2 (CD86), and ICOSL (CD278); and a growing list of inhibitory receptors, namely CTLA-4 (CD152), PD-1 (CD279), BTLA (CD272), B7-H4, B7S3, and BTNL2; the corresponding ligands for such inhibitory receptors are B7-1/B7-2, PDL-1(CD274)/PDL-2 (CD273), HVEM (CD258), and three as yet unknown ligands. A newly described inhibitory ligand expressed on APCs, VISTA, inhibits T cell function via an unknown receptor on T cells. In addition, B7-H3 (CD276) is thought to serve both as a coactivating and as a coinhibitory receptor.

Activating molecules
CD28/B7-1, B7-2
General considerations
CD28 is the prototypic costimulatory receptor on T cells and is involved in several key immune responses which include (a) activation of naïve T cells, (b) Th1 and Th2 differentiation and proliferation, (c) enhancement of T cell survival, (d)promotion of cytokine production via stabilization of cytokine mRNA, and (e) regulation of peripheral maintenance of Tregs.

The engagement of CD28 is important for the productive activation of naïve T cells and for preventing the induction of apoptosis and anergy. As such, reagents to inhibit CD28 have been sought after in transplantation to inactivate or delete alloreactive T cells during their initial encounter with cognate antigen. CD28 binds B7-1, which is inducible on many cell types including T cells, and B7-2, which is constitutively expressed on APCs and further upregulated upon APC activation. The same ligands bind CTLA-4 with greater affinity than CD28, but CTLA-4 ligation inhibits rather than activates T cell responses. The importance of CTLA-4 is evidenced by the development of lymphoproliferation and autoimmunity in CTLA-4 deletion mice. Because CTLA-4 is only expressed in T cells after activation, the function of B7 family members is to initially enhance T cell responses via CD28 and then inhibit them via CTLA-4.

Activated T cells retain CD28 expression in mice and humans. However, a subset of CD8+ T cells that are negative for CD28 accumulate in humans during aging and chronic HIV infection. This has been correlated with vaccine unresponsiveness and the progression of HIV disease. These cells have an effector memory phenotype, retain strong alloreactivity, and are resistant to CD28 blockade, thus constituting a possible barrier to the induction of transplant tolerance. Importantly, T cells that have lost CD28 expression have recently been shown to be susceptible to inhibition by the blockade of adhesion molecules, suggesting there may be a therapeutic approach to control such cells.

CD28 exists as a dimer on the surface of T cells and localizes to the area of TCR engagement in microclusters at the immunologic synapse that forms with MHC/antigen on APCs. These microclusters retain TCR-activated PKCθ, leading to sustained signals for T cell activation. The biology of CD28 signaling is complex. Of the CD28 ligands, B7-1 is mostly expressed as a dimer, while B7-2 is mostly expressed as a monomer on the cell surface. CD28 engagement results in the activation of two main pathways via PI3/Akt/mTOR and NF-κB. These pathways control cell survival, and also appear to play a central role in T cell differentiation. The mTORC1 component of mTOR is necessary for Th1 and Th17 differentiation, while mTORC2 is required for Th2 differentiation. Furthermore, deficiency of mTOR results in inducible T regulatory cells (iTregs) rather than T effector cell differentiation. The activation of already differentiated Th1 cells in the absence of mTOR results in anergy induction. Finally, mTOR appears to negatively regulate the acquisition of memory by CD8+ T cells via mTORC1. These functional consequences of mTOR inhibition are relevant to transplantation as mTOR is the target of the immunosuppressive drug sirolimus.

The engagement of CD28 by its ligands, B7-1 and B7-2 enhances T cell survival via upregulation of the anti-apoptotic molecule Bcl-x_L, promotes proliferation and cytokine production via the stabilization of cytokine mRNA, ensures optimal telomere activity, and enhances glucose metabolism. Activated T cells require increased glucose metabolism for their function, which is achieved by the expression of the glucose transporter Glut1. CD28 also regulates the strength of signal delivered to the activated T cell, which along with the type of cytokines in the microenvironment, appears to specify the differentiation of activated naïve T cells.

Another essential role of CD28 is through regulating thymic development and peripheral maintenance of Tregs. Indeed, CD28-deficient mice, B7-1/B7-2-deficient mice, and wildtype mice treated with CD28 inhibitors have reduced numbers of Tregs in the thymus and the periphery. CD28 is also required for the suppressive function of Tregs, as mice with conditional deletion of CD28 in Tregs develop severe autoimmunity that predominantly affects the skin and lungs. This has important implications in the therapeutic use of CTLA-4-Ig in transplantation, as reduced activation of CD28-expressing T effector cells may unintentionally reduce the numbers of Tregs. In addition to a cell-intrinsic control of T cells by CD28, this receptor can induce reverse signaling by B7 family members on APCs. The engagement of CD28 by dendritic cells has been shown to promote the production of IL-6 and IFN-γ in a B7-1- and B7-2-dependent manner in the mouse (Figure 4.2). IL-6, for instance, facilitates the proliferation of conventional T cells and their escape from Treg-mediated suppression; IL-6 also drives Th17 differentiation under certain conditions.

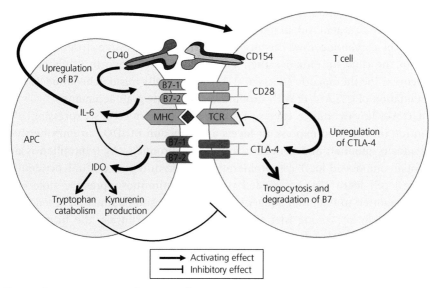

Figure 4.2 Consequences of CD28 and CTLA-4 engagement. Antigen recognition by the TCR and concomitant CD28 engagement by low levels of B7 ligands results in expression of CD154 which, upon binding to CD40, further upregulates MHC and B7 molecules on APCs to enhance T cell activation. CD28 binding to B7 results in B7-dependent production of IL-6 by dendritic cells that promotes T cell proliferation. Activated T cells then upregulate CTLA-4 whose association with phosphatases inhibits TCR signals. In addition, given the higher affinity of CTLA-4 for B7 family members, CTLA-4 can outcompete CD28 for B7-1 and B7-2, and can also physically capture these ligands by trogocytosis, rendering the APCs less able to positively costimulate T cells. Finally, signaling of CTLA-4 to B7 results in the upregulation and activation of IDO, that suppresses T cell responses, and in inhibition of IL-6 synthesis.

Targeting the CD28/B7 axis in transplantation

CD28 has been targeted extensively in transplantation and is a great example of the translation of a therapeutic target from bench to bedside (Li et al., 2009). Two main approaches have been used to inhibit CD28, namely (i) targeting of its ligands B7-1 and B7-2 and (ii) reagents that block the CD28 receptor itself.

Two principal methods have been used to block B7-1 and B7-2: blocking antibodies to these ligands and CTLA-4-Ig, a fusion protein containing the extracellular domain of CTLA-4 with the Fc portion of an IgG. CTLA-4-Ig was generated on the premise that having a higher affinity for B7-1 and B7-2 than CD28, CTLA-4-Ig would block further interactions of B7 with CD28. Thus, anti-B7 antibodies and CTLA-4-Ig block the ability of B7 ligands to engage CD28, resulting in anergy or apoptosis of T cells upon antigen encounter. However, these reagents also block the ability of B7 ligands to bind to CTLA-4 on already activated T cells, thus preventing any inhibitory effect of T cell-intrinsic CTLA-4. Furthermore, as CD28 signals are important for Treg homeostasis and function, reagents that prevent CD28 engagement may also reduce the "fitness" of Tregs. It is perhaps not surprising that while CTLA-4-Ig or anti-B7 antibodies can prolong allograft survival in animal models of transplantation, they have failed to induce tolerance in more stringent rodent models or in nonhuman primates. There has been interest in combining these agents with immunosuppressive drugs currently used in the clinic to enhance their efficacy. While calcineurin inhibitors can antagonize the therapeutic effects of CTLA-4-Ig in fully mismatched models, the combination of CTLA-4-Ig with sirolimuscan promote graft acceptance.

CTLA-4-Ig can induce reverse signaling on dendritic cells expressing B7, resulting in increased expression levels and function of IDO, an enzyme that degrades tryptophan and generates kynurenin products. As tryptophan is an essential amino acid for T cell proliferation and kynurenins can independently induce T cell death, IDO is regarded as a potent immunosuppressive molecule. IDO is required to maintain allogeneic pregnancies and its function is required for CTLA-4-Ig to prolong islet allograft survival. In contrast, the humanized versions of CTLA-4-Ig (abatacept, or the higher affinity mutant belatacept) were not able to induce IDO, perhaps because the Fc portion of these molecules was mutated to reduce FcR binding. Both abatacept and belatacept are approved for clinical use, the latter now being used in some centers for the prophylaxis of kidney transplant rejection in combination with basiliximab induction, mycophenolatemofetil, and corticosteroids. Belatacept appears to be relatively safe and prolongs renal allograft survival with superior renal function for up to 5 years compared to calcineurin inhibitors, despite a higher incidence of acute rejection and infection episodes early on. As well, there may be an increased risk of lymphoma in EBV-mismatched donor-recipient transplant pairs.

Targeting of B7-1 and B7-2 may have different consequences. While originally described to bind CTLA-4 more avidly than B7-2, a new interaction has been reported between B7-1 and PD-L1, in which B7-1 can serve as a coinhibitory receptor on T cells. This interaction is functional *in vivo*, where the use of an antibody that only blocks the B7-1/PD-L1 interaction accelerated chronic rejection of heart allografts in a single class II mismatch model. A more recent approach to target CD28 has been to develop antibodies to the CD28 receptor itself. These reagents have the advantage of preserving CTLA-4/B7 and B7-1/PD-L1 interactions, thus gaining both the intrinsic coinhibitory effects of CTLA-4 and B7-1 on T cells and the natural ability of endogenous CTLA-4 to induce IDO in dendritic cells. Targeting CD28 would nevertheless retain the potential caveat of reducing Treg homeostasis. Unfortunately, the generation of antibodies that block CD28 has been challenging, as the dimer nature of CD28 on the T cell surface makes most bivalent antibodies agonistic thus providing an unintended positive costimulatory signal. Indeed some antihuman CD28 antibodies have been shown to activate T cells, resulting in severe transient multiorgan failure in volunteers of a phase I study. Recently, antagonistic monovalent anti-CD28 antibodies have been generated and tested in nonhuman primates. *In vivo*, these antibodies delayed acute rejection when administered as a monotherapy and synergized with calcineurin inhibitors to prevent acute and chronic rejection of cardiac and renal allografts to induce donor-specific hyporesponsiveness. This correlated with the accumulation of Tregs in the periphery and in the graft and with increased expression of IDO mRNA, suggesting that the theoretical advantages of CD28 targeting over B7 targeting hold true *in vivo*.

ICOS/ICOSL
General considerations
ICOS is a CD28 family member that also coactivates T cells (Simpson et al., 2010). Because its expression level on naïve T cells is very low, most of its costimulatory function occurs in activated T cells, where it is expressed on unpolarized T cells as well as Th1, Th2, Th17, T follicular helper (T_{FH}) cells, and Tregs. ICOS is also expressed on B cells and the most prominent feature of patients that are genetically deficient for ICOS is the development of common variable immunodeficiency, with defects in germinal center formation and classswitch recombination to IgA, IgE, and certain isotypes of IgG, thus supporting an essential role for ICOS in B cell responses. Indeed, ICOS-deficient mice lack T_{FH} cells, the T cell subtype specialized in B cell help, and germinal center formation. Importantly, ICOS expression can be regulated post-transcriptionally by Roquin, a member in the RING-type ubiquitin ligase family. Mice with an altered form of Roquin that cannot degrade ICOS mRNA (*sanroque* mice) consequently display elevated levels of ICOS, leading to enhanced germinal center formation, T_{FH} differentiation, and lupus-like disease.

In addition to its role in T_{FH} cell development, engagement of ICOS by its ligand is important for the differentiation and effector function of Th1, Th2, and Th17 cells and promotes their proliferation, survival, and production of effector cytokines, although there is some controversy as to its role on mouse versus human Th17 differentiation and on whether the effects on Th2 cells are at the level of differentiation or expansion of already differentiated cells. ICOS has also been implicated in T cell memory as both ICOS-deficient and CIVD patients have reduced numbers of memory cells, but it is not completely clear whether this is due to decreased generation or maintenance of memory. Finally, ICOS also appears important in maintaining Treg homeostasis, controlling IL-10-producing Tregs and peripheral tolerance, although it is not required for iTreg differentiation.

Targeting ICOS/ICOSL in transplantation

ICOS blockade or ICOS deficiency results in prolonged cardiac allograft survival, correlating with decreased intra-graft T cell activation and cytokine expression, and reduced alloantibody production. The timing of ICOS blockade may be critical for effectiveness, as either blockade of ICOS early after transplantation or having a genetic absence of ICOS is much less effective at prolonging allograft survival than delaying blockade, perhaps because of compensation by CD28 on T cells initially. In combination with anti-CD154, anti-ICOS appears to prevent chronic rejection in mouse models. In contrast, in a model of murine kidney allograft transplantation where little acute rejection is observed, ICOS blockade has been shown to accelerate rejection, supporting a role for ICOS in tolerance induction. Whether this is due to a function of ICOS in Tregs remains to be investigated.

TLT-2, B7-H3

While the ligand B7-H3 is broadly expressed on hematopoietic and nonhematopoietic cells at the mRNA level, protein distribution is restricted to activated APCs and T cells, suggesting tight post-transcriptional regulation (Yi and Chen, 2009). Mouse B7-H3 contains a single isoform with a single extracellular immunoglobulin domain, whereas the human genome contains an additional isoform comprising a tandem repeat of the immunoglobulin domain. Recent work has identified Triggering Receptor Expressed on Myeloid Cells (TREM)-like transcript 2 (TLT-2) as a receptor for B7-H3, although this interaction remains controversial. TLT-2 is expressed on activated T cells and B7-H3-Ig can bind to activated T cells independently of other known CD28 family members. B7-H3 may function as both an activator and an inhibitor of T cell responses. The expression of B7-H3 on an EL-4 lymphoma resulted in enhanced tumor elimination by T cells and B7-H3-deficient dendritic cells stimulated reduced T cell alloresponses compared to wildtype dendritic cells *in vitro*. In contrast, recombinant mouse and human B7-H3 inhibited anti-CD3-mediated proliferation and cytokine production, and B7-H3-deficient mice developed earlier and more severe disease in models of airway inflammation and EAE than control mice. These conflicting results may be due to the binding of B7-H3 to two receptors with opposite function, much like B7-1 and B7-2 binding to both CD28 and

CTLA-4. In transplantation, the absence of B7-H3 was shown to synergize with sirolimus to prevent acute rejection of cardiac and islet allografts and also reduced the incidence of chronic heart allograft vasculopathy, suggesting that B7-H3 acts as an activating costimulatory molecule.

Inhibitory molecules
CTLA-4/B7-1, B7-2

CTLA-4 is structurally related to CD28 and binds B7-1 and B7-2, but with even higher affinity particularly for B7-2 (Bour-Jordan et al., 2011). In contrast to CD28, CTLA-4 is not expressed in naïve T cells but is induced upon T cell activation, and mediates cell-cycle arrest to terminate immune responses. Most CTLA-4 molecules are present in endocytic vesicles as CTLA-4 is rapidly endocytosed in a clathrin-dependent manner when it reaches the cell surface. Underscoring the potent inhibitory function of this molecule, mice deficient in CTLA-4 die at 3–4 weeks of age of fulminant lymphoproliferative disorder. The inhibitory function of CTLA-4 can be explained by at least five properties of CTLA-4 (Figure 4.2). Firstly, the higher affinity of CTLA-4 for B7-1 and B7-2 may simply block these ligands from binding CD28. Furthermore, CTLA-4 can physically capture and remove B7 molecules from APCs in a process of trans-endocytosis or "trogocytosis," resulting in B7 degradation, and rendering APCs less able to costimulate T cells. Thirdly, engagement of CTLA-4 can result in the activation of several phosphatases that antagonize TCR signals. This may lead to reduced formation of signaling microclusters on T cells leading to diminished T cell adhesion. A "reverse-stop signaling model" has been suggested in which CTLA-4 augments T cell mobility and decreases T cell activation, limiting the time of contact of T cells with APCs by inhibiting the TCR signals that promote strong adhesion, as longer contacts are necessary for productive T cell responses. Fourthly, as noted before, CTLA-4 can induce reverse signaling by B7 onto dendritic cells driving increased expression and function of IDO that in turn reduces T cell proliferation and promotes death of T cells. Finally, CTLA-4 is highly and constitutively expressed in Tregs and has been shown to play a role in their suppressive function, as its selective elimination from Foxp3-expressing Tregs results in lymphoproliferation and animal death.

In transplantation, blockade of CTLA-4 or B7-1 and B7-2 has been shown to accelerate cardiac allograft rejection in CD28-deficient mice, whereas its agonistic cross-linking with single-chain anti-CTLA-4Fv expressed on the surface of allogeneic tumor cells can reduce tumor elimination, thereby confirming the inhibitory role of CTLA-4 in alloresponses. Developing reagents to harness the inhibitory potential of CTLA-4 for therapeutic use has proven challenging as all currently described antibodies for human and mouse CTLA-4 are blocking and are therefore capable of enhancing T cell responses *in vivo*, rather than agonistic, and are therefore inhibitory. Blocking CTLA-4 antibodies have been developed for antitumor immunotherapy with Ipilimumab gaining FDA approval for melanoma in 2011, 3 months prior to approval of the B7-blocking CTLA-4-Ig belatacept for transplantation.

CTLA-4 is required for the induction of transplantation tolerance in several models, including tolerance after generation of mixed chimerism following bone marrow transplantation and peripheral tolerance induced with anti-CD154 and DST, or with anti-CD45RB antibodies. In addition, blockade of CTLA-4 after induction of tolerance can precipitate acute rejection in several mouse models, suggesting that CTLA-4 is not only important for the induction but also for the maintenance of transplantation tolerance.

PD-1/PDL-1, PDL2; B7-1/PDL-1

PD-1 is expressed on Tregs, CD4+, CD8+, B cells, NK cells, and macrophages after activation and in a sustained manner in chronically stimulated "exhausted" CD8+ T cells (Francisco et al., 2010). The PD-L1 and PD-L2 ligands for PD-1 are expressed on activated APCs. PD-L1 is also present on a subset of activated T cells and Tregs as well as constitutively on parenchymal cells such as heart, lung, kidney, and placenta and is inducible on endothelial cells. Importantly, PD-L1 can also serve as a ligand for B7-1 on activated T cells, with B7-1 serving as a coinhibitory receptor for T cells. These various possible interactions complicate interpretations from use of antibodies or fusion proteins of these family members. The generation of antibodies that can block engagement of B7-1 but not PD-1 by PD-L1 has recently helped clarify the functional consequences of these interactions *in vivo*.

PD-1 engagement results in reduced proliferation and cytokine production by T cells and PD-1-deficient mice display lymphoproliferation, although milder than that observed in CTLA-4-deficient mice. The autoimmune phenotype depends on the background strain, with BALB/c mice deficient in PD-1 developing cardiomyopathy, while C57Bl/6 mice develop lupus-like glomerulonephritis and arthritis. PD-1 ligation has also been recently shown to affect the stability of T cell/dendritic cell contacts by inhibiting TCR-mediated stop signals and enhancing T cell motility.

In transplantation, anti-PD-L1 has been shown to augment acute and chronic cardiac allograft rejection, in a manner that depends on PD-L1 binding to B7-1 rather than to PD-1. Similarly, the prolongation of allograft survival reported with a PDL1-Ig fusion protein and its ability to synergize with anti-CD154 or rapamycin for the induction of tolerance needs to be revisited to determine whether it is due to the engagement of PD-1 or B7-1. Differential effects of anti-PD-L1 and anti-PD-L2, which are known to depend on expression of CD28, may similarly require further teasing to distinguish effects of blockade of PD-1 from that of B7-1. Nevertheless, PD-1 can play an important inhibitory role and is thought to mediate hyporesponsiveness in chronically activated "exhausted"' CD8+ T cells. Interestingly, blockade of PD-1 can restore exhausted CD8+ T cells' function to eliminate chronic viral infections and exacerbate GVHD in an adoptive splenocyte transfer model.

Transgenic overexpression of PD-1 in T cells resulted in the increased prolongation of cardiac allografts mismatched for minor alloantigens while blockade of PD-1 precipitates the rejection of cardiac allografts after establishment of tolerance. Collectively, these suggest that PD-1 plays an important role in the maintenance of graft survival and tolerance. In addition to inhibiting the function of conventional T cells, engagement of PD-1 may also increase T cell regulation. PDL1-Ig can enhance the conversion of naïve T cells into iTregs and enhance their suppressive function, whereas lack of PDL-1 on APCs prevents this conversion. Thus, therapeutic targeting of PD-1 could harness two mechanisms of tolerance, namely the induction of regulation and coinhibition of conventional T cells.

BTLA, CD160, HVEM
BTLA is another CD28 family member with coinhibitory properties (Murphy and Murphy, 2010) (Figure 4.3). BTLA lacks the cysteine dimerization domain contained in CD28 and CTLA-4 and is therefore present as a monomer on the

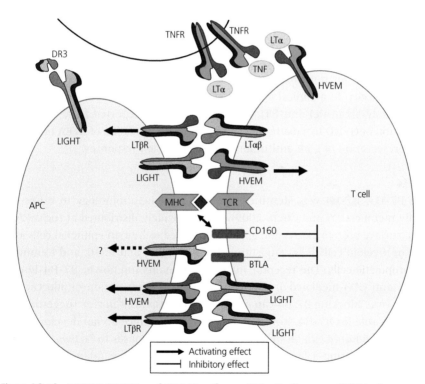

Figure 4.3 The LIGHT, HVEM, and CD160 pathway. Naïve T cells express HVEM whereas activated T cells express LIGHT, LTαβ, BTLA and CD160. HVEM can serve as a coactivator of T cells upon engagement of LIGHT or of soluble LTα. HVEM can also serve as a ligand for BTLA and the GPI-anchored CD160 that can both coinhibit T cells. Adding to the complexity of this pathway, LIGHT can also serve as a ligand for LTβR and can also bind DR3. LTα can also serve as a ligand for TNFR1 and TNFR2 (both labeled as TNFR in this figure), and TNFRs can also engage TNF.

cell surface. BTLA is expressed on B cells, on dendritic cells and some NK cells and on anergic and activated T cells but not Tregs. Its expression remains sustained in Th1 cells, suggesting that it may selectively suppress Th1 responses. It has also been shown to suppress innate immune responses. BTLA is one of the only members of the immunoglobulin family whose ligand, HVEM, is not in the same family but is a member of the TNFR family. CD160, an alternative receptor for HVEM, is a GPI-anchored member of the immunoglobulin family that also appears to transduce inhibitory signals to T cells. BTLA-deficient mice have increased susceptibility to autoimmunity and show enhanced T and B cell responses.

Costimulatory receptors appear to work in concert to mediate effects. In partially mismatched models of heart allografts, the blockade or absence of BTLA resulted in accelerated allograft rejection. Surprisingly, targeting of BTLA in a model of fully mismatched cardiac allografts prolonged allograft survival, correlating with enhanced expression of PD-1. Similarly, rather than accelerating rejection, anti-BTLA cooperated with CTLA-4-Ig to induce donor-specific tolerance to islet allografts. This may be due to a role of BTLA in maintaining the survival of $CD4^+$ T cells as blockade or genetic deficiency of BTLA resulted in decreased survival of donor T cells in a model of GVHD. It is also conceivable that anti-BTLA antibodies may have some degree of agonistic ability *in vivo*. Cyclosporin A but not sirolimus has been reported to reduce upregulation of BTLA in T cells. In a clinical application, the administration of a nondepleting (presumably agonistic) anti-BTLA mAb was recently reported to result in the prevention of GVHD in a manner dependent on the expression of BTLA on T cells with preservation of graft antitumor and antipathogen responses.

B7-H4

Like B7-H3, B7-H4 was identified by DNA sequence homology to other B7 family members (Yi and Chen, 2009). Though widely distributed at the mRNA level, surface protein expression appears restricted to human epithelial cells and human myeloid cells following stimulation with IL-6 and IL-10, and to mouse hematopoietic cells. The receptor for B7-H4 remains unknown. B7-H4-Ig can inhibit anti-CD3-mediated T cell activation and the generation of alloreactive CTLs *in vitro*. Blocking B7-H4 can enhance T cell responses *in vivo*, suggesting an inhibitory role for B7-H4. However, B7-H4-deficient mice do not develop autoimmunity and only exhibit mildly enhanced Th1 responses to *Leishmania major* infection, indicating a less prominent role for B7-H4 than other coinhibitory molecules. Interestingly, B7-H4 has also been reported to be a negative regulator of innate immunity by inhibiting the proliferation of neutrophil progenitors.

In transplantation, blockade or genetic ablation of B7-H4 has been reported to accelerate the rejection of fully mismatched cardiac allografts in CD28-deficient but not wildtype mice, and induce cardiac allograft rejection in B7-1/B7-2 double-deficient mice that otherwise accept heart transplants long term. The latter studies indicate that the inhibitory effect of B7-H4 is independent of CTLA-4 activity. Finally, the prolongation of allograft survival by CTLA-4-Ig was dependent on the recipient but not donor B7-H4.

B7S3

B7S3 is a new member of the B7 family with two different spliced isoforms; B7S3 is expressed in hematopoietic and nonhematopoietic cells. The human genome appears to contain a single B7S3 homolog whereas the mouse genome comprises 10 related family members. The receptor of B7S3 remains to be defined. B7S3-Ig was found to bind to APCs constitutively and to T cells after activation, and was shown to prevent T cell activation *in vitro*, suggesting an inhibitory function for this molecule. Its role in transplantation remains to be investigated.

BTNL2

Butyrophilin-like 2 (BTNL2) is another new B7 family member that is highly expressed in lymphoid tissues and in the intestine. Mutations in BTNL2 have been linked to higher susceptibility to sarcoidosis and myositis. Generation of a BTNL2-Ig fusion molecule identified its receptor on activated T and B cells, but distinct from known CD28 family members. BTNL2-Ig inhibited T cell activation *in vitro*, suggesting a role of BTNL2 as a negative costimulatory molecule.

VISTA

V-domain Ig Suppressor of T cell Activation (VISTA) is the most recent B7 family member identified to date and exhibits homology to PD-L1. VISTA is expressed on hematopoietic cells and VISTA-Ig or VISTA-expressing APCs inhibited T cell proliferation *in vitro*, whereas a blocking anti-VISTA mAb induced exacerbated EAE in mice. Overexpression of VISTA by tumor cells was also shown to inhibit antitumor responses, identifying VISTA as another negative costimulatory molecule.

TNFR/TNF superfamily

The TNFR superfamily has more than 20 members; they can be soluble or membrane-bound. The intracellular domains of these receptors associate with TNF receptor-associated factor (TRAF) adaptors and activate MAP kinases and the transcription factor NF-κB. While TNFR, Fas and TRAIL contain a death domain in their cytoplasmic tail that mediates apoptosis, other family members without the death domain support T cell activation and survival. CD40 and its ligand, CD40L (CD154), was the first costimulatory pair identified in this family. Other members in this family include CD27/CD70, CD30/CD30L, OX40/OX40L, 4-1BB/4-1BBL, GITR/GITRL, and HVEM/LIGHT. No coinhibitory pairs have been identified so far within this family, with the exception of the cross-family pairing of HVEM with the inhibitory members of the Ig family BTLA and CD160.

Of all these receptors, only CD27 and HVEM are expressed by naïve T cells, whereas all other members are induced following T cell activation. However, memory cells and Tregs constitutively express several TNFR superfamily members. Thus, these molecules may control effector and memory responses rather than initial T cell priming.

CD40/CD154

CD40 is expressed on dendritic cells, B cells, and macrophages at low levels and upregulated upon activation (Elgueta et al., 2009). It can also be induced in parenchymal cells such as epithelial, endothelial cells, and fibroblasts. Its ligand, CD154, is expressed on activated T cells, NK cells, eosinophils, and platelets. CD40 signaling on dendritic cells results in increased expression of B7-1 and B7-2, thus, enhancing their antigen presentation to T cells. CD40 is also essential for T-dependent B cell response, as CD40 engagement triggers B cell proliferation, differentiation, germinal center formation, antibody isotype switching, and affinity maturation, and therefore is critical for the generation of memory B cells and long-lived plasma cells.

Genetic ablation of CD154 or blockade of CD40/CD154 interactions can markedly prolong allograft survival in rodents, as does a short course of anti-CD154 in models of cardiac, renal, and pancreatic islet allograft transplantation. However, chronic rejection often develops, suggesting an incomplete control of alloimmunity. Several investigators have combined anti-CD154 with other immunosuppressive regimens, such as CTLA-4-Ig or sirolimus, with increased efficacy, though still failing to induce donor-specific tolerance. Importantly, addition of anti-CD154 mAb can enable a nonmyeloablative conditioning regimen to induce stable mixed chimerism and donor-specific tolerance of skin allografts. Combining anti-CD154 with donor-specific transfusion (DST) can also induce donor-specific tolerance in models of heart or pancreatic islet allografts and long-term allograft survival in very stringent models such as fully mismatched skin allografts. The immunosuppressive effect of DST may be due to T cell inactivation following indirect presentation of apoptotic donor cells by recipient dendritic cells in the absence of CD40-CD154 interaction. In fact, anti-CD154 mAbs/DST therapy has the ability to promote several pathways of T cell tolerance, including deletion of activated T cells (especially CD8$^+$ T cells), conversion of conventional T cells into iTregs, and increased suppressive function of nTregs. This treatment also prevents the maturation of dendritic cells, further reducing T cell priming in rejection. Interestingly, CsA can block the tolerogenic effect of anti-CD154 mAb, perhaps because its inhibition of IL-2 prevents the expansion of Tregs and its blockade of NF-AT activation abolishes the induction of T cell anergy.

Anti-CD154 therapy was also very effective in nonhuman primates transplanted with kidney or pancreatic islet allografts, although cessation of therapy eventually resulted in graft rejection. Initial phase I clinical trials in patients were halted due to unexpected thromboembolic events related to platelet expression of CD154. Given the remarkable effects of targeting CD154 in animal models of transplantation, pharmaceutical companies are actively pursuing alternatives to target the CD40/CD154 pathway, including blocking antibodies to CD40, anti-CD154 antibodies that do not promote platelet aggregation, and CD154 RNA inhibition approaches.

CD27/CD70

CD27 is one of two members of the TNFR family expressed on naïve T cells (Denoeud and Moser, 2011). It is also expressed on B cells and NK cells. Its ligand, CD70, is expressed on APCs and upregulated on activated T and B cells. CD27 signaling is thought to be important in T cell activation, T-dependent antibody production by B cells and NK-mediated immunity against viral infections. The use of CD27-deficient mice has revealed a more important role for CD27 on CD8$^+$ than CD4$^+$ T cells for effector function and memory development following viral infection. Although CD27 does not have a death domain, it can recruit death pathways that can promote apoptosis of T and B cells and transgenic expression of CD70 in B cells results in profound depletion of naïve T cells from secondary lymphoid organs and animal death by opportunistic infections. Human memory B cells express CD27 that binds to CD70 to develop into plasma cells. Thus, blockade of the CD27-CD70 pathway may also inhibit memory B cell responses.

In transplantation, blockade of CD70 has been shown to prolong cardiac allograft survival in wildtype mice and induce long-term acceptance in CD28-deficient recipients, without signs of chronic rejection. Although anti-CD70 mAb had little effect on CD4-mediated rejection, it prevented CD8-mediated rejection as well as reduced development of CD8$^+$ memory T cells. Addition of anti-CD70 to anti-CD154 and anti-LFA-1 therapy during primary allogeneic skin transplantation has recently confirmed the ability of the CD27 pathway to reduce the formation of memory T cells, resulting in better acceptance of secondary donor cardiac allografts. Similarly, sensitization with primary cardiac allografts in CD27-deficient recipients resulted in prolonged survival of secondary donor hearts transplanted 40 days later, correlating with reduced memory T cell formation. Whether targeting of this pathway could also inactivate already differentiated wildtype memory T cells remains to be clarified. The role of CD27/CD70 in Tregs is also not well understood.

CD30/CD30L

CD30, another member of the TNFR family, is absent from naïve T cells and is differentially expressed in activated T cell subsets, with Th2 cells expressing higher levels than Th1 cells, and Tregs expressing CD30 constitutively. Its binding partner, CD30L, is expressed on APCs and parenchymal cells. CD30 appears to be shed from effector and memory cells and its presence in the urine of kidney transplant recipients has been proposed to be a prognostic factor for acute rejection. Soluble levels of CD30 in the blood have also been associated with rejection of kidney, pancreatic islet, heart, lung and liver allografts in animals and humans. CD30 has been shown to trigger the apoptosis of memory CD8$^+$ T cells following transplantation of allogeneic pancreatic islets in the immune privileged site of the testes. Tregs-mediated killing of memory CD8$^+$ T cells in a cardiac transplant model was also shown to be CD30-dependent. Similarly, Tregs isolated from CD30-deficient mice were less effective at suppressing GVHD than wildtype Tregs.

OX40/OX40L

OX40 is also expressed on activated T cells, memory T cells and Tregs (Demirci and Li, 2008). In addition to enhancing T cell activation, OX40 promotes T cell differentiation into Th1 and Th2 phenotypes and is required for the generation of T cell memory, possibly by sustaining T cell survival via a maintained expression of Bcl-2, Bcl-x$_L$ and survivin. In addition, memory T cells generated in the absence of OX40 appear defective in their ability to produce IFN-γ. Agonistic engagement of OX40 also prevents Tregs from suppressing conventional T cells and reduces the differentiation of naïve T cells into iTregs and IL-10-producing regulatory cells. However, unlike CD28, OX40 is not necessary for the thymic development of nTregs and OX40-deficient T cells have normal suppressive capacity. OX40 signaling has also been shown to restore effector function to anergic T cells. Therefore, OX40 can potentially promote immune responses both by enhancing effector T cell activation and preventing regulation, and may also reverse tolerance.

Blockade of OX40, but not of other costimulatory molecules, prevented the activation of alloreactive T cells in mice double deficient for CD28 and CD154 or in wildtype mice treated with anti-CD154 and CTLA-4-Ig, and promoted acceptance of fully allogeneic skin grafts. These data demonstrate that expression of OX40 is independent of CD28 and CD40 signaling and that OX40 is the main costimulatory pathway that can drive T cell activation in the absence of CD28 and CD40 engagement. In addition, because skin allograft rejection can be affected by both CD4 and CD8$^+$ T cells, and CD8$^+$ T cells that resist blockade of CD28 and CD40L are notoriously difficult to control, OX40 blockade may be able to restrain both T cell subsets. Conversely, OX40 signals at the time of transplantation have been shown to prevent heart allograft acceptance mediated by anti-CD154 mAb, or islet allograft rejection in CD154-deficient mice, and to promote alloantibody production in a CD40-independent manner. Following establishment of tolerance, OX40 signals did not precipitate acute but rather chronic rejection. Interestingly, blockade of OX40 but not of other costimulatory molecules has also been shown in combination with CD28 and CD154 blockade to prolong skin allograft rejection mediated by memory T cells, and the combination of OX40 and CD28 blockade also prolonged cardiac allograft survival in pre-sensitized recipients. These results suggest that inhibiting OX40 may successfully control alloreactive memory T cells that are currently thought to be the main barrier to transplantation tolerance in larger animals that develop alloreactive T cell memory through heterologous immunity following infections, or through prior sensitization as a result of pregnancies, blood transfusions, or previous transplantations (Demirci and Li, 2008).

4-1BB/4-1BBL

4-1BB is a member of the TNFR family primarily expressed on activated CD8+ T cells and to a lesser extent on activated CD4+ T cells and NK cells (Lee and Croft, 2009). It is also constitutively expressed on Tregs. Its ligand is expressed on activated DCs, B cells, and macrophages. Due to its preferential costimulation of CD8+ T cells, mice deficient in 4-1BB have defects in the generation of CTLs following viral infections. However, 4-1BB can also promote the activation of CD4+ T cells and Th2 differentiation. In transplantation, agonistic anti-4-1BB mAb has been shown to accelerate rejection of skin and heart allografts whereas blocking 4-1BB prolonged survival of intestinal allografts whose rejection is dependent on CD8+ T cells. 4-1BB also appears to play a role in promoting memory formation of CD8+ T cells. Similar to OX40, ligation of 4-1BB has been shown to reduce the suppressive function of nTregs, but a specific agonistic antibody of 4-1BB has been reported to drive the generation of suppressive CD8+ T cells *in vivo* and tip the Th17/Treg balance towards Tregs, thereby ameliorating EAE in mice. The molecular mechanisms underlying these effects remain to be further defined.

GITR/GITRL

GITR is also expressed on activated T cells, B cells, NK cells and Tregs, and is also found on macrophages (Azuma, 2010). GITRL is expressed on DCs and parenchymal cells. GITR can serve as a coactivator of T cell responses, but can also trigger apoptosis of the cells in which it is expressed. GITR can reduce suppression, although it is not clear if this is only due to the activation of conventional T cells that then escape suppression or also to direct inhibition of the suppressive function of Tregs. Consistent with these *in vitro* findings, blockade of GITR engagement using a GITR-Ig fusion protein, when in combination with anti-CD154, has recently been shown to prolong skin allograft survival in a Treg-dependent manner.

HVEM/LIGHT

In contrast to most other TNFR family members, HVEM is highly expressed on naive T cells, but its expression decreases during T cell activation and is restored to high levels as cells become quiescent (Murphy and Murphy, 2010). This is in fact the opposite expression kinetics to one of its binding partners, BTLA. HVEM is also expressed on B cells and NK cells. HVEM can bind to two ligands in the TNF family, LIGHT and the soluble LTα and to two receptors in the immunoglobulin family, BTLA and CD160. As reviewed above, HVEM serves as a ligand for the BTLA and CD160 receptors through which it drives coinhibitory signals to T cells. In contrast, engagement of HVEM as a receptor by the LIGHT ligand coactivates T cells. To complicate matters, LIGHT also binds to LTβR and Decoy receptor 3 (DR3) while LTβR in turn binds to the membrane-bound LTαβheterotrimer, and LTα can bind to TNFR1 and TNFR2 (Figure 4.3). The LTαβ-LTβR together with the TNF-TNFR systems control multiple physiologic processes, including T cell homeostasis, inflammation, differentiation, and development and maintenance of lymphoid organs, the latter via the activation of the noncanonical NF-κB pathway. Focusing on the interaction of HVEM with LIGHT (Murphy and Murphy, 2010), in bone marrow transplantation, transfer of HVEM-deficient or LIGHT-deficient donor cells did not give rise to GVHD, unlike transfer of wildtype cells. Blocking anti-HVEM antibody reduced disease severity conferred by wildtype donor cells and facilitated stable hematopoietic chimerism. In an islet transplant model, blockade of HVEM/LIGHT pathway using LTβR-Ig synergized with CTLA-4-Ig to prolong graft survival. Interpretation of these data, however, has to be made cautiously given the complex interactions of these family members and the ability of HVEM to serve both as a coactivating receptor and a coinhibitory ligand.

TIM family

The T cell immunoglobulin mucin (TIM) family was discovered in 2001 during the search for asthma susceptibility genes and molecules differentially expressed on Th1 and Th2 cells. The TIM family contains eight genes in mice, of which three, TIM-1, TIM-3, and TIM-4, are conserved in humans. Besides their costimulatory functions, TIM proteins also function as phosphatidylserine receptors to recognize and clear apoptotic cells (Yeung et al., 2011).

TIM-1, TIM-4, phosphatidylserine

TIM-1 is preferentially expressed on differentiated Th2 cells; but it is also expressed on B cells, mast cells, and NKT cells. Of note, TIM-1 is also known as Kidney Injury Molecule 1 (KIM-1), which is found on renal tubular epithelium following acute kidney injury. TIM1 was initially found to bind to TIM-4, but recent studies have challenged this notion. TIM-1 signaling can costimulate T cell proliferation and increase IL-4 production*in vitro*. Several antibodies to TIM-1 have been generated that bind to the extracellular IgV domain. The 3B3 antibody, which exhibits a high affinity for TIM-1, enhances immune responses *in vivo*, exacerbates EAE, and prevents tolerance. In contrast, antibodies with a lower affinity, such as RMT1-10, inhibit allergen-induced airway inflammation and EAE. In transplantation, anti-TIM-1 antibody 3B3 converted Tregs into Th17 cells *in vitro*, augmented T effector cells, and antagonized tolerance induction in an islet transplant model. In contrast, RMT1-10 has been shown to prolong cardiac allograft survival in mice, and synergized with sirolimus to induce tolerance in a manner that was dependent on Tregs. In a T-bet-deficient model that lacks Th1 responses and resists tolerance induction by anti-CD154 and CTLA-4-Ig, RMT1-10 has been shown to restore tolerance. Interestingly, the tolerogenic effect of RMT1-10 appears to depend on B cells. In this model, TIM-1 expression identified a subset of B cells that express IL-4 and IL-10 and may mark a Breg population, as transfer of these cells could induce donor-specific tolerance. IL-4 was essential for TIM-1 expression on B cells and for TIM-1-mediated IL-10 production by B cells. The opposite effects of the anti-TIM-1 antibodies may be due to their differential affinities for TIM-1, and underscore the potential challenge in targeting these molecules either to enhance or attenuate immune responses.

TIM-3, galectin-9, phosphatidylserine
TIM-3 was initially found on Th1 cells but has now been described on Th1, Th17, CD8+ T cells, DCs, macrophages, and mast cells. Its ligand, the S-type lectin galectin-9, is expressed on Tregs, B cells, mast cells, and parenchymal cells and is upregulated by IFN-γ. TIM-3 is also a phosphatidylserine receptor. TIM-3 acts as a coinhibitory receptor for Th1 and Th17 cells, partly by inducing caspase-dependent T cell apoptosis. A blocking anti-TIM-3 antibody has been shown to induce accelerated cardiac allograft rejection, associated with increased alloantibody production, Th1/Th17 polarization, and inhibition of iTreg induction. Consistent with galectin-9 expression on Tregs, blockade of TIM-3 has been shown to reduce suppression by Tregs and prevent tolerance induction. Administration of soluble galectin-9 has resulted in prolonged skin and cardiac allograft survival in mice, with reduced production of Th1 and Th17 cytokines and promotion of Tregs, demonstrating the therapeutic potential of this approach.

Phosphatidylserine, TIM-4
TIM-4 is not expressed on T cells but rather on APCs, including dendritic cells, macrophages, and peritoneal B-1 cells. Unlike other TIM family members, the cytoplasmic tail of TIM-4 lacks any known signaling domains, and therefore may not mediate signaling to APCs. However, binding of TIM-4 to its putative receptor on T cells promotes Th2 responses. Intriguingly, TIM-4-Ig has been shown to inhibit naïve T cells but enhances the function of pre-activated T cells in a mechanism that is not well understood. The role of TIM-4 in alloresponses remains to be elucidated.

Summary and relevance to clinical transplantation

Adaptive immune responses are influenced by the presence of infection, injury, and inflammation. Transplantation generates numerous inflammatory responses, which affect transplant rejection and ultimately survival by the coordinated events of innate and adaptive immunity. Costimulatory molecules at the very core of T cell priming, differentiation, memory response, development of Tregs, and generation of B cells help. The concept of blocking costimulatory pathways to induce donor-specific tolerance remains promising, but recent studies have revealed extreme complexity of their regulation. In addition to optimal targeting of "positive" costimulatory receptors, reagents may have unwanted effects on Tregs that express many of the same costimulatory receptors expressed on effector T cells. Use of reagents to block costimulation of memory T cells could potentially exacerbate recurrence of infections. An additional challenge is to understand the role of costimulatory molecules expressed by parenchymal cells and the specific consequences of blocking them, particularly those that dampen allogeneic responses. Finally, there is a paucity of therapeutic options to harness coinhibitory molecules to suppress T cell responses.

References

Azuma, M., Role of the glucocorticoid-induced TNFR-related protein (GITR)-GITR ligand pathway in innate and adaptive immunity. Critical reviews in immunology, 2010. 30(6): p. 547–557.

Bour-Jordan, H., et al., Intrinsic and extrinsic control of peripheral T-cell tolerance by costimulatory molecules of the CD28/ B7 family. Immunological reviews, 2011. 241(1): p. 180–205.

Demirci, G. and X.C. Li, Novel roles of OX40 in the allograft response. Current opinion in organ transplantation, 2008. 13(1): p. 26–30.

Denoeud, J. and M. Moser, Role of CD27/CD70 pathway of activation in immunity and tolerance. Journal of leukocyte biology, 2011. 89(2): p. 195–203. Epub 2010 Aug 10.

Elgueta, R., et al., Molecular mechanism and function of CD40/CD40L engagement in the immune system. Immunological reviews, 2009. 229(1): p. 152–172.

Francisco, L.M., P.T. Sage, and A.H. Sharpe, The PD-1 pathway in tolerance and autoimmunity. Immunological reviews, 2010. 236: p. 219–242.

Lee, S.W. and M. Croft, 4-1BB as a therapeutic target for human disease. Advances in experimental medicine and biology, 2009. 647: p. 120–129.

Li, X.C., D.M. Rothstein, and M.H. Sayegh, Costimulatory pathways in transplantation: challenges and new developments. Immunological reviews, 2009. 229(1): p. 271–293.

Murphy, T.L. and K.M. Murphy, Slow down and survive: enigmatic immunoregulation by BTLA and HVEM. Annual review of immunology, 2010. 28: p. 389–411.

Simpson, T.R., S.A. Quezada, and J.P. Allison, Regulation of CD4 T cell activation and effector function by inducible costimulator (ICOS). Current opinion in immunology, 2010. 22(3): p. 326–332.

Yeung, M., M. McGrath, and N. Najafian, The emerging role of the TIM molecules in transplantation. American journal of translational, 2011. 11 (10): p. 2012–2019.

Yi, K.H. and L. Chen, Fine tuning the immune response through B7-H3 and B7-H4. Immunological reviews, 2009. 229(1): p. 145–151.

CHAPTER 5

Major histocompatibility complex

Raja Rajalingam, Qiuheng Zhang, J. Michael Cecka, and Elaine F. Reed

Department of Pathology and Laboratory Medicine, David Geffen School of Medicine at UCLA, Los Angeles, USA

CHAPTER OVERVIEW

- The major histocompatibility complex (MHC) is a cluster of genes that encode cell surface molecules, including HLA antigens in humans, and HLA genes are highly polymorphic among individuals.
- Structurally and functionally, the MHC is divided into three classes.
- HLA class I molecules are widely expressed, whereas HLA class II molecules are confined to APCs; both present antigens to T cells to trigger immune responses.
- HLA differences (mismatches) between donor and recipient are the key trigger of rejection.
- HLA matching can improve graft survival in most solid organ transplants.
- HLA molecules are targets of alloantibodies. Most alloantibodies are directed against mismatched donor HLA molecules, but antibodies against non-HLA molecules are being identified and can be of clinical significance.

Introduction

The human major histocompatibility complex (MHC) is located on chromosome 6p21.3 and contains about 224 functional genes and pseudogenes. Nearly 40% of the genes encode molecules that are involved in the immune response, including the human leukocyte antigens (HLAs) that are major barriers to transplantation. HLA genes are highly polymorphic and exhibit marked linkage disequilibrium. Differences in HLA molecules between a recipient and a donor provoke T cell, B cell, and natural killer (NK) cell responses. Therefore, HLA molecules are key targets of rejection responses in allogeneic transplantation. Matching HLA antigens of the donor with that of the recipient prolongs graft survival in most solid

---

Transplant Immunology, First Edition. Edited by Xian Chang Li and Anthony M. Jevnikar.
© 2016 John Wiley & Sons, Ltd. Published 2016 by John Wiley & Sons, Ltd.
Companion website: www.wiley.com/go/li/transplantimmunology

organ and all stem cell transplants; however, the polymorphic nature of these antigens makes finding good matches rare. Many patients develop antibodies to donor HLA antigens and sensitization is a major obstacle for transplantation. Recently developed solid-phase assays that define HLA class I and class II antibodies with exquisite specificity and sensitivity provide great insights into the virtual crossmatch to facilitate transplantation in sensitized patients as well as to guide the management of patients undergoing desensitization therapies. The development of *de novo* antibodies that arise following transplantation also affects long-term graft outcomes. This chapter provides an overview of the human MHC molecules and their importance in clinical transplantation.

Structure and function of MHC

Genomic organization of MHC

The human MHC can be physically divided into three regions: MHC class I, class II, and class III genes. The general MHC structure is conserved among most species studied, although there are some differences in the organization and iteration of genes. The human MHC class I region is composed of highly polymorphic HLA class I genes (HLA-A, -B, -C), nonclassical HLA class I genes (HLA-E, -F, -G), class I-like genes (MICA, MICB), and other genes apparently not related to the immune system (Figure 5.1). Key functions of classical class I molecules are presentation of peptide antigens to CD8+ T cells and serving as inhibitory ligands for NK cell receptors. The products of nonclassical genes and class I-like genes are not involved in antigen presentation to T cells, but serve as ligands for NK cell receptors. For example, HLA-E binds a restricted set of peptides derived from the signal peptides of HLA-A, B, C, and G antigens. NK cells utilize the CD94/NKG2A receptor to bind HLA-E molecules to inhibit NK cells from eliciting killing activities. HLA-G molecules are expressed on the trophoblast and can inhibit NK cell-mediated lysis through interaction with the receptors ILT2 and ILT4. Stress-induced products of class I-like genes MICA and MICB bind NKG2D receptors on NK cells, which activates NK cells to kill stressed or damaged cells.

The human MHC class II region contains genes that encode antigen-presenting molecules (HLA-DR, -DQ, -DP), antigen-processing molecules (HLA-DM, -DO), immune proteasome genes (LMP), and the TAP transporters that associate with classical class I antigen presentation. HLA-DR, DQ, and DP molecules present antigens to CD4+ T lymphocytes. The DM and DO genes are not expressed on the cell surface, but form heterotetrameric complexes that are involved in peptide exchange and load onto DR, DQ, and DP molecules. The HLA-DR region contains one functional gene for the α-chain (DRA), but has one or two functional genes for the β-chain (DRB1, DRB3, DRB4, DRB5), depending on the HLA-DRB1 allele type (Figure 5.2). Based on the DRB1 allele type and the DRB gene content, human MHC haplotypes can be divided into

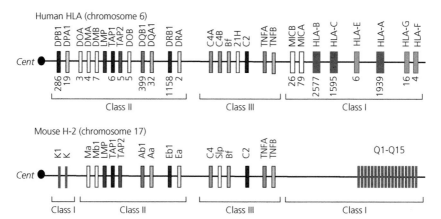

Figure 5.1 Genetic map of the human and mouse major histocompatibility complexes (MHCs). Partial schematic map of human MHC on chromosome 6 (upper panel) and mouse H-2 genes on chromosome 17 (lower panel). Illustrations are not drawn to scale. The centromere (circle) and major HLA and H-2 genes (boxes) are indicated in order. The number of distinct proteins (alleles) encoded by each human MHC gene is indicated under each locus. source: Data from IMGT/HLA database, April 2014, http://www.ebi.ac.uk/imgt/hla/stats.html.

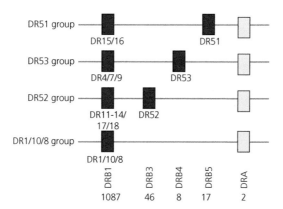

Figure 5.2 Human MHC class II DR region is variable in gene content. Based on the DRB1 allele type, human MHC haplotypes fall into four groups: DR51, DR52, DR53, and DR1/10/8 that vary in DRB gene number (blue boxes). The serological specificities encoded by each DRB gene are provided under each locus. The number of alleles encoded by each DR gene is indicated. source: Data from IMGT/HLA database, April 2014, http://www.ebi.ac.uk/imgt/hla/stats.html.

four types: DR51 group (encodes DR15 or DR16 and DR51 molecules), DR52 group (encodes DR11, DR12, DR13, DR14, DR17 or DR18 and DR52 molecules), DR53 group (encodes DR4, DR7 or DR9 and DR53 molecules), and DR1/10/8 group (encodes DR1, DR10 or DR8 molecules). The MHC class III region is the most dense region of the human genome and contains many immune and non-immune related genes that are highly conserved (Figure 5.1).

MHC genes evolve through duplication, followed by diversification, co-evolution, and sequence exchange. The classical class I region of chimpanzees, the closest relatives of humans, has a genomic organization very similar to that of humans; however, the nucleotide sequence similarity between humans and chimpanzees, which is about 99% across the genome, drops to 86% in the MHC class I region as a result of the extensive polymorphism in the region. The mouse MHC, known as the H-2 system, is located on chromosome-17 and has a similar regional organization as the human MHC, except for an additional classical class I locus, centromeric to the class II region (Figure 5.1). The number and sequence of mouse class I loci differ substantially, but the structure and function of mouse MHC molecules are comparable to those of the human HLA. Also, unlike primates, the mouse lacks MICA/B-related genes in its MHC; however, a related gene family, MILL, is located near the leukocyte receptor complex on chromosome-17.

HLA gene polymorphism

The focus, for HLA in transplantation, has been the classical class I and class II HLA molecules and alleles. The most notable feature of these HLA regions is the high degree of polymorphism exhibited by its gene products, which likely reflects some survival benefit in its diversity as well as its ability to present countless peptides from pathogens. Early population studies using serological typing methods identified an unprecedented number of HLA antigens at each locus. However, DNA sequencing reveals even more extensive polymorphism as the serologically defined antigens include multiple allelic variants that differ at one or more nucleotide residues. To date, 8576 distinct HLA class I molecules and 2649 class II molecules have been recognized (IMGT/HLA database, version 3.16, April 2014).

The differences among HLA proteins are localized primarily to the antigen-binding domains of these molecules, which bind peptides and interact with T-cell receptors. The high degree of HLA polymorphism is presumably the result of positive selection for human survival by enhancing the diversity in the repertoire of HLA-bound peptides. HLA class I polymorphisms are predominantly found in the first 180 amino acids of the heavy chain and the HLA class II polymorphisms are found in the first 90–95 amino acids of the α and/or β chains. The extensive allelic diversity at these loci is generated by point mutation, recombination, and gene conversion. Most substitutions are shared by more than one HLA allele and thus demonstrate a patchwork pattern of sequence polymorphism, indicating the presence of segmental exchanges.

HLA haplotypes and inheritance

The HLA alleles present on each parental chromosome is called an HLA haplotype, and these are inherited in a Mendelian fashion (Figure 5.3) and are co-dominantly expressed. Each parental chromosome provides a haplotype or

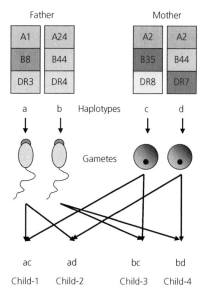

Figure 5.3 HLA haplotype segregation in a family. Each child inherits one HLA haplotype from each parent. Because each parent has two different haplotypes (paternal = ab and maternal = cd), four different haplotypic combinations are possible in the offspring (ac, ad, bc, bd). Therefore, a child has a 25% chance of having HLA-identical or zero haplotype matched sibling donor, and a 50% chance of having a one-haplotype matched sibling donor. All children have one-haplotype matched to each parent unless recombination has occurred.

linked set of HLA genes to the offspring. The child carries one representative antigen from each of the class I and class II loci of each parent. A child is, by definition, a one-haplotype match to each parent unless recombination has occurred. Statistically, there is a 25% chance that siblings will share the same parental haplotypes (two-haplotype match or HLA-identical), a 50% chance that they will share one haplotype (one-haplotype match), and a 25% chance that neither haplotype will be the same (zero-haplotype match). Haplotypes are usually inherited intact from each parent, although crossover between the A and B locus occurs in about 2% of the offspring, resulting in a recombination. The HLA region demonstrates strong linkage disequilibrium across HLA-A, B, C, DR, and DQ. Linkage disequilibrium is a phenomenon where alleles at adjacent HLA loci are inherited together more often than would be expected by chance. For example, if HLA-A1 and HLA-B8 occur at gene frequencies of 16 and 10%, respectively, in a population the probability of finding them together should be 1.6%. However, the observed occurrence of the HLA-A1-B8 combination is significantly higher than the predicted incidence (about 8%). Existing data suggest that positive selection operates on the haplotype and that the linked loci confer a particular selective advantage for the host.

HLA class I and class II molecules

HLA class I and class II molecules are expressed on distinct cell populations. The HLA class I molecules are expressed by all nucleated cells in the body; they present endogenous peptides (such as viral peptides) to CD8+ cytotoxic T cells, which in turn respond to the infected cells. However, the level of HLA class I expression varies by class I loci, alleles, as well as tissue types. Furthermore, expression of class I molecules can be downregulated by pathological events such as malignant transformation, viral infections, and stress conditions or upregulated by pro-inflammatory cytokines. HLA class II molecules on the other hand present exogenous peptides (i.e., bacterial peptides) to CD4+ helper T cells, which regulate the effector function of other immune cells. Thus, HLA class II molecules are expressed on selected cell types, especially on antigen-presenting cells (APCs). The expression levels of both class I and class II HLA molecules, and expression of HLA class II molecules on other cell types can be induced in response to cytokines including TNF-α and INF-γ.

HLA structure

The basic structure of HLA antigens is to perform the antigen presentation function. Although the class I and class II HLA molecules differ structurally, both have a platform formed by beta-pleated sheet and a groove bordered by alpha helices oriented distally from the plasma membrane of the cell surface. Most of the polymorphic residues are clustered in and around the edges of the groove. The fine structure within the groove includes pockets that accommodate peptides (Figure 5.4). Accommodation of different amino acid side chains serves to anchor residues with specific characteristics, which confers a rudimentary specificity to the HLA allele. Not all HLA antigens can bind the same peptides. Class I molecules are loaded primarily with intracellular degradation products in the endoplasmic reticulum and class II molecules are loaded primarily with peptides derived from endocytosed extracellular proteins. The T-cell receptor recognizes this compound ligand, making contact with both the HLA molecule and the peptide antigen fragment. Exposure to diverse pathogens has probably driven and selected HLA polymorphisms that provide a survival advantage and, therefore, ethnic populations living in distinct geographical regions, such as Caucasians, Africans, and Asians, tend to show different constellations of common HLA allotypes.

Cellular responses to HLA alloantigens

Allogeneic HLA antigens provoke strong immune responses. It has been estimated that the frequency of T cells that respond to allogeneic HLA antigens may be hundreds of times greater than that responding to nominal antigens. These strong responses are responsible for making HLA antigens a major barrier to transplantation of tissues and organs between individuals. Two basic types of response have been observed primarily, one involving the "direct" presentation

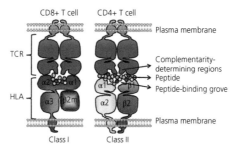

Figure 5.4 Structure of HLA molecules. HLA class I and class II molecules present peptide antigens to CD8+ and CD4+ T cells, respectively. The HLA class I molecule is a heterodimer of a membrane-spanning heavy α chain (encoded by HLA-A, -B or -C gene) bound noncovalently to a non-MHC gene (located in chromosome 15) encoded light β2-microglobulin (β2m) chain, which does not span the membrane. The α chain folds into three domains: α1, α2, and α3. The α1 and α2 domains form an antigen-binding groove. The HLA class II molecule is composed of two transmembrane glycoprotein chains, α (encoded by DRA, DQA1 or DPA1) and β (encoded by DRB1, DQB1 or DPB1). Each chain has two domains, and the two chains together form a compact four-domain structure similar to that of HLA class I molecule. The α2 and β2 domains, like the α3 and β2-microglobulin domains of the HLA class I molecule, have amino acid sequence and structural similarities to immunoglobulin C domains. The α1 and β1 domains of class II molecules form the peptide-binding cleft. The major difference between class I and class II is that the ends of the peptide-binding grove are more open in HLA class II molecules than in HLA class I molecules. As a result, the HLA class I can accommodate only short peptides (~9 amino acids long) and the ends of the peptide are substantially buried within the class I molecule. In contrast, the class II groove has open ends and can accommodate longer peptides (12–20 amino acids long). The T-cell receptor (TCR) recognizes the complex of HLA and its bound peptide.

of donor HLA antigens to the recipient's T cells and the other the "indirect" presentation of donor HLA antigens that have been processed by the recipient's APCs and presented to the recipient's T cells via recipient HLA molecules. Indirect presentation proceeds in the same way as the presentation of exogenous nominal antigens in that donor HLA antigens are taken up by host APCs and antigenic peptides are loaded into the recipient's HLA class II molecules for presentation to T cells. Less well-understood is the "semi-direct" presentation pathway, which shares features "with direct presentation of pathogenic peptides by self-APC" and involves the transfer of donor cell membrane components, including donor MHC/donor peptide complexes, to the recipient APC.

In addition to T and B lymphocytes, NK cells, a third population of lymphocytes, are also involved in alloimmune responses. Historically, NK cells were thought of as components of innate immunity. However, it is now clear that NK cells use a highly specific target cell recognition receptor system, consisting of a multitude of inhibitory and activating receptors. Killer cell immunoglobulin-like receptors (KIRs) are the key receptors of human NK cells. Fourteen distinct KIRs have been identified, and among those eight are the inhibitory type and six are the activating type. The number and type of KIR genes present varies substantially between individuals. Inhibitory KIRs recognize distinct motifs of polymorphic HLA class I (HLA-A, B, or C) molecules. Upon engagement of their specific HLA class I ligands, inhibitory KIR dampen NK cell reactivity. In contrast, activating KIRs are believed to stimulate NK cell reactivity when they sense their (unknown) ligands. KIR and HLA gene families map to different human chromosomes (19 and 6, respectively), and their independent segregation produces a wide diversity in the number and type of inherited KIR–HLA combinations, likely contributing to overall immune competency. In allogeneic transplantation, recipient NK cells expressing an inhibitory receptor can be activated to mediate target cell killing when the allograft lacks the relevant HLA class I ligand for that inhibitory receptor.

HLA typing

Traditionally, HLA antigens were defined using serological microcytotoxicity techniques that relied on the availability of viable lymphocytes and a panel of carefully selected antisera that recognized distinct HLA antigens. During the past 15 years, DNA-based typing techniques have replaced serological methods in clinical applications. DNA typing methods provide a more precise definition of the HLA system and improve the reliability of the typing. The oligonucleotide reagents required for DNA-based HLA typing are synthetic and easily standardized and manufacture controlled. Furthermore, DNA typing approaches proved invaluable in confirming homozygosity. The methods most widely used for HLA typing and histocompatibility testing are based on the recognition of locus-specific polymorphisms in genomic DNA by sequence-specific primers (SSPs) or by hybridization of sequence-specific oligonucleotide probes (SSOPs) with DNA that has been selectively amplified by the polymerase chain reaction (PCR) (Figure 5.5). Using the extensive DNA sequence data available, oligonucleotide primers and probes that specifically hybridize to sites that are unique to an HLA locus, allele, or group of alleles have been developed and are commercially available for HLA typing.

Three basic techniques used in conjunction with PCR are reverse sequence-specific oligonucleotide (rSSO) probe hybridization method, SSP directed amplification method, and sequencing-based typing (SBT) method. The rSSO typing is a commonly used method of HLA typing that utilizes a liquid bead-based Luminex® technology (Figure 5.5). A biotinylated locus-specific amplicon is generated from the sample genomic DNA by PCR and subsequently denatured. This product is combined with a single cocktail of color-coded polystyrene beads. Each bead is coated with a unique allele- or group-specific oligonucleotide probe. The beads presenting complementary probes to the amplicon will hybridize. Amplicons annealed to the conjugated probes are detected via streptavidin phycoerythrin (SAPE) chemistry. This chemical tag, bound to the biotinylated amplicon, is excited by one of the two lasers on the Luminex 100™ flow-based instrument. The second laser identifies the associated bead color. The combined

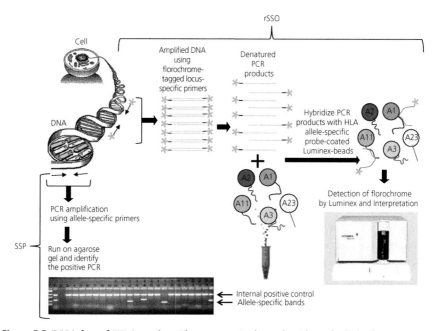

Figure 5.5 DNA-based HLA typing. The reverse single nucleotide probe hybridization (rSSO) method using Luminex bead arrays is depicted in the upper panel. DNA samples are PCR amplified and the amplicons are enzymatically labeled with a biotin molecule during the PCR reaction. The PCR products are hybridized with immobilized probe arrays of Luminex color-coded polystyrene beads. Amplicons annealed to the polystyrene beads are detected via streptavidin phycoerythrin chemistry. This chemical tag, bound to the biotinylated amplicon, is excited by one of the two lasers on the Luminex flow-based instrument. The second laser identifies the associated bead color. The combined data are interpreted by computer software, identifying positive signal beads and their respective color for HLA allele assignment. Sequence-specific primer typing (SSP).The lower panel is a picture of an agarose gel electrophoresis showing the pattern of allele/group-specific PCR products corresponding to amplification of HLA class I or class II genes. Each PCR well included a unique set of primers that were designed to have perfect matches with a single allele or group of alleles and produce a product with a particular known size. Each PCR reaction includes a positive internal control primer pair, which amplifies a conserved gene segment (i.e., Human β-globulin gene), which is present in all human DNA samples and is used to verify the integrity of the PCR reaction.

data are interpreted by computer software, identifying positive signal beads and their respective color for allele group assignment.

The SSP method is a simple PCR-based technique, which uses sequence-specific primers for DNA-based HLA typing. SSP depends on DNA amplification using group- or allele-specific primers and detecting an amplified product of the correct size by gel electrophoresis. The size is determined by running an agarose gel that separates the PCR products according to their size. The assignment of alleles merely consists of determining whether amplification has occurred or not, that is, visualization and detection of the appropriate sized amplicon by agarose gel electrophoresis.

SBT is the most comprehensive method employed for a complete HLA typing. The SBT method provides the highest resolution possible, which is important for identifying compatible genetically unrelated hematopoietic stem cell donor and recipient pairs, as well as for discovering new alleles. SBT uses a strategy that involves locus- or group-specific amplifications of the polymorphic exons followed by direct sequencing of the PCR products. Bi-directional sequencing is performed and the sequences of both strands are imported into sequence alignment and analysis software for allele assignment. Because of the sharing of sequences between HLA alleles, some genotypes with particular allele combinations result in ambiguous results. These ambiguities are resolved by performing additional allele- or group-specific PCR amplifications, hybridization with informative probes, or by direct sequencing amplified products. Next generation sequencing (NGS) will solve the problem of typing ambiguities through the combination of clonal amplification, which provides phase information and the capacity to sequence larger regions of the HLA genes at a lower cost compared to current methods.

HLA nomenclature

The HLA nomenclature can be daunting as the change from serological typing (which defines antigens) to DNA typing (which defines alleles) resulted in some conflicts. The standard DNA nomenclature is illustrated in Figure 5.6 and includes distinct fields (separated by a colon) for an antigen, allele group, and designation for silent substitutions (those which do not result in a change in the protein) and differences in noncoding regions. In the clinical setting, HLA typing for hematopoietic stem cell transplants is reported at the allele level (B*15:01 in the example, Figure 5.6) and HLA typing for solid organ transplants is reported at the antigen level (B62). This usually is the first two digits after the asterisk, but because the DNA nomenclature uses allele groups that are related by nucleotide sequence similarities, there are a few exceptions.

Anti-HLA antibodies in transplantation

Patients who become sensitized to donor HLA antigens through pregnancies, prior transplantation, and blood transfusions or other exposures, or patients who produce antidonor HLA antibodies following their transplant, present formidable challenges in transplantation. Circulating donor-specific anti-HLA antibodies in transplant patients may damage the graft to varying degrees, ranging from catastrophic hyperacute rejection to transplant glomerulopathy in kidney allografts to a shortened graft survival time in most solid organs. For many years, antibodies directed against donor HLA antigens have been avoided through crossmatch testing, using patient serum and donor lymphocytes to determine whether there are circulating antibodies against the donor.

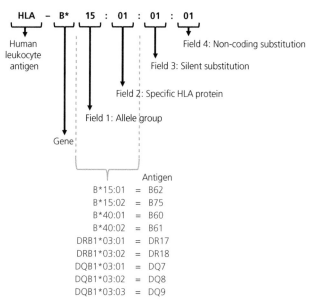

Figure 5.6 HLA nomenclature. With the ever increasing number of HLA alleles described, the WHO nomenclature committee for factors of the HLA system decided recently to introduce colons (:) into the allele names to act as delimiters of the separate fields. The first field specifies a group of alleles and is equivalent to the serologically defined antigen. The number used in the first field directly corresponds to the antigen name with some exceptions because the DNA nomenclature uses allele groups that are related by nucleotide sequence similarities (some are listed in blue). The second field specifies a group of alleles that encode a distinct HLA protein. Field three denotes synonymous mutations within the coding region of the gene. The fourth field represents genetic variations in noncoding regions.

For sensitized candidates, this test identifies incompatible donors whose organs would not be suitable for the patient. By excluding potential donors who are incompatible with broadly sensitized recipients, successful transplantation is possible; however, patients who develop antibodies that are reactive with many of the more common HLA antigens have limited opportunities for transplantation with a compatible donor. Patients who produce new anti-HLA antibodies against their donor following transplantation are at increased risk of graft failure unless their response can be controlled or abrogated. The effect of anti-HLA antibodies on different transplanted organs may differ in severity, in the specific pathologic lesions, and ultimately the degree of damage they cause to the organ, but emerging evidence shows that donor-specific antibodies can damage any transplanted organ including the liver in liver transplants.

Antibodies may be produced against donor HLA antigens that differ from the patient's own antigen by as minute as a single amino acid. On the other hand, a single HLA antibody may be reactive with a number of different HLA antigens. Many of the epitopes recognized by HLA antibodies have been tentatively identified by comparing amino acid sequence differences and similarities among HLA antigens that are members of *cross-reacting groups* (CREGs). For example, the epitope that is associated with the amino acids arginine at position 163 and glutamic acid at position 166, which are found in HLA-A11, A25, A26, A43 and A6601 and in no other HLA antigens. Some antibodies eluted from A25 react with each of these HLA antigens, because their target epitope is affected by these particular amino acids at these exposed positions on the surface of the HLA molecule. The range of antibody specificities that can be produced by an individual is unpredictable, but data suggest that it may be influenced by the specific epitope differences in the alloantigen exposure.

Methods to detect and characterize HLA antibodies

Tests for antibodies against HLA antigens fall under two categories: cell based and solid-phase. The primary cell-based test, namely, the micro-cytotoxicity test, developed in 1964, was used for many years to identify HLA antigens, for crossmatching and to identify sensitized patients. The test combined the patient or reference serum with patient lymphocytes and a rabbit complement. Cells that were killed by complement-binding antibodies were identified by vital dye exclusion and a substantial degree of cell death indicated a positive reaction (Figure 5.7). The key feature of the micro-cytotoxicity test was that it required only one microliter of serum, which allowed laboratories to share anti-HLA reagents and to characterize the HLA antigens serologically. The same test was used to identify sensitized patients by testing the patient's serum against a panel of lymphocytes from potential donors. The test was modified at many laboratories by changing incubation times and washes or by adding anti-human globulin reagents to increase its sensitivity and reduce false-positive reactions. In the 1980s, indirect flow cytometric measurement of antidonor antibodies was introduced. This increased the sensitivity of the test many fold (Figure 5.7).

Solid-phase technologies for antibody detection and characterization began to appear in the 1990s and have now evolved to permit precise identification of the HLA antibodies, even in broadly reactive sera (Figure 5.8). These new methods employ affinity-purified HLA antigens, isolated from cells or produced by recombinant DNA technologies, which are chemically attached to solid supports (primarily microbeads that can be differentiated through internal dyes). The solid-phase tests have made "virtual" crossmatches possible for most patients, because individual HLA reactivities can be measured. The virtual crossmatch compares the antibody specificities present in the patient's serum with those in a potential donor's HLA type to assess crossmatch compatibility (Figure 5.9). The Organ Procurement and Transplantation Network (OPTN) has established a mechanism to enter "unacceptable" HLA antigens for transplant candidates based on antibody identification using solid-phase tests, which are used to virtually crossmatch donors for organ allocation in the United States. Similar

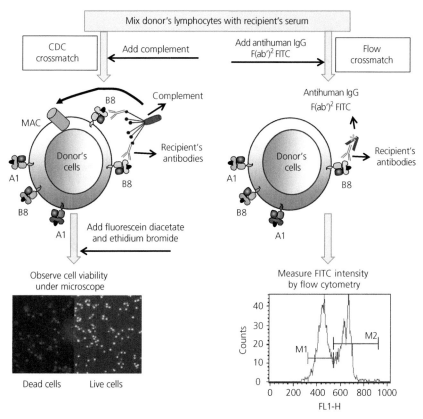

Figure 5.7 Lymphocyte crossmatching. Left panel: the complement-dependent lymphocytotoxicity assay tests the capacity of the transplant recipient's serum to kill donor T and B lymphocytes in the presence of complement. Dead lymphocytes (red fluorescence) are discriminated from live lymphocytes (CFDA, green fluoresence) by incorporation of a vital dye (propidium iodide) and scored as 1 (<20%), 2 (20–40%), 4 (40–60%), 6 (60–80%), or 8 (>80%) killing. A score of 4 or greater is considered positive. Right panel: Binding of recipient anti-HLA antibodies to donor T cells labeled with anti-CD3 phycoerythrin (PE) and B cells labeled with anti-CD19 PE mAbs are detected by a fluorescent secondary antihuman Fitc-conjugated antihuman IgG F(ab′)2antibody. The amount of antibody bound to the cell corresponds to the fluorescence intensity which is determined using a flow cytometer. The amount of antihuman IgG antibody bound to lymphocytes treated with normal human control IgG (median fluorescence intensity) is subtracted from the median fluorescence intensity of the recipient serum to determine the result. A score of greater than 50 MCS for the Tcell flow crossmatch and greater than 100 MCS for the B cell flow crossmatch is considered positive.

approaches have been established in Europe and in the United Kingdom to streamline organ allocation to sensitized patients. The virtual crossmatch facilitates the allocation of crossmatch-compatible deceased donor kidneys to sensitized patients who previously would have undergone crossmatch testing before declining the offer.

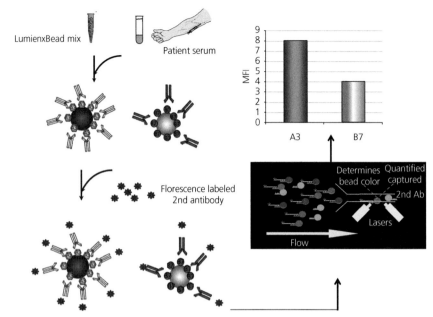

Figure 5.8 Luminex detection of HLA antibodies using single HLA antigen coated beads. The Luminex bead-based antibody identification technology consists of a series of 100 polystyrene beads with single HLA molecules attached. Each bead is internally labeled with different ratios of two red fluorochromes giving each bead a unique signal. The patient's serum is mixed with the single antigen bead mix and the binding of anti-HLA antibodies is detected using a secondary phycoerythrin (PE) labeled antihuman IgG antibody. The luminex beads are passed through two laser detectors in a single profile. One detector excites the red fluorochrome in the beads, whereas the other detector excites the PE bound to the second antibody. The degree of PE fluorescence binding is expressed as mean fluorescence intensity (MFI), which corresponds to the specificity and strength of the HLA antibody.

Assessing sensitization before and after transplantation

As a patient's sensitization status may change while awaiting transplantation, monitoring sensitization status in transplant candidates and providing up-to-date antibody profiles is important for the life-saving organ transplants (heart, lung, liver, intestine). With improved tests to identify and characterize the antibody specificities for sensitized patients and the improving accuracy of virtual crossmatches, it is often possible to expand the potential donor pool for the sensitized candidates for these organs, permitting importation of organs recovered at distant hospitals and improving the chances for identifying a compatible organ. Importantly, anti-HLA antibodies developed after organ transplants play a role in acute and chronic allograft rejection, highlighting the need to detect these antibodies in a clinically relevant manner. Thus, post-transplant assessment of anti-HLA antibodies is useful in identifying patients at risk for acute and/or chronic rejection. The development of antidonor HLA antibodies is

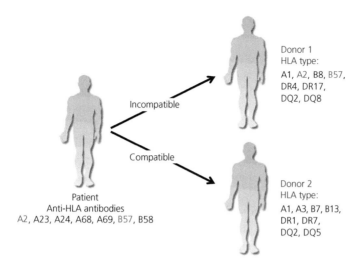

Figure 5.9 Virtual crossmatch. The virtual crossmatch uses the antibody specificities identified in a patient's serum by solid-phase flow and/or luminex single antigen bead arrays and the donor HLA type to predict compatibility. An actual crossmatch uses patient serum and donor lymphocytes to detect donor-reactive antibodies. Donor-specific antibodies and their target are indicated in red types.

positively associated with chronic rejection of heart, renal, lung, and liver allografts. The frequency of rejection episodes and the production of antidonor HLA antibodies were found to be associated with an increased risk of developing transplant vasculopathy, the hallmark of chronic rejection. When renal transplant patients were examined prospectively for the development of anti-HLA antibodies, a strong association between the production of donor specific antibodies (DSA), antibody-mediated rejection (AMR), and early graft dysfunction was detected. Additionally, in a multicenter large-scale prospective study, the presence of HLA antibodies was confirmed in patients with well-functioning grafts and this detection predicted later graft failure. These studies demonstrate that assessment of DSA production after transplantation may identify patients at risk for AMR, early graft dysfunction, and/or the development of chronic rejection.

The use of post-transplant antibody assessment is beneficial because it provides a means to monitor the patient in a less invasive manner than protocol biopsy; it is less expensive and can be repeated often. Post-transplant antibody monitoring is important to graft survival because the development of antidonor HLA antibodies is an early indicator of a response against the allograft while complement activation (as shown by C4d deposition) is a secondary event as are other noncomplement mediated mechanisms of AMR. The development of anti-donor HLA antibodies may also reflect an inadequate level of immunosuppression or non-adherence.

Non-HLA antigens in organ transplantation

Although the immune response to HLA antigens plays a central role in allograft rejection, evidence shows that non-HLA antigens also contribute to the pathogenesis of acute and chronic rejection, which limit long-term graft survival of solid organ transplants. The clinical relevance of non-HLA antigens has been suggested by the observation that among recipients of HLA-identical sibling transplants the ten-year graft survival was significantly better for patients without HLA antibodies compared with patients with HLA antibodies. Some sensitized patients also develop antibodies against non-HLA endothelial or epithelial antigens. Much of the direct evidence for the role of non-HLA antigens comes from studies of patients with tissue-reactive antibodies that are not directed against HLA antigens.

Anti-endothelial cell antibodies (AECAs) primarily target autoantigens, including vimentin and cardiac myosin (CM) in heart, collagen V (Col V) and K-α1 tubulin in lung, agrin, and angiotensin II receptor type I (AT1) in kidney transplantation. It is unclear whether the appearance of these autoantibodies is the cause of graft dysfunction or is a response to graft damage from other injuries. Patients who develop these antibodies during graft loss may be at risk of AMR in a subsequent transplant. AECAs are not generally detectable in crossmatch testing nor by current solid-phase antibody tests. Limited availability and cost of testing has hampered the understanding of their role in graft injury.

Anti-MICA antibodies

MICA is encoded by a highly polymorphic gene located in the HLA class I region with at least 76 alleles. MICA antigens have a restricted tissue distribution and are expressed on epithelium, endothelium, keratinocytes, and fibroblasts. Their expression levels can be induced in response to cellular stress mediated by ischemia reperfusion injury as well as cytokines such as IL-2, IL-4, and IL-15.

Alloantibodies against MICA have been reported to be associated with acute and chronic vascular rejection of renal and heart transplants. In a large multicenter study, presensitization to MICA was associated with increased graft loss in renal recipients transplanted with donors' who were well-matched for HLA. MICA antibodies have been shown to mediate complement-dependent cytotoxicity against endothelial cells, suggesting that these antibodies can cause complement-mediated damage of the allograft. Most studies reporting a role for MICA in transplantation have been indirect and circumstantial because the donor specificity of the antibodies was not ascertained.

It should be noted that current crossmatching techniques that use lymphocytes, will fail to detect AECAs. To address this issue, flow-cytometry crossmatch tests have been developed using primary cultured endothelial cells to detect AECAs. The XM-One assay uses Tie-2 antibody-coated magnetic beads to select precursor EC directly from donor blood. Studies are needed to confirm if this crossmatch method is useful for identifying clinically relevant AECA.

Summary

The need for accurate, high resolution typing of HLA and more precise methods for quantitation of HLA antibodies in transplant patients are on the rise. The major impetus for this is to facilitate transplantation of highly sensitized patients through virtual HLA crossmatching. There are numerous methodological innovations on the horizon that will help achieve this goal. NGS coupled with advances in automation as well as data analysis will improve typing and resolution of HLA. Future technologies and data analysis tools that improve the identification of the epitopes recognized by alloantibodies should also be valuable in understanding the immunogenicity of HLA molecules and identifying acceptable mismatches.

The mechanisms by which antibodies alter or reduce graft survival are still not fully understood. There is a complex interaction between the complement cascade and intracellular signaling pathways activated within the cells of the graft following antibody binding, which either contributes to rejection or induces accommodation. Also, there is a growing appreciation for the role antibody plays in other effector mechanisms, in particular leukocyte recruitment, for which we have no direct therapeutic strategies. Focusing on the pathways involved in antibody, complement, and non-T-effector cell processes will offer an enhanced perspective as to the molecular mechanisms of accommodation and chronic rejection. Revelation of these pathways will help in the identification of targeted drug therapy to improve the success of transplantation.

With a growing number of patients who are awaiting re-transplantation, the importance of antigraft antibodies (HLA and non-HLA) will continue to increase as more sensitized patients are added to waiting lists. The identification of these antibodies is a complex part of post-transplant antibody production monitoring. As the problem of antibody-mediated graft injury becomes better appreciated, resolving such problems will greatly improve long-term transplant outcomes.

Further reading

van Bergen J, Thompson A, Haasnoot GW, Roodnat JI, de Fijter JW, Claas FH, Koning F, Doxiadis II. KIR-ligand mismatches are associated with reduced long-term graft survival in HLA-compatible kidney transplantation. Am J Transplant 2011, **11**(9):1959–1964.

Bjorkman PJ, Saper MA, Samraoui B, Bennett WS, Strominger JL, Wiley DC. Structure of the human class I histocompatibility antigen, HLA-A2. Nature 1987, **329**:506–512.

Breimer ME, Rydberg L, Jackson AM, Lucas DP, Zachary AA, Melancon JK, Von Visger J, Pelletier R, Saidman SL, Williams WW, Jr., et al. Multicenter evaluation of a novel endothelial cell crossmatch test in kidney transplantation. Transplantation 2009, **87**:549–556.

Cecka JM, Kucheryavaya AY, Reinsmoen NL, Leffell MS. Calculated PRA: Initial results show benefits for sensitized patients and a reduction in positive crossmatches. Am J Transplant 2011, **11**:719–724.

Colvin RB, Smith RN. Antibody-mediated organ-allograft rejection. Nat Rev Immunol 2005, **5**:807–817.

Djamali A, Kaufman DB, Ellis TM, Zhong W, Matas A, Samaniego M. Diagnosis and management of antibody-mediated rejection: Current status and novel approaches. Am J Transplant. 2014, **14**(2):255–271.

Gloor JM, Winters JL, Cornell LD, Fix LA, DeGoey SR, Knauer RM, Cosio FG, Gandhi MJ, Kremers W, Stegall MD. Baseline donor-specific antibody levels and outcomes in positive crossmatch kidney transplantation. Am J Transplant 2010, **10**:582–589.

Klein J, Sato A: The HLA system. First of two parts. N Engl J Med 2000, **343**:702–709.

Klein J, Sato A. The HLA system. Second of two parts. N Engl J Med 2000, **343**:782–786.

Loupy A, Lefaucheur C, Vernerey D, Prugger C, Duong van Huyen JP, Mooney N,Suberbielle C, Frémeaux-Bacchi V, Méjean A, Desgrandchamps F, Anglicheau D, Nochy D, Charron D, Empana JP, Delahousse M, Legendre C, Glotz D, Hill GS, Zeevi A, Jouven X. Complement-binding anti-HLA antibodies and kidney-allograft survival. N Engl J Med 2013, **369**(13): 1215–1226.

Opelz G. Non-HLA transplantation immunity revealed by lymphocytotoxic antibodies. Lancet 2005, **365**:1570–1576.

Parham P. MHC class I molecules and KIRs in human history, health and survival. Nat Rev Immunol 2005, **5**:201–214.

Porcheray F, DeVito J, Yeap BY, Xue L, Dargon I, Paine R, Girouard TC, Saidman SL, Colvin RB, Wong W, et al. Chronic humoral rejection of human kidney allografts associates with broad autoantibody responses. Transplantation 2010, **89**:1239–1246.

Reed EF, Rao P, Zhang Z, Gebel H, Bray RA, Guleria I, Lunz J, Mohanakumar T, Nickerson P, Tambur AR, Zeevi A, Heeger PS, Gjertson D. Comprehensive assessment and standardization of solid phase multiplex-bead arrays for the detection of antibodies to HLA-drilling down on key sources of variation. Am J Transplant. 2013, **13**(11):3050–3051.

The MHC sequencing consortium. Complete sequence and gene map of a human major histocompatibility complex. Nature 1999, **401**:921–923.

Wiebe C, Gibson IW, Blydt-Hansen TD, Karpinski M, Ho J, Storsley LJ, Goldberg A, Birk PE, Rush DN, Nickerson PW. Evolution and clinical pathologic correlationsof de novo donor-specific HLA antibody post kidney transplant. Am J Transplant 2012, **12**(5):1157–1167.

Zhang X, Reed EF. Effect of antibodies on endothelium. Am J Transplant 2009, **9**:2459–2465.

CHAPTER 6

T cells and the principles of immune responses

Jonathan S. Maltzman[1], Angus Thomson[2], and David M. Rothstein[2]

[1]Department of Medicine, University of Pennsylvania, Philadelphia, PA, USA

[2]Department of Medicine, Surgery and Immunology, Starzl Transplant Institute, University Pittsburgh, Pittsburgh, USA

CHAPTER OVERVIEW

- T cells must be activated first before becoming effector cells.
- T cell activation is controlled by multiple signals, which include signals from the TCR, costimulatory molecules, and cytokine receptors.
- There are distinct phases of T cell response including proliferation, differentiation, apoptosis, and memory generation, all of which are tightly regulated by multiple mechanisms.
- T cells exhibit either effector or regulatory properties, both are required for immunity and homeostasis of the immune system.
- The balance of effector and regulatory responses determines outcomes of organ transplants.

Introduction

T cells are central to productive immune responses. The importance of T cells is underscored by the fact that mice lacking T cells exhibit gross immunodeficiency and fail acutely to reject allografts. In general, productive T cell activation is controlled by three distinct sets of signaling pathways, which are delivered by T cell receptors (TCRs), costimulation, and cytokine receptors. These signaling pathways collectively control activation, differentiation, and effector function of T cells during primary immune responses. Activated T cells then undergo phases of contraction and memory transition in which most activated T cells die of apoptosis, leaving behind a small proportion of cells as memory cells. This transition from short-lived effector T cells to long-lived memory T cells is tightly regulated by selective cytokines, costimulatory molecules, and certain metabolic

---

Transplant Immunology, First Edition. Edited by Xian Chang Li and Anthony M. Jevnikar.
© 2016 John Wiley & Sons, Ltd. Published 2016 by John Wiley & Sons, Ltd.
Companion website: www.wiley.com/go/li/transplantimmunology

pathways. Some activated T cells are also converted to regulatory cells that prevent overstimulation of the immune system and maintain immune homeostasis. This chapter will describe the principles of T cell responses and how such responses are targeted to promote transplant survival.

T cell activation

The TCR: A receptor for every possible antigen

T cells must be activated before becoming effector cells. T cell activation begins with engagement of the TCR by antigens. Most T cells in the periphery express a TCR consisting of an alpha and beta chain, and a small subset of T cells express a TCR composed of gamma and delta chain. The αβ TCR recognizes antigenic peptides of 8–25 amino acids in length that are held in a special cleft of the major histocompatibility complex (MHC) molecules expressed on the surface of antigen-presenting cells (APCs). MHC molecules are highly polymorphic, endowing APC the capacity to present a variety of antigens. The TCR repertoire is also diverse, and this diversity is generated in the thymus during T cell development through random combinatory recombination of multiple "Variable" (V), "Diversity" (D) (β chain only), and "Joining" (J) region gene segments, each available between 3 and 20 different versions in the genome. Diversity is further enhanced by imprecise joining of the VDJ segments, addition of DNA to fill in the "gaps," and finally by noncovalent pairing of different TCR α and β chains. With up to 10^{13} possible TCRs, each T cell has an almost unique TCR (although in any given individual, only ~10^8 different specificities can be detected). In the periphery, a foreign antigen is recognized by T cells expressing high affinity receptors capable of initiating T cell activation. This property forms the basis of both T cell responses against pathogens as well as alloantigens.

Division of labor: CD4 and CD8 define two major T cell subsets

A majority of peripheral T lymphocytes express either CD4 or CD8 on their cell surface. These molecules bind to nonpolymorphic regions of MHC class II and class I molecule, respectively, thus stabilizing the TCR-MHC/antigen interactions. As a result, CD4 cells recognize antigens presented in the context of MHC class II while CD8 cells recognize antigens presented in the context of MHC class I molecules. As such, CD4 cells play a predominant role in initiating immune responses, and subsequently provide helper function to CD8 cells, other CD4 cells, and B cells. In contrast, MHC class I molecules are ubiquitously expressed on all nucleated cells and primarily present peptides derived from intracellular proteins. Thus, CD8 cells play a particular role in immune surveillance for virally infected or malignant cells and function primarily as cytotoxic cells. However, segregation of class I and II peptide processing is not absolute. Through a process called "cross-presentation," exogenously derived peptides can be loaded onto class I molecules, allowing presentation and activation of potentially responsive CD8 T cells.

In some models, CD4 and CD8 cells must simultaneously recognize cognate antigens on a single APC in order for CD4 T cells to provide help for optimal generation of cytotoxic CD8 T cells and memory cells. It was subsequently found that antigen presentation to CD4 cells could activate dendritic cells (DCs) through CD154–CD40 interactions, "licensing" DCs to activate CD8 cytotoxic T cells. It is also now apparent that CD4 help is not required for initial CD8 cell activation or CD8 memory cell generation. Rather, CD4 help is necessary for subsequent expansion and survival of CD8 memory cells upon re-exposure to antigen. CD4 T cells are a major source of Interleukin-2 (IL-2), a necessary growth factor for CD8 cell expansion. Activated CD4 T cells also provide help to B cells, including in their proliferation, Ig class switching, affinity maturation, and development of B cell memory and finally in plasma cell responses.

MHC class II restricted CD4+ T cells are necessary and sufficient for rejection of heart or islet allografts through both the direct and indirect pathways. Rejection responses are redundant. CD4 T cells can mediate rejection even in the absence of CD8 cytotoxic cell either through direct effector function (Fas Ligand, cytokines), enlistment of activated innate cells, or by providing "help" to B cells that leads to antibody affinity maturation and IgG class switching. However, in certain circumstances such as allogeneic skin transplants, CD8+ cells alone are sufficient for rejection. It should be noted that isolated MHC class II mismatches can give rise to direct or indirect CD4 allo-responses and CD8 responses via (indirect) cross-presentation. Moreover, isolated MHC class I differences can give rise to indirect CD4 cell responses. In total, the adaptive immune system that protects against pathogens contains redundancies that are difficult to completely circumvent in clinical transplantation.

T cell activation: Signal 1

The TCR alpha- and beta-chains are transmembrane proteins, which possess short cytoplasmic tails that cannot transduce signal by themselves. The TCR is therefore dependent on its association with CD3 and its transmembrane molecules (gamma, delta, epsilon, and TCRζ), which collectively form a multimeric complex through which TCR signals can be transmitted. Indeed, CD3 was an early target in clinical solid organ transplantation using the now discontinued, mouse antihuman monoclonal antibody OKT3.

TCR cross-linking triggers a series of intracellular phosphorylation cascades involving tyrosine and serine/threonine kinases (Figure 6.1). Tyrosine phosphorylation is the earliest detectable biochemical event following TCR ligation. It plays a critical role initiating many signaling cascades—through alteration of enzyme activity and by providing docking sites for proteins containing SH2 (src homology-2) domains, which recognize phosphorylated tyrosine residues. Assembly of signaling proteins occurs by virtue of SH2 and a variety of other

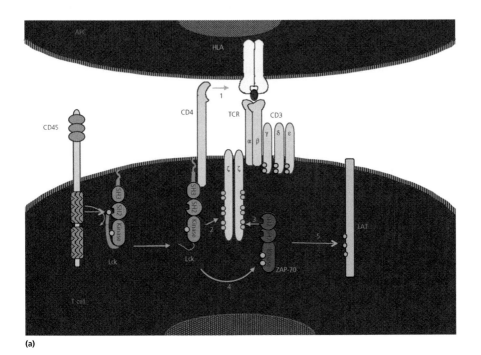

(a)

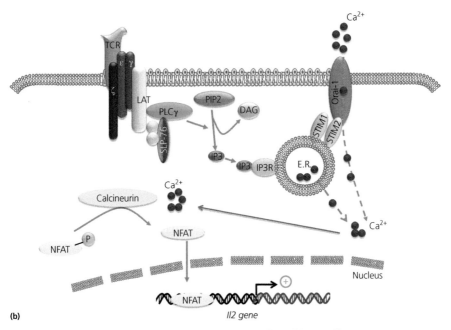

(b)

Figure 6.1 Sequential signal transduction events mediated by T cell receptor (TCR) crosslinking. (a) The TCR complex is composed of the αβ TCR, CD3 molecules (γδε), and TCR ζ- ζ containing 10 ITAMs. Active LCK phosphorylates ITAM tyrosines creating binding sites for ZAP-70, which when activated leads to the phosphorylation of downstream molecules such as LAT. (b) LAT, GADS, and SLP-76 form a scaffold for PLCγ1, which when activated results in IP3 and DAG generation. Increased IP3 leads to increased cytoplasmic calcium through activation of IP3R, STIM, and ORAI. Increased cytoplasmic calcium concentration activates the calcineurin phosphatase, which dephosphorylates NFAT allowing nuclear translocation and gene regulation.

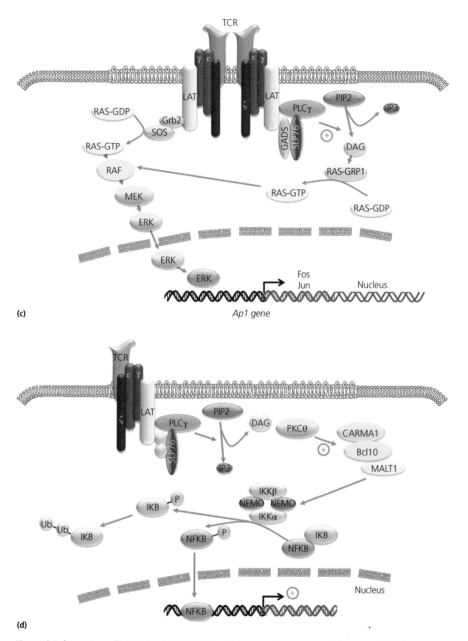

Figure 6.1 (Continued) (c) The RAS/MAPK pathway can be activated through DAG-dependent and DAG-independent pathways (d) DAG also binds to and activates PKCϑ, which catalyzes the formation of the CARMA1/Bcl10/MALT1 complex and activates the IKK complex. Phosphorylation of IkB leads to its binding to ubiquitin, targeting this protein for degradation. This subsequently releases NFkB that can then translocate to the nucleus and regulate transcription.

protein–protein interaction motifs. Such intermolecular interactions allow enzymes and substrates to associate, to regulate enzyme activity, and to define the specificity of particular signaling cascades. Assembly of signaling cascades is aided by "adaptor" or "scaffolding" molecules that lack intrinsic catalytic activity, but allow the binding and bridging other signaling molecules needed for signaling.

TCR signaling is complex and the following text contains details that provide insight into the hurdles faced in clinical transplant. T cells use a number of pathways for activation, but are not all targeted to prevent or treat rejection. The central theme of T cell signaling involves phosphorylation by kinases and dephosphorylation by phosphatases. The src family protein tyrosine kinase (PTK) Lck is brought into the TCR region upon co-receptor (CD4 or CD8) binding to a nonvariable region of MHC expressed on APC (Figure 6.1a). The tyrosine phosphatase CD45 plays a key role in T cell activation by maintaining Lck in a "ready state" by dephosphorylating the inhibitory tyrosine 505 site. Once activated, Lck phosphorylates members of the CD3/TCR zeta complex on pairs of tyrosine residues found in a very specific sequence termed an immunotyrosine activation motif or ITAM (YxxL $(x)_{7-12}$ YxxL/I). Phosphorylation of both tyrosines in an ITAM results in a binding site for the tandem SH2 domains found on another PTK called "ZAP-70." ZAP-70 also associates with the TCR complex, where it can also be activated by Lck through tyrosine phosphorylation. Once at the cell surface, ZAP-70 phosphorylates a number of downstream signaling molecules initiating pathways leading to an increase in intracellular calcium and activation of the classical NFAT, NF-κB, Ras/MAPK, and PI3K pathways.

Activated ZAP-70 phosphorylates multiple tyrosines of the transmembrane adaptor, linker of activated T cells (LAT) (Figure 6.1b). Phosphorylation of LAT leads to the recruitment of the adaptors GADS and SLP-76, which along with phospholipase C gamma 1 (PLCγ1) nucleate a multimolecular "signalosome" that includes several other signaling proteins such as Vav, Nck, and the Tec PTK, Itk. PLCγ1 activation, mediated through membrane localization and phosphorylation by Itk, results in the hydrolysis of phosphatidylinositol 4,5 bisphosphate (PIP2) into inositol 1,4,5 triphosphate (IP3) and diacylglycerol (DAG). Cytosolic IP3 binds IP3 receptors on the endoplasmic reticulum (ER) leading to the release of calcium stores, an increase in intracellular calcium concentration, and activation of the ER calcium sensors STIM1 and STIM2. STIM1 and STIM2 then transduce a signal to the transmembrane calcium channel Orai, leading to an influx of calcium from outside the cell (Figure 6.1b).

Calcineurin inhibitors (CNIs) are widely used in clinical transplantation and have provided considerable insights in intracellular signaling. Elevated intracellular calcium levels activate the serine/threonine phosphatase calcineurin. The target of calcineurin is the nuclear factor of activated T cells (NFAT) family of transcription factors. Dephosphorylation of NFAT by calcineurin exposes a nuclear localization sequence, allowing translocation of NFAT to the nucleus where it critically regulates multiple genes including IL-2. Thus, blocking NFAT activity provides a potent mechanism for immunosuppression in transplantation. Cyclosporine A (CsA), the prototypical member of this group, and tacrolimus (historically referred to as FK506) bind to immunophilins, namely, cyclophilin and FKBP12, respectively. CsA complexed with cyclophilin or FK506 bound to FKBP12 inhibits the calcineurin activity required for the dephosphorylation of NFAT, which is required for nuclear entry. Thus, the immunosuppressive effect of CNIs is primarily due to the inhibition of NFAT activity and decreased transcription of IL-2/IL-2R as well as many other NFAT-regulated genes.

DAG is the second metabolic product of PIP2 hydrolysis and initiates a number of downstream pathways (Figure 6.1c). One effect of DAG is to activate the Ras/MAPK pathway through direct activation of Ras guanyl nucleotide-releasing protein (RASGRP). Ras may also be activated through a DAG-independent pathway initiated by the recruitment of the adapter molecule Grb2 to tyrosine phosphorylated LAT. In turn, Grb-2 binds to another guanine neucleotide exchange factor (GEF), son of sevenless (SOS). These GEFs (SOS and RASGRP) promote exchange of GDP for the higher energy GTP molecule, thereby "recharging" Ras catalytic activity. Activated Ras begins a cascade of serine/threonine phosphorylation reactions, activation of multiple transcription factors by phosphorylation, and eventually increased transcription of several genes required for efficient IL-2 production. Currently, no inhibitors of the RAS/MAPK pathway are used in solid organ transplantation.

In addition to the activation of the Ras pathway, DAG also activates the NF-κB (nuclear factor κ-B) pathway (Figure 6.1d). In a resting T cell, NF-κB family members are sequestered in the cytoplasm through their interaction with an IκB (inhibitor of NFκB). DAG-mediated activation of PKCΘ initiates the formation of a multimolecular complex (composed of MALT1, CARMA1, and Bcl10) that phosphorylates IκBα through activation of the IκB kinase complex (IKK), composed of IKKα, IKKβ and the regulatory subunit NEMO. Phosphorylation of IκBα results in ubiquitination of this protein, a generalized targeting system for cellular protein degradation. This releases NF-κB, allowing it to enter the nucleus and regulate gene transcription. Inhibitors of PKCΘ are not currently available outside of clinical trials, but may be of benefit in transplant immunosuppression as its expression is restricted to T cells.

Amplification signals through phosphatidylinositol 3′-hydroxyl kinase (PI3K)

Stimulation of T cells through both the TCR and costimulatory signals also results in tyrosine phosphorylation mediated by activation of the lipid kinase, PI3K (Figure 6.2). PI3K acts to modify the same membrane lipid, PIP2, as does PLCγ1. However, rather than cleaving PIP2 into DAG and IP3, PI3K is a lipid kinase that phosphorylates PIP2 resulting in PIP3, which creates a binding site on the inner leaflet of the cell membrane for a number of signaling proteins that contain

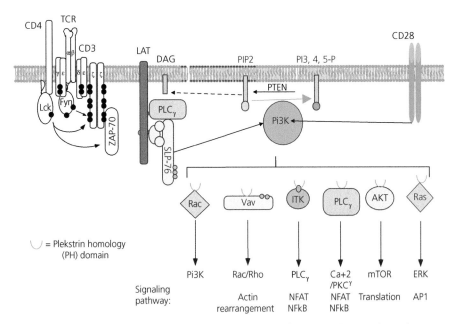

Figure 6.2 PI3K-mediated pathways. PI3kinase activated by TCR and CD28-dependent pathways mediates the phosphorylation of PIP2 (PI4,5-P) to PIP3 (PI3,4,5-P) on the inner surface of the plasma membrane, which leads to recruitment of multiple signaling proteins containing PH domains promoting the activation of a number of different signaling pathways. The signal can be terminated through PTEN-mediated dephosphorylation of PIP3 back to PIP2.

pleckstrin homology (PH) domains. This not only localizes these molecules near the cell membrane but also generally results in increased enzymatic activity. Signaling molecules regulated by PH domains include VAV (involved in cytoskeletal rearrangements affecting cell motility and immune synapse formation), RAS (activates the Erk pathway, discussed earlier), ITK (promotes PLCγ activity), and PLCγ itself. PI3K activates the serine/threonine kinase, protein dependent kinase 1 (PDK1), which in turn phosphorylates AKT initiating a host of other signals involved in cell growth and survival (Figure 6.3).

AKT also regulates the activity of the mammalian target of rapamycin (mTOR), a serine/threonine protein kinase also involved in regulation of cell growth, proliferation, metabolism, and survival (Figure 6.3). mTOR has distinct functions depending on its association with two different binding partners. mTOR complexed to Raptor (TORC1 complex) regulates cell proliferation by promoting protein translation through activation of ribosomal S6K and inhibition of the translational repressor, 4EBP1. mTOR complexed with Rictor (TORC2) promotes cell survival through feedback activation of AKT and its downstream survival pathways. Rapamycin and everolimus are small molecule inhibitors that bind FKBP12 to form a complex that inhibits mTOR, with a preference for TORC1 (Figure 6.3). mTOR inhibitors including new inhibitors of both TORC1

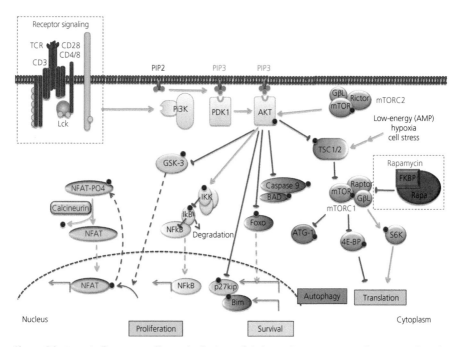

Figure 6.3 AKT influences cell survival via multiple pathways. TCR and CD28-mediated activation of PI3K generates PIP3 and recruitment and activation of the serine-threonine kinase PDK1. PDK1 phosphorylates and activates membrane localized AKT. AKT-mediated phosphorylation of downstream targets can be either activating (indicated with a green arrow) or inhibitory (indicated in red). Multiple pathways initiated by AKT phosphorylation lead to increased survival, proliferative capacity, and metabolic fitness, and regulates protein translation and energy utilization. The latter is regulated through mTOR combined in the mTORC1 complex. This pathway is normally regulated by TSC1/2, which senses energy demands vs. availability. mTOR (TORC1) is inhibited by rapamycin bound to its binding protein FKBP12. mTOR is also found in a distinct complex TORC2, which promotes AKT activity.

and TORC2 complexes currently under evaluation are potent immunosuppressive agents that inhibit proliferation and promote apoptosis of activated T cells. However, parenchymal cells also use mTOR for cell cycling, which accounts for antiproliferation effects on nonlymphoid cells and tissue.

Sequential signaling is required for T cell triggering

Peptide antigen recognition by T cells presents the immune system with logistical problems. APCs express a multitude of MHC-peptide complexes on their cell surface, thus maximizing immune system surveillance for tumor antigens or potential pathogens. However, only a small number of MHC-peptide complexes will contain the antigen of interest for a given T cell. T cells overcome this by being highly motile, "crawling" over the surface of APCs to "scan" for their cognate antigen (Figure 6.4). This requires adhesion molecules such as Lymphocyte Function Associated antigen-1 (LFA-1; a heterodimer comprising CD11a and

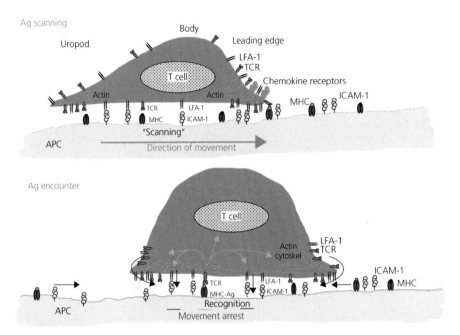

Figure 6.4 Encounter with antigen alters T cell cytoskeleton and adhesion. T cells normally scan the surface of APCS for cognate interaction. This occurs through the rapid formation and release of low-affinity adhesive interactions between LFA-1 that interacts with the actin cytoskeleton. Initial triggering of the TCR by cognate MHC: peptide triggers inside-out signals that augment LFA-1 avidity and cause an arrest of T cell motility. This allows the TCR to sample additional MHC: peptide complexes allowing sequential signaling required for full blown T cell activation. Surface molecules on both the T cell and APC undergo spatial rearrangement resulting in the formation of a stable contact and an immune synapse.

CD18), an integrin that can rapidly associate as well as disassociate from its ligand. TCR encountering its proper antigen induces a conformational change in LFA-1 (termed "inside-out signaling"), which markedly increases its affinity for its ligand, intercellular adhesion molecule-1 (ICAM-1/CD54) on APCs (Figure 6.5). This results in a "stop signal" to slow the T cell dramatically and allows efficient sampling of the DC for additional cognate antigen. This "stop signal" may be variably regulated by several key molecules. For example, CTLA-4 signaling on activated CD4 cells inhibits the stop signal to counte-regulate further antigen responsiveness. Since LFA-1 plays a key role in both T cell stopping and immune cell migration through the endothelium, it is perhaps not surprising that anti-LFA-1 is a potent experimental tolerogenic agent, but it may also effectively target memory as well as naïve T cells.

Signal 2: Costimulation
Costimulatory molecules are discussed in great detail in Chapter 4. The limited discussion here serves to integrate these pathways and provide an appreciation of the complexity of immune responses and the therapeutic role of costimulatory

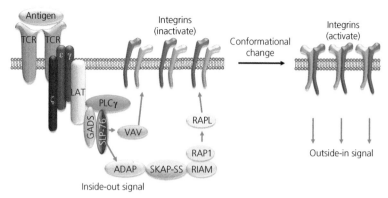

Figure 6.5 Integrin signaling involves both inside-out and outside-in components. Crosslinking of the TCR initially leads to the formation of the LAT-GADS-SLP-76 anchored signalosome. The signalosome recruits an ADAP-SKAP55-RIAM complex leading to the activation and relocalization of RAP1 to the plasma membrane. SLP-76-associated VAV contributes to actin reorganization allowing integrin mobility in the plasma membrane. RAP1 recruits RAPL that binds to integrin cytoplasmic tails resulting in clustering and in a conformational change that increases avidity. Binding of high-affinity integrins to their ICAM-1 ligand on the target cell then initiates an additional "outside-in" signaling cascade that augments TCR signaling.

blockade. The initial concept of T cell costimulation or "second signal" was based on studies of T cell expressed CD28 interacting with its ligands, CD80/CD86, primarily on activated DCs and B cells, but may also include cytokine-activated epithelial cells. This second signal was found to boost IL-2 production and cell survival. Moreover, in the absence of costimulation, T cells were rendered anergic, meaning that they did not respond with normal proliferation after antigen re-exposure, even when proper costimulation was subsequently provided (Figure 6.6). The degree to which CD28 costimulation provides a quantitative TCR signaling boost as compared to providing qualitatively distinct signals remains an area of active investigation. It is clear however that CD28 costimulation promotes activation of PI3k, which phosphorylates membrane phospholipids to create binding sites for signaling proteins that contain PH domains (Figures 6.2 and 6.3). Overall, engagement of CD28 enhances TCR signaling.

CD80 and CD86 could bind to an alternate receptor, namely CTLA-4, which is upregulated on activated T cells (Figure 6.6). In contrast to providing positive signaling as in CD28, CTLA-4 possesses a potent inhibitory effect. Several mechanisms for CTLA-4 inhibitory function have been proposed, including inhibition of proximal TCR signaling through association with phosphatases PP2A and SHP-2, competition with CD28 for B7 binding, interference with clustering of signaling molecules, and by altering T cell conjugate formation with APCs. In addition, CTLA-4 is constitutively expressed on regulatory T cells (Treg) where it is required for their suppressive action in part through its ability to induce

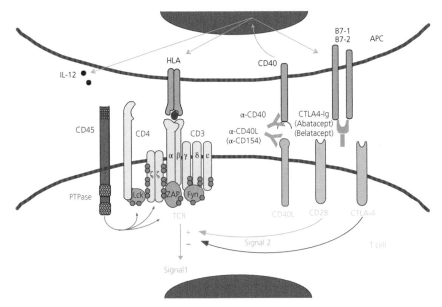

Figure 6.6 T cell activation requires costimulatory signals. The TCR and CD4 or CD8 coreceptor recognize MHC-peptide on an APC, thereby activating signaling cascades termed "Signal 1." Ligation of CD28 and CD40L on the T cell generates a "second" costimulatory signal 2. Activated T cells express CTLA-4, which can produce an inhibitory signal. CTLA4-Ig interferes with both CD28 costimulation and CTLA4-mediated inhibition. Anti-CD40 or anti-CD154 promotes tolerance by interfering with CD40-CD154 signaling.

B7-mediated production of IDO (indoleamine 2,3-dioxygenase), an enzyme that catabolizes extracellular tryptophan required by proliferating effector T cells. CTLA-4 remains an exciting target to promote tolerance.

The biological insights from CD28/CTLA4 have been translated into therapeutic strategies. Based on CTLA-4 having a much higher avidity for its ligands than does CD28, a fusion protein was generated using the high-affinity CD80/CD86-binding region of CTLA-4 fused to Ig, namely CTLA4-Ig (Figure 6.6). With its higher avidity, CTLA4-Ig can effectively block CD28 interactions with CD80/CD86 to block "signal 2." CTLA4-Ig was shown to be potent in small animal models and induced allograft tolerance. Belatacept is a second-generation humanized version of this fusion protein that has been modified to achieve even higher affinity for its B7 ligands, and was recently clinically approved for kidney transplantation. This agent has been shown to be effective as an immunosuppressive agent that may be administered monthly and without CNI. However, Belatacept has not proved effective for the clinical induction of tolerance (a state of immune quiescence after drug withdrawal). The variable ability of reagents to induce tolerance in humans and rodents may relate to memory T cells and the heterologous immune response. In this regard, memory T cells are less dependent on CD28 costimulatory signals and more resistant to costimulatory blockade than naïve T cells.

In addition to CD28 and CD80/CD86, another set of costimulatory molecules have been defined, which includes CD40/CD154, and members in this set belong to the TNF/TNFR superfamily. CD40 signaling leads to maturation of DCs and upregulation of both CD80/86 costimulatory ligands and MHC class II. CD40 blockade inhibits both an important step in DC maturation and T cell costimulation, as well as the elaboration of inflammatory cytokines such as IL-1 and IL-12. Moreover, CD40 is a major pathway required for B cell expansion, Ig class switching and memory cell generation. Consistent with this, CD40 blockade inhibits alloantibody production and the less appreciated but important APC function of B cells. Anti-CD40L (CD154) mAbs are extremely potent in rodent transplant models and in producing long-term transplant survival. Human trials were halted due to the development of serious thromboembolic side effects.

Our insight into costimulation has evolved to be ever more complex with both positive and negative effects on immune responses. Having at least three (Immunoglobulin, TNF/TNF-R, and T cell immunoglobulin and mucin domain (TIM)) gene superfamilies being involved as well as the distribution of molecules and ligands differing on different cell types and in different stages of activation adds to this complexity. Costimulatory signals can influence effector differentiation, survival, and proliferation of responding T cells. As noted, signals may be stimulatory or inhibitory and it appears that most costimulatory molecules and their ligands are involved in bidirectional signaling. Costimulatory blockade may act directly or indirectly on T cells or APCs and inhibition of either member of ligand pairs may lead to an effect. Importantly, their differential expression on different types of T cells may allow for a fine-tuned control of the immune response. The challenge will be to try to identify strategies that target costimulatory pathways, which can inhibit T effector and T memory cells, while promoting Treg or other regulatory cell types (e.g., Bregs and monocyte derived suppressor cells).

Signal 3: Cytokine signaling and T effector cell differentiation

Cytokines are small, potent, biological response modifying protein molecules secreted by T cells and many other cell types. Cytokine classes include ILs, chemokines, and interferons. They function in autocrine, paracrine, and endocrine fashion and play an important role in leukocyte activation, differentiation, proliferation, survival, and migration. Cytokines have pleiotropic effects on parenchymal cells, resulting in activation and changes in the micro-environment of the transplanted graft. A more complete description of cytokines and cytokine receptors can be found in Chapter 3.

T cells and other leukocytes secrete and respond to cytokines and response is via surface receptors that are generally multichain proteins. Secretion of cytokines from hematopoietic cells is often modulated by the activation state. For example, IL-2 is a T cell growth and survival factor with enhanced expression following activation of T cells. It can also increase death of activated T cells through its effects on cell cycle proteins involved in apoptosis. The high affinity form of the IL-2 receptor is a heterotrimeric protein composed of α, β and γ chains. Similarly to IL-2, the α chain of its receptor (CD25) is induced following activation of T lymphocytes and can be targeted in clinical transplantation by basiliximab. The gamma chain of the IL-2 receptor (CD132) is also known as the common gamma chain (γc) as it is a component of many (IL-4, IL-7, IL-9, IL-15, IL-21) receptors. The γc chain associates with JAK3, a member of the Janus Kinase (JAK) family (Figure 6.7). Ligation of receptors results in dimerization with the association of JAKs that phosphorylate tyrosine residues on the cytoplasmic tail of these receptors. Tyrosine phosphorylation then recruits members of the signal transducer and activator of transcription (STAT) family to the complex. STAT proteins are then in turn phosphorylated by the active JAK kinase and STATs to form homo- and hetero-dimers, capable of entering the nucleus, to bind to DNA and regulate transcription of target genes. Different Type I receptors use different JAK/STAT combinations resulting in alternate transcriptional

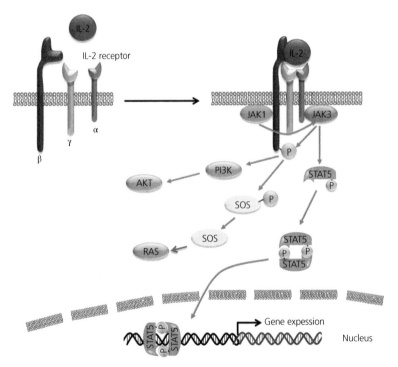

Figure 6.7 Interleukin 2 (IL-2) receptor utilized Janus kinases/Signal Transducer and Activator of Transcription (JAK/STAT) signaling. The IL-2 receptor is composed of three transmembrane proteins, α, β and γ. Ligation of IL-2 brings these chains together JAK and recruiting STAT proteins. Phosphorylated STATs dimerize and translocate to the nucleus where they regulate transcription of target genes. Tyrosine phosphorylated IL-2R chains also serve as docking sites for PI3K that activates the AKT (Figure 6.3) and adaptor proteins such as SHC and GRB-2 that bind SOS, which activates the Ras pathway (Figure 6.1c).

programs. Genetic absence of JAK3 leads to severe immunodeficiency. JAK3 inhibition with toficitinib is FDA approved as an immunosuppressive approach and is currently undergoing clinical trials in transplantation and autoimmunity.

T cell differentiation to effector cells

Following activation, T cells proliferate rapidly and develop into effector T cells with cytotoxic and other functions. However, depending on the "balance" of signals, CD4+ T cells may differentiate into different phenotypes of "helper" or effector cells, each with different patterns of cytokine expression and functions. These subtypes are committed by epigenetic changes, that is, DNA modifications that are inherited by progeny after cell division. Thus, extrinsic cytokine and DC-mediated signals during initial antigen presentation induce the expression of key transcription factors that trigger T cell differentiation into different subtypes, which to date have largely been defined by their broad patterns of cytokine expression. For example, T helper type 1 cells (Th1) are induced by IL-12-mediated activation of STAT4, which results in the expression of the T-bet transcription factor. T-bet drives the production of IFN-γ and TNF-α, prototypic cytokines of Th1 cells (Figure 6.8). Such cells are involved in

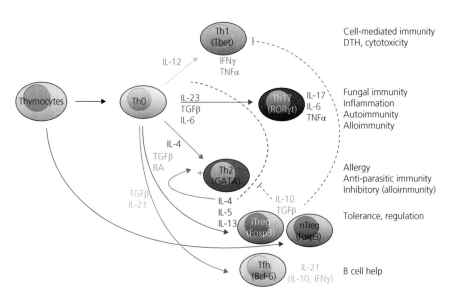

Figure 6.8 CD4 cells differentiate into multiple functional "helper" subsets. Following initial activation, stimulation conditions and the cytokine milieu determine differentiation through modulation of master regulatory transcription factors. Cytokines that promote (solid arrows) and inhibit (dashed arrows) differentiation to various subsets are shown. The function of each population is shown in the column on the right.

cell-mediated immune responses against intracellular pathogens and tumors and are particularly damaging in allograft rejection. In contrast, Th2 cells are driven by STAT6-mediated induction of the GATA3 transcription factor, leading to the secretion of IL-4, IL-5, and IL-13. These cells are normally induced in response to parasitic infections and allergic diseases such as asthma. While these can augment antibody production and isotype shifting, a bias towards a Th2 response under some conditions can be protective in transplantation (or less aggressive than a Th1 response). While not absolute, generally stronger TCR signaling and the presence of IL-12 and TNFα favor a Th1 response. Costimulatory molecules can also favor differentiation down one pathway or another and cytokines produced by one subset can inhibit differentiation down the alternative pathway, that is, IL-4 produced by Th2 cells inhibits Th1 differentiation while IFNγ produced by Th1 cells inhibits Th2 differentiation.

Multiple additional Th subsets have been described more recently. Th17 cells express the RORγT transcription factor and respond to fungi and extracellular bacteria. Generation of Th17 requires expression of IL-23 and the IL-23 receptor. Th17 cells play a major inflammatory role in several autoimmune diseases including inflammatory bowel disease (IBD), and experimental autoimmune encephalomyelitis (EAE) (a rodent model of multiple sclerosis). While the role of Th17 cells in acute allograft rejection is less clear, becoming predominant only in animals where Th1 pathways are impaired, Th17 cells may have a particular role in chronic rejection. A final subset, T follicular helper (Tfh) cells, require the BCL6 transcription factor and are involved in affinity maturation and antibody isotype switching by B cells in the germinal centers, through the expression of IL-21. It is currently uncertain whether Tfh cells represent a distinct lineage, or represent a specialized state of other previously defined lineages. For example, in addition to the specialized expression of IL-21, Tfh cells can produce IFNγ and IL-4, more typical of Th1 and Th2 cells, respectively. Until recently, the Th1, Th2, Treg, and Th17 cells were considered to strictly identify distinct lineages. It has been discovered that plasticity exists within the lineages. For example, some Th17 cells express the prototypical Th1 cytokine IFNγ. Moreover, Foxp3+ iTregs and Th17 cells in particular, appear to be able to transdifferentiate into one another under certain conditions.

In transplant settings as alluded to above, the Th1 response and possibly the Th17 response are considered more destructive than Th2 cells, per se. However, all can cause graft injury. The "deviation" of T effector differentiation has been considered as an approach to promote allograft tolerance. While experimental agents including costimulatory blockade can reduce Th1 and augment Th2 differentiation, rigorous examination has revealed that Th2 cytokines are not required for tolerance and Th1 or Th17 cytokines are not required for rejection. The redundancy of response again presents a formidable challenge to clinical translation.

Progression from naïve to memory T cells

In a primary immune response, T lymphocytes are activated, expand exponentially, and differentiate to effectors. Following expansion, there is a contraction phase during which 90–95% of antigen specific cells die (Figure 6.9). Long-lived memory T cells with altered activation and metabolic requirements are derived from the remaining cells. A hallmark of the adaptive immune system is the generation of memory cells, which are defined by their ability to respond "faster and greater" to rechallenge with antigen. Thus the generation of memory T cells is a major goal of vaccination. This section will describe mechanisms involved in contraction, memory T cell generation, and maintenance.

Programmed cell death or apoptosis following robust immune responses is critical to maintain immune system homeostasis and, of course, is the central mechanism of thymic tolerance. One mechanism that contributes to apoptosis during the contraction phase is cytokine withdrawal. Multiple cytokines that signal through γc receptors (most prominently IL-2, IL-7, and IL-15) promote lymphocyte survival through altered expression of members of the Bcl-2 family of proteins. Bcl-2 family members are either anti-apoptotic or pro-apoptotic, and the balance of these proteins determines cell survival versus apoptosis (Figure 6.10). The pro-apoptotic Bcl-2 family members (e.g., Bak and Bax) insert into the outer leaflet of the mitochondrial membrane where they multimerize to form pores that permit the release of Cytochrome c into the cytosol.

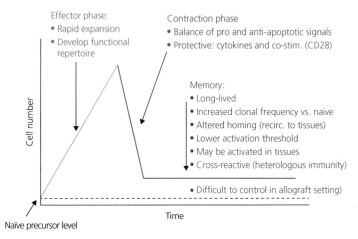

Figure 6.9 Kinetics of an immune response. Naïve T cells exist at a low frequency for any given antigen. Following exposure, naïve cells rapidly expand and differentiate into effector T cells. In many cases, the immune response clears the pathogen leading to decreased antigen load. Approximately 95% of effector cells die during an active contraction mediated by lack of antigen, cytokine withdrawal, and activation-induced cell death. However, approximately 5% of the expanded population survives as long-lived memory T cells with altered patterns of activation and homing.

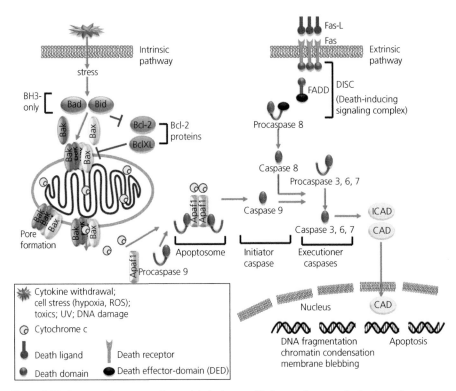

Figure 6.10 Apoptosis occurs via multiple intracellular pathways. Activation of caspases 3, 6, and 7 initiate a final common pathway of DNA fragmentation leading to apoptosis. Caspase 3 may be activated by either intrinsic or extrinsic pathways. The intrinsic pathway can be activated by cytokine withdrawal and other toxic insults/cell stresses, which are sensed by BH3-only proteins of the Bcl-2 family and lead to the insertion of proapoptotic Bcl-2 family members (Bak/Bax) into the mitochondrial membrane releasing cytochrome C into the cytosol. This is counteracted by anti-apoptotic members of the bcl-2 family (bcl-2, BCL-xl). Cytoplasmic cytochrome C binds Apaf-1, inducing the formation of the apoptosome and activation of caspase 9. Caspase 9 can then activate caspase 3. The extrinsic pathway is initiated by ligation of the trimeric death receptors of the TNFR family such as FAS on activated T cells. Binding by Fas-L leads to recruitment of the death effector domain containing Fas-associated death domain (FADD) protein to the death domain in the FAS cytoplasmic tail. FADD recruits and activates Procaspase 8. Caspase 8 may activate caspase 3 directly or indirectly through the intrinsic pathway ultimately resulting in DNA fragmentation.

Pro-apoptotic molecules are antagonized by anti-apoptotic Bcl-2 family members such as Bcl-2 and Bcl$_{XL}$, which prevent this pore formation and stabilize the mitochondrial membrane. A third set of (BH3-only) Bcl-2 proteins, including Bid, Bad, and Bim, act to integrate signals and control triggering of apoptosis. These proteins inhibit the anti-apoptotic Bcl-2 proteins and promote the insertion and/or multimerization of pro-apoptotic proteins in the mitochondrial membrane. A wide variety of cell stressors including hypoxia, oxidative stress

(ROS), UV irradiation, and DNA damage promote apoptosis through activation of BH3-only proteins. Cytokine withdrawal favors expression/activation of pro-apoptotic Bcl-2 proteins that then trigger apoptosis.

Once released into the cytoplasm, cytochrome c binds to Apaf -1, resulting in the formation of a complex with Apaf-1 and pro-caspase 9, known as the "apoptosome." This activates caspases that are proteases normally present as inactive "pro"- forms. Association of procaspases allows for a pro-caspase pro-tealytic cleavage cascade to their active forms. In the apoptosome, clustering results in the activation of the "initiator caspase-9," which can cleave and acti-vate caspase 3 and other downstream "executioner caspases" (e.g., caspase 6 and 7) to ultimately result in apoptosis, with membrane blebbing and DNA fragmentation. Targeting the inhibitor of caspase-activated DNAse (ICAD), releases CAD (caspase-activated DNAse) that enters the nucleus and cleaves DNA—the *sine qua non* of apoptosis. As the immune response is initiated, cell activation leads to elaboration of cytokines that act as growth factors, promot-ing both T cell proliferation and survival, which greatly expands T cell numbers (Figure 6.9). As the immune response resolves, many T cells compete for a limited pool of cytokines. The resulting apoptosis thus restores cytokine and T cell balance.

Programmed cell death of peripheral T cells is also mediated by the activation of a family of death receptors by a process referred to as activation-induced cell death (AICD) (Figure 6.10). AICD has been more completely described through the TNF-receptor family member Fas (APO-1, CD95), and other family members (TNF-R1 and TRAIL-death receptor (DR4, DR5)), which are upregulated upon T cell activation. Ligand binding (with Fas-L, TNFα, and TRAIL), results in receptor trimerization and formation of the death-inducing signaling complex (DISC), which includes the "death domain" (DD)-containing protein FADD (Fas-associated death domain-containing protein). "Death effector domains" (DEDs) allow recruitment of a similar domain on procaspase 8 to allow activation. Clustering within the DISC results in cleavage of procaspase 8, release of active caspase 8, and a cascade of executioner caspase activation as in the mitochon-drial pathways described. Active caspase 8, like caspase 9, is an "initiator cas-pase" that can directly cleave and activate the executioner caspases. In addition, caspase 8 can cleave and activate the BH3-only protein Bid, which promotes apoptotic Bcl-2 family members to form mitochondrial pores, enhancing apop-tosis through the mitochondrial pathway. Caspase-8 is regulated endogenously by Flice-inhibitory protein (c-FLIP), a key checkpoint protein, which is influ-enced in T cells by IL-2 and cell cycle. While over-expression of c-FLIP blocks apoptosis and limits tolerance, under-expression in the absence of IL-2 blocks tolerance. Finally, the blockade of receptor-mediated apoptosis through caspase-8 triggers a recently described form of regulated necrosis termed necroptosis in parenchymal cells. The role of this pathway in T cell homeostasis has not been defined.

The importance of apoptosis in allograft tolerance is exemplified by studies using Bcl-XL transgenic mice, in which T cells are resistant to apoptosis. These mice are resistant to tolerance induced by costimulatory blockade. Alloresponsive cells that are not inhibited by costimulatory blockade are also not limited by apoptosis/AICD and these cells contribute to rejection. As noted, costimulation provides TCR-activated T cells with proliferative as well as survival signals. Therefore, stimulation in the face of costimulatory blockade is likely to promote apoptosis of alloreactive cells in wild type, but not in apoptosis-resistant animals. Important perhaps to consider therapeutically, conventional immunosuppressive agents such as sirolimus promote apoptosis of alloreactive cells, while CNIs prevent initial T cell activation-induced apoptosis and removal of potentially alloreactive T cells.

While a majority of expanded CD4 and CD8 T cells undergo apoptotic cell death, approximately 5–10% survive and become long-lived memory T cells (Figure 6.9). It is unclear whether memory cells are derived from activated T cells in a stochastic manner or whether this is predetermined. Regardless, the expression of CD127 (IL7Rα) and the lectin KLRG1 during contraction may be used to define populations of effector cells destined for death (IL7Rαlo/KLRG1hi) as compared to memory generation (IL7Rα+/KLRG1lo). Following contraction, a population of long-lived memory T cells can be identified through the use of cell surface markers, for example CD44hi in mice and CD45RO+in humans (see Table 6.1). As noted previously, CD4 helps promote proliferation of CD8 memory cells upon re-exposure to antigen, and may do so by making cells more resistant to AICD mediated by TRAIL.

Table 6.1 Characteristics of naïve and memory T cells.

	Naïve	Central memory	Effector memory
Response rate	Slow	Rapid	Rapid
Cell surface phenotype	CD44^{lo}	CD44^{hi}	CD44^{hi}
	CD45RO$^-$	CD45RO$^+$	CD45RO$^+$
		CCR7$^+$	CD45RA$^{+/-}$
		CD62L$^+$	CCR7$^-$
			CD62L$^-$
Costimulation	CD28:CD80/CD86		
Trafficking	Restricted to secondary lymphoid tissue	Lymphoid	Non-lymphoid
Survival	TCR-dependent	Long-lived cytokine-dependent	Long-lived cytokine-dependent

TCR, T cell receptor.

Memory cells express an array of cell surface receptors that are distinct from naïve T cells. Interestingly, memory T cells can be further subdivided into the so-called central memory (T_{CM}) and effector memory (T_{EM}) T cells. The populations differ phenotypically, in their migration patterns as well as functionally. T_{CM} express high levels of the chemokine receptor CCR7 and L-selectin (CD62L). This combination of receptors allows T_{CM} to migrate from the blood into the secondary lymphatic tissues through high endothelial venules and traffic to T cell zones in the secondary lymphoid organs. These provide a reservoir for the reactivation of the immune response upon re-encounter of an antigen. In contrast, T_{EM} express is found in tissues. They express effector cytokines at a steady state and are thought of as being poised to respond quickly to antigenic re-exposure.

Memory T cells have altered metabolic demands and are primed for a more rapid response to antigen re-exposure; they also have differences in costimulatory requirements for activation. For example, memory T cells are much less dependent on CD28 costimulation than naïve T cells, and a sub-population of human CD8 T cells does not express CD28 at all. Costimulation via alternate cell surface receptors such as ICOS, CD2, and OX40 may supply the necessary costimulatory signals to these cells (see Chapter 4). Possibly, as a consequence of this decreased dependence on costimulatory signals, memory T cells do not require secondary lymphatic tissue (lymph nodes and spleen) for their re-activation. Rather, they can directly recognize an antigen and mount an immune response in the allograft.

Pre-existing alloreactive memory T cells present an important obstacle to successful transplantation. It is estimated that approximately 50% of the cells initially responding to transplanted tissue are memory cells. Alloreactive memory T cells may have been generated in response to presensitization (blood transfusion, previous transplant and pregnancy), heterologous immunity (through cross-reactivity with a pathogen), or through expansion in a lymphopenic environment occurring especially after depletive therapy through a process known as lymphopenia-induced proliferation. These cells are less responsive than naïve cells to lymphodepletion strategies, costimulatory blockade, and other conventional immunosuppressive and tolerance-inducing therapies. Thus, they present a potent barrier to transplant tolerance. Development of optimal approaches to dealing with memory T cells in a transplant setting is an area of active investigation in many laboratories.

Regulatory T cells

The primary function of a subset of CD4+ T cells termed Tregs is to dampen immune responses. While a number of regulatory cells, including CD4 T cells, CD8 T cells, and "double negative" T (DNT) cells, have been described the most

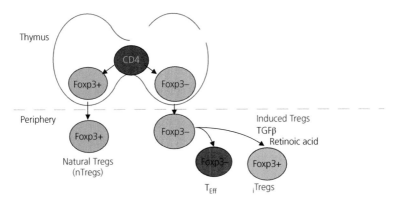

Figure 6.11 Regulatory T cells may arise directly from the thymus or may be induced in the periphery. Regulatory T cells (Tregs) expressing the transcription factor Foxp3 may arise as CD4 single positive cells during development in the thymus and are termed "natural Tregs" (nTregs). Alternatively, stimulation of CD4+Foxp3- conventional T cells in the presence of TGFβ or Retinoic acid can lead to induction of Foxp3 and differentiation into induced Tregs (iTregs).

investigated form are CD4 Tregs that express the transcription factor Foxp3. The potency of these cells is underscored by the severe systemic autoimmunity exhibited in humans and mice that lack normal Foxp3. The so-called natural regulatory T cells (nTregs) develop as a distinct lineage in the thymus and express high affinity TCRs that may be directed toward self (Figure 6.11). nTreg can comprise approximately 10% of peripheral CD4 T cells in steady state and interestingly exhibit an "activated" phenotype, with constitutive expression of CD25, CTLA-4, and other T cell activation markers. Their detailed mechanisms of action are not fully defined, but they involve cell–cell interactions (e.g., CTLA-4), metabolic/growth factor deprivation (tryptophan and adenosine degradation and IL-2 consumption), and inhibitory cytokines (IL-10 and TGFβ) (Figure 6.12). Foxp3+ Treg can also be induced *in vitro* by activation in the presence of TGFβ and/or retinoic acid. Such induced Treg (iTreg) can be generated from the 90% of cells that are not Foxp3+, but iTreg do not express identical patterns of mRNA as nTreg do and do not appear to be as stable as nTreg *in vivo*. There is, for example, observed transdifferentiation between Treg and Th17 cells. Thus, iTregs may not be as robust as nTreg. It is important to note that there are less well-defined Tr1 Tregs that lack Foxp3 expression and are primarily suppressive through high-level expression of IL-10.

In animal transplant models, many experimental agents require Tregs for the induction and/or maintenance of tolerance. However, this does not necessarily imply that Treg are specifically induced by successful therapy. Treg are important for establishing an immunological set point and their depletion enhances the immune response. Thus, depletion of Tregs prevents tolerance mediated by a variety of agents. Moreover, Treg are antigen-responsive *in vivo*, and may expand any time the effector response is sufficiently limited to prevent

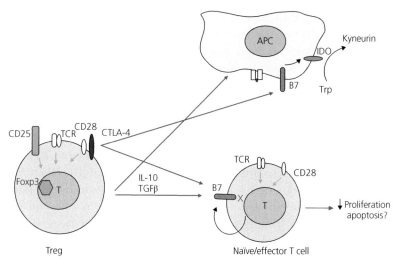

Figure 6.12 Treg inhibit activation and proliferation of effector T cells. Regulatory T cells activated through TCR signaling inhibit conventional T cells (Tconv) by a variety of mechanisms. Cytokines IL-10 and TGFβ inhibit DC maturation and elaboration of inflammatory cytokines and may also inhibit activation and differentiation of Teff cells down inflammatory pathways. CTLA-4 may directly bind to B7 molecules expressed by activated CD4 cells and induce a negative signal. CTLA-4 ligation of B7 on APCs results in the production of IDO an ecto-enzyme that breaks down Tryptophan in the surrounding environment. Proliferating Tconv are sensitive to Trp depletion.

rejection. This expansion of antigen-specific Tregs within the total pool may play an important role in maintaining tolerance as depletion of Treg can disrupt established tolerance. In murine models, nTreg identified by their Foxp3 expression, can be isolated for *ex vivo* expansion. Alternatively, conventional (nonregulatory) CD4 cells can be used to generate iTreg and expand *in vivo*. Both nTreg and iTreg expanded *in vitro* can inhibit GVHD, allograft rejection, or autoimmunity suggesting that this may be useful in transplantation. There are numerous reports that iTreg can be induced by various tolerogenic agents *in vivo*, but these reports are dependent on specific TCR-transgenic mouse models that express specific TCRs with high affinity for antigen that predispose to Treg development once cognate antigen is present. When polyclonal responses are examined, Foxp3+ Treg have not been convincingly demonstrated via specific immune responses, in the presence or absence of tolerogenic agents. Alternative approaches may be able to expand nTreg *in vivo* through augmented survival and proliferation. These include rIL-2 complexed with anti-IL-2 (to prolong half-life and limit engagement of the IL-2R on CD8 and NK cells) and Flt3-L (to expand DCs that secondarily expand Tregs). Whether expansion for Tregs is sufficiently specific to pursue clinical trials remains to be established.

The situation is more complicated in humans than in mice. As Foxp3 is a transcription factor, it cannot be examined in live cells by current technology.

Efforts to purify Treg thus depend on the high-level expression of surrogate's markers including CD25 as well as the low expression of the IL-7Rα (CD127). It is noteworthy that Foxp3 is expressed acutely after activation of human Tconv cells; and therefore, it is not the complete specific marker for Treg observed in rodents. This must be considered while assessing Treg levels in allograft recipients in the absence of functional studies that actually show "regulation". Finally, conventional immunosuppressive agents can affect Tregs. Tregs are highly dependent on IL-2 and CD28 signaling. While CNIs and CTLA4-Ig are effective agents for inhibition of Tconv cells, they are largely detrimental to Tregs. Tregs do appear to be partially resistant to Rapamycin. Similarly, anti-IL-2Rα mAbs are widely used in the clinic to inhibit activated T effector cells in transplantation, but they can reduce the number of Tregs in the periphery. Thus, despite continued enthusiasm for the identification, expansion, and use of Tregs, the issues outlined have collectively delayed the clinical use of *ex vivo* expansion and transfer of Tregs into humans for transplant prolongation.

Summary

There is no doubt that T cells are central to transplant rejection as well as immunological tolerance, but they exist in a complex environment in which they instruct other cells as well to respond to multiple signals. The balance of harmful versus beneficial response is related not only to the identity of the T cells but also to the context in which responses occur, a theme that is shared with other cells of the immune system. Thus the diversity of T cells and their complex biology provides a great challenge to clinical transplantation in selecting therapeutic targets.

Further reading

Afzali, B., G. Lombardi, and R. I. Lechler. (2008). Pathways of major histocompatibility complex allorecognition. Current opinion in organ transplantation 13:438–444.

Chiffoleau, E., P. T. Walsh, et al. (2003). Apoptosis and transplantation tolerance. Immunological reviews 193: 124–145.

Kanno, Y., G. Vahedi, et al. (2012). Transcriptional and epigenetic control of T helper cell specification: Molecular mechanisms underlying commitment and plasticity. Annual review of immunology 30: 707–731.

Lechler, R. I., W. F. Ng, and R. M. Steinman. (2001). Dendritic cells in transplantation—friend or foe? Immunity 14:357–368.

Li, X. C., D. M. Rothstein, and Sayegh M. H (2009). Costimulatory pathways in transplantation: challenges and new developments. Immunological reviews 229(1): 271–293.

Morelli, A. E., and A. W. Thomson. (2007). Tolerogenic dendritic cells and the quest for transplant tolerance. Nature reviews immunology 7:610–621.

Rudensky, A. Y. (2011). Regulatory T cells and Foxp3. Immunological reviews 241(1): 260–268.

Smith-Garvin, J. E., G. A. Koretzky, et al. (2009). T cell activation. Annual review of immunology 27: 591–619.

Steinman, R. M., and J. Idoyaga. (2010). Features of the dendritic cell lineage. Immunology reviews 234:5–17.

Surh, C. D., and J. Sprent (2008). Homeostasis of naive and memory T cells. Immunity 29(6): 848–862.

Wu, L., and Y. J. Liu. 2007. Development of dendritic-cell lineages. Immunity 26:741–750.

CHAPTER 7

Ischemia and reperfusion injury

Yuan Zhai, Yoichiro Uchida, Bibo Ke, Haofeng Ji, and Jerzy W. Kupiec-Weglinski

Dumont-UCLA Transplantation Center, Division of Liver and Pancreas Transplantation, Department of Surgery, David Geffen School of Medicine at UCLA, Los Angeles, USA

CHAPTER OVERVIEW

- Ischemia reperfusion injury is inevitably associated with organ transplantation.
- Organ injury is the result of inflammatory responses involving multiple innate and adaptive immune cells.
- Organ injury is perpetuated by the release of pro-inflammatory cytokines and activation of innate immune cells.
- The innate immune sensors (TLR, RLR, NLR) are involved in ischemia reperfusion injury.
- Identification of new molecular pathways (Tim-1/4, inflammasome) provides targets for new drugs to reduce organ damage.

Introduction

Ischemia reperfusion injury (IRI) is an inevitable consequence of organ procurement and implantation procedure. IRI remains one of the key problems in clinical transplantation. The tissue damage surrounding donor organ, removal, storage, and engraftment contributes to poor graft outcomes, such as primary graft nonfunction, late dysfunction, and higher incidence of acute and chronic rejection. IRI also compromises the quality of organ transplants, further contributing to the shortage of available organs for transplantation. Hence, preventing or minimizing the adverse consequences of IRI will not only improve transplant outcomes but also increase the number of patients that can be successfully treated by transplantation. Despite its importance, the mechanism of IRI remains understudied, and effective strategies that prevent or reduce IRI in the clinic are very much limited.

Transplant Immunology, First Edition. Edited by Xian Chang Li and Anthony M. Jevnikar.

IRI, regardless of organs transplanted, is a multifaceted process that involves elements of "warm" and "cold" ischemia injury. The "warm" injury phase occurring *in situ* in low or no blood flow states is dominated by innate cell-derived cytotoxic molecules. The process of "cold" injury, occurring during *ex vivo* preservation of organs, is dominated by damage to endothelial, epithelial, and other parenchymal cells that disrupt the microcirculation (Ikeda et al., 1992). Although "warm" and "cold" ischemia affects different cellular constituents in the graft, inflammation represents a common pathway in organ damage. The essential role of pro-inflammatory responses in the development of IRI in transplant recipients has been well established. Although mechanistic details continue to be debated, the central role of inflammation in a self-amplified cascade that leads to parenchymal cell damage through a complex interaction of cytokines, chemokines, and reactive oxygen species (ROS), as well as by promoting the infiltration and activation of innate immune cells, is well recognized. Indeed, prevention of local immune cell activation often mitigates IRI in the transplanted organ.

Here, we discuss our current understanding of IRI in immune activation, as well as the conversion of an immunologically quiescent organ to a highly inflammatory one. Although we focus on IRI cascade in the liver, the organ-specific differences are emphasized. Most of the mechanistic studies were performed in a mouse model of segmental hepatic IRI. A more clinically relevant model, combining cold and warm IRI components, followed by orthotopic liver transplantation has been recently established and also discussed.

Mechanism of organ injury

There are two major stages of IRI, as depicted in Figure 7.1, with distinct mechanisms of tissue damage (Zhai et al., 2011). The initial ischemic injury is caused by the loss of blood supply to the organ. This process induces hypoxia, metabolic disturbances, and consequently cellular necrosis. The subsequent alterations in local pH, glycogen consumption, and adenosine triphosphate (ATP) depletion further amplify tissue damage. The reperfusion injury that follows the restoration of blood supply involves a panel of cytotoxic mechanisms, mediated by intense tissue inflammation and activation of innate as well as adaptive immune cells. These ultimately lead to additional organ injury. In the presence of ATP depletion and profound metabolic disorders, cellular programs that usually result in apoptosis can be subverted to necrosis in ischemic organs. In the case of the liver, TNF-α seems to be critical to IRI, as administration of TNF blocking antibodies or use of TNF-R1 KO mice prevented liver IRI in both rat and mouse models. However, TNF-α, by itself, is not sufficient to induce hepatocyte death, as TNF-R1 activation (by secreted TNF-α) triggers both pro- and anti-apoptotic pathways. NF-kB is a key regulator of hepatocyte response to inflammatory

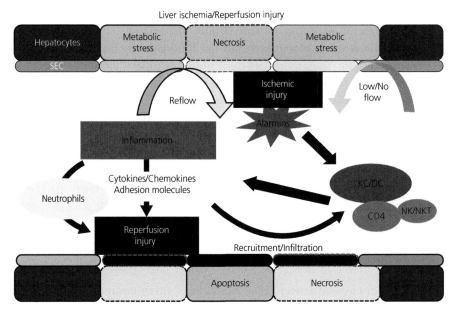

Figure 7.1 Stages of liver ischemia and reperfusion injury (IRI). The ischemic injury, a localized process of metabolic disturbances, results from glycogen consumption, lack of oxygen supply, and adenosine triphosphate depletion. In the reperfusion injury, an immune activation-mediated amplification process, damage associated molecular patterns (alarmins) produced during the initial cellular insult, trigger liver non-parenchymal cells to generate the pro-inflammatory milieu, which damage the liver tissue directly or indirectly by activating neutrophils and recruiting immune cells from the circulation.

stimulation as its activation upregulates multiple cytoprotective genes and prevents hepatocyte death, while its suppression sensitizes hepatocytes to TNF-α-induced cell death. Thus, NF-kB activation plays a dual role in liver IRI in a cell-type specific manner, that is, its activation in non-parenchymal cells (NPCs) promotes local inflammation, whereas its activation in parenchymal cells prevents the hepatocellular injury. Hence, organ IRI in transplant recipients may require cell-specific regulation of NF-kB signaling.

In addition to inflammation, hepatocytes are also under various stress. One of the critical consequences of NF-kB inhibition in hepatocyte TNF-α signaling is prolonged MAP kinase c-Jun N-terminal kinase (JNK) activation, which is critical for the activation of caspase 8, a key protease in the apoptosis cascade. TNF-α induces a transient JNK activation, which is mediated in part by the ROS-dependent pathway whereas NF-kB activation increases antioxidant SOD2 to suppress ROS and JNK activation. It has been shown that JNK antagonizes NF-kB mediated anti-apoptotic function during TNF-α signaling by promoting proteasomal elimination of c-FLIP-long. The roles of ROS and JNK pathways in liver IRI have been well studied. Overexpression of SOD1 has blocked ROS production, prevented JNK activation, and protected liver IRI. Treatment with pharmacological inhibitors of JNK activation ameliorated signs of liver damage due to cold and warm IR in rats, decreased the hepatic cell death and improved animal survival. CD40 activation may also contribute to inflammation-induced organ injury. Hepatocyte CD40 expression can be further upregulated by TNF-α and pro-inflammatory cytokines. CD40 ligation by T cell-derived CD154 or its agonist Abs has been shown to trigger hepatocyte apoptosis, particularly when NF-kB activation is inhibited. This pro-apoptotic effect of CD40 signaling is associated with hepatocyte FasL induction via sustained JNK activation.

At the present time, there are few clinical strategies that specifically target IRI apart from minimizing cold ischemic times and more recently, the introduction of pulsatile perfusion in kidney transplantation. Most recently, there have been studies supporting the use of normothermic rather than hypothermic perfusion of organs, pioneered in lung transplants. This leads to less expression of pro-inflammatory mediators that are usually generated by anaerobic hypothermic conditions, and a more favorable pattern of cytokine expression within the organ. While the results in lung transplants look very promising, it is not clear yet if this approach will benefit other transplants. Cell death which is a prominent feature of IRI may be targeted directly. There are also emerging new classes of drugs that can target apoptosis molecules more selectively, as well as regulated forms of necrosis such as necroptosis by necrostatins. Collectively, these may all help to preserve organ integrity and function following storage.

Toll-like receptors (TLRs) in innate immune activation during IRI

There are many types of immune cells involved in IRI in the liver and other organs, as shown in Figure 7.2, which include Kupffer cells (KCs), dendritic cells (DCs), neutrophils (PMNs), T cells, and NK/NKT cells. In the initial stage, liver resident KCs and DCs become activated by the damage-associated and/or pathogen-associated molecular pattern (DAMP/PAMP) molecules. These danger molecules or "alarmins," induced during cellular stress, facilitate local inflammation milieu, the hallmark of IRI, which propagates the inflammation response to the whole organ. In the second stage, activated circulating monocytes and PMNs are recruited into the organ to sustain local immune response and to further amplify tissue destruction.

The Toll-like receptor (TLR) system which is highly conserved plays a key role in the pathophysiology of IRI in many organ systems. TLR4 activation has been shown to mediate liver IRI via interferon regulatory factor-3 (IRF-3)-dependent MyD88-independent mechanism (Zhai et al., 2004). Although in a neonatal murine model of small-bowel IRI, TLR2 KO mice sustained greater intestinal damage, TLR2 deficiency was protective in renal IRI, and involved both MyD88-dependent and MyD88-independent pathways. A more recent

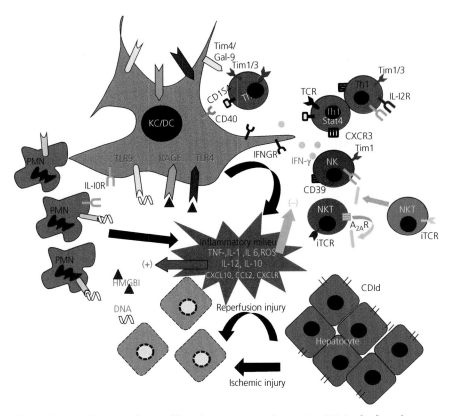

Figure 7.2 A mechanistic scheme of liver immune activation against IRI. In the first phase, organ ischemia induces necrotic cell death, providing diverse "danger" molecules, such as HMGB1 and DNA fragments to activate Toll-like receptors 4 (TLR4), receptor for advanced glycation end-products and TLR9 signaling on Kupffer cells/dendritic cells (KCs/DCs) and neutrophils. T cells, particularly CD4 Th1 effectors, may also facilitate innate activation via CD154-CD40 pathway. In the second phase, IFN-γ produced by T cells, NKT and NK cells enhances local innate activation. In addition, CD1d and CD39 activate NKT and natural killer (NK) cells, respectively. The immune activation cascade progresses via positive and negative regulatory loops. Pro-inflammatory milieu further activates and recruits circulating immune cells to promote cytotoxicity against liver parenchymal cells. IL-10 counter-regulates sustained proinflammatory activation, whereas adenosine receptor 2A inhibits NKT cell activation. Type II NKT cells may also downregulate IFN-γ production by type I NKT cells.

study points to TLR4-and MyD88-mediated signaling in renal IRI. These studies enable comparison of liver IRI with renal IRI, such that both depend on TLR4, with liver injury dominated by the MyD88-independent and renal IRI mediated by the MyD88-dependent pathway. TLR signaling has also shown to be important in myocardial IRI, as TLR4 deficiency decreased infarct size and tissue inflammation. Interestingly, the absence of TLR4 on kidney cells provided greater protection against renal IRI than loss of TLR4 in recipient immune cells, highlighting the importance of these receptors on the transplanted organs in IRI.

This is consistent with the ability of tubular epithelial cells, for example, to interact via TLR4, with HMGB1 and alarmins that are released from necrotic parenchymal cells. Most recently, there have been studies that indicate that programmed forms of necrosis are activated in organs, particularly with blockade of caspase-8-induced apoptosis and c-FLIP. This has been termed "necroptosis" and is regulated through RIPK1 and RIPK3 serine kinases, which can be therapeutically targeted with drugs to modulate necroptosis. Loss of RIPK3 in kidneys in a mouse model results in resistance to IRI, reduced HMGB1 release, and enhanced survival when used as donor kidneys or hearts in fully allogeneic transplants. Such results also suggest that modification of donor livers, kidneys, and hearts that alter death or interaction with TLR may be a useful strategy to reduce IRI.

Certain evidence suggests that protection against IRI after disruption of TLR4 pathway is mediated through STAT3 and PI3K/Akt-dependent mechanisms (Figure 7.3). Thus, defective STAT3 or PI3K/Akt signaling has been shown to activate host innate immune responses to trigger tissue damage. Moreover, phosphatase and tensin (PTEN) homolog deletion on chromosome 10 can counter-regulate PI3K activity in cell survival and growth, whereas macrophage PTEN deficiency can enhance PI3K activity and decrease TLR4-mediated cytokine expression. Indeed, PI3K/Akt activation provides negative feedback mechanism to suppress TLR4-driven inflammatory gene programs, promote anti-apoptotic Bcl-2/Bcl-xL function, and hence reduce local cell apoptosis. Importantly, activation of PI3K/Akt signaling and depression of PTEN activity appears to be STAT3-dependent. Moreover, the serine/threnine kinase glycogen synthase kinase 3β (Gsk3β) pathway has been also shown to be essential, as its inactivation mitigated liver IRI pathology in a PI3K-dependent fashion. Pharmacological intervention to target these pathways may be useful to attenuate IRI.

The pathogenic role of endogenous damage-associated molecular patterns (DAMP) that are released during IRI to trigger the activation of TLRs has been the focus of intense study, recently. The two broadly categorized endogenous TLR ligands include those released from necrotic cells, such as heat shock proteins (60, 70, Gp96), high-mobility group box-1 (HMGB1), Interleukin-33 (IL-33), and DNA/RNA-complexes; and those derived from degraded extracellular matrix, that is, heparan sulfate, hyaluronan, fibrinogen, fibronectin A domain, and tenascin C. Liver nonparenchymal TLR4 is the main target for HMGB1 (Tsung et al., 2005). Hepatocyte TLR4, detectable in low copies seems to have a marginal role in early liver inflammation. Of note, HMGB1 biology is becoming increasingly complex, with many issues regarding the molecular nature of HMGB1 (oxidized, reduced), TLR4 binding (direct stimulation or by enhancing LPS activity), and putative role of other binding moieties, such as RAGE (receptor for advanced glycation end products). RAGE is essential in liver IRI by regulating MIP-2 production via Egr-1-dependent mechanism, as well as

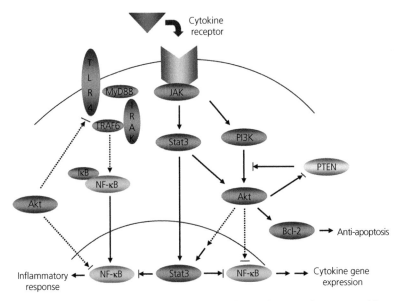

Figure 7.3 TLR4–STAT3–PI3K/Akt cross-regulation in the mechanism of IR-triggered liver inflammation and damage. Defective STAT3 or PI3K/Akt signaling activates innate immune response, whereas phosphatase and tensin (PTEN) deficiency enhances PI3K activity and depresses TLR4-mediated local inflammation. MyD88 blockade activates PI3K/Akt while downregulating NF-κB to suppress the inflammatory phenotype. PI3k/Akt may also negatively regulate TLR4 to inhibit IkB phosphorylation and NF-kB translocation.

by influencing cell death and TNF-α production via Egr-1-independent mechanism. The role of RAGE in kidney injury is less well defined, but it appears that TLR binding has a greater impact in IRI. Interestingly, RAGE blockade has led to higher TNF-α expression levels in the late (18 h) phase of liver reperfusion.

PMN-derived neutrophil elastase (NE) may also contribute to TLR4 activation (Figure 7.4). Activated KCs and hepatocytes produce pro-inflammatory cytokines, including TNF-α, as do cells in small bowel, and kidney tubular cells. TNF-α drives hepatocyte apoptosis and triggers chemokine-mediated endothelial expression of adhesion molecules, with the resultant transmigration of PMNs from the vascular lumen into liver parenchyma. NE stimulates pro-inflammatory CXCL-1/CXCL-2 by infiltrating PMNs. Inhibition of NE depresses CXC chemokine programs, prevents PMN/ macrophage recruitment, and suppresses local inflammation. However, it is plausible that NE not only accelerates IR-mediated damage in a feedback mechanism with recruited PMNs, but may also serve as a putative endogenous TLR ligand causing TLR4 upregulation on both KCs and hepatocytes.

TLR9 is an intracellular sensor involved in both microbial and sterile inflammation. It detects bacterial and endogenous DNA, and serves to sense necrotic cell death that triggers innate immune activation. TLR9 expressed in PMNs, appears to be essential for IR-induced ROS, IL-6 and TNF-α expression. DNA

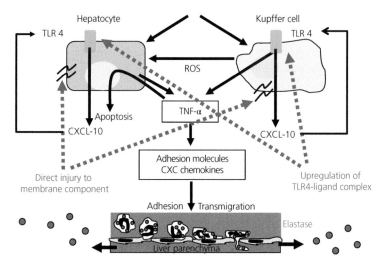

Figure 7.4 Neutrophil elastase and TLR4-mediated inflammation response in liver IRI. TNF-α promotes hepatocyte apoptosis and activated pro-inflammatory chemokine programs, leading to transmigration of PMNs from the vascular lumen into liver parenchyma. NE accelerates IR-stressed inflammation and may serve as an endogenous TLR4 ligand to further enhance TLR4 signaling in KCs and hepatocytes.

released from necrotic hepatocytes can induce pro-inflammatory gene pattern incultured hepatocytes via TLR9 (Bamboat et al., 2010a). As TLR9 signals through MyD88, a question arises as to why TLR4-mediated damage in the liver can also be MyD88-independent? It is possible that MyD88-independent activation of KC and DC by DAMPs in the early phase of organ injury (1–6 h) depends on the direct cytotoxicity of soluble TNF-α enriched inflammatory milieu. In later stages of IRI (>12 h), however, newly recruited and activated PMNs may require MyD88 signaling.

The role of other TLR family members in innate immune activation and IRI remains to be elucidated. For example, TLR3, which recognizes necrotic cell-derived RNA products, has been shown to sustain inflammation in a murine gastrointestinal ischemia model. These results need to be examined in other organ systems. Thus, different TLRs operate at distinct stages and in different cell types during the course of IRI in transplant recipients.

Non-TLRs in innate immune activation in IRI

The role of non-TLR innate receptors, such as nucleotide-binding domain (NOD)-like receptor (NLR) and RIG-I-like receptor (RLR), in modulating cytokine/chemokine programs and regulating local immune responses has only recently come under intense study in transplantation. Unlike TLRs, which are imbedded in the cell surface, non-TLR molecules recognize PAMP within the cytosol. However, similar to TLRs, they may also trigger local inflammation and immune activation. Cells undergoing death by pyroptosis via inflammasomes also release pro-inflammatory mediators similarly to other forms of necrosis. One member of the NLR family, namely, NLRP3 (NLR family, pyrin domain containing (3) has been involved in PMN recruitment to sites of hepatic necrosis in a model of sterile inflammation. As NALP3 silencing attenuated liver damage, reduced production of IL-1β, IL-18, TNF-α, and IL-6, diminished HMGB1 levels and decreased local cell infiltration (Zhu et al., 2011); inflammasome signaling may be essential in liver and other forms of IRI. Certainly, inflammasome-mediated injury is a key component of renal IRI as well as chronic forms of inflammatory organ injury in general. ATP released from necrotic liver cells may activate NLRP3 inflammasome to generate an "inflammatory microenviron-ment," which in turn alerts circulating PMNs to adhere within liver sinusoids. Crosstalk between TLR and inflammasome pathways in IRI and organ damage clearly warrants further analysis. As well, potential therapeutic strategies may include antibody neutralization of IL-1β and other mediators of inflammasome-related cell death.

IL-10 and innate immune activation

Under normal circumstances, activation of innate immune cells in IRI is a self-limiting process as injury needs to be controlled by the host. Thus, IRI and innate activation is linked to the activation of regulatory mechanisms that suppress tissue inflammation. Regulatory mechanisms include the production of contrain-flammatory cytokines including, but not limited to TGFβ, IL-4, IL-10, and IL-13 (Zhai et al., 2011) and, most recently, IL-37. IL-37 was recently shown to block IL-18-mediated death of kidney epithelial cells and prevent kidney IRI using transgenic expression within the kidney. During IRI in the liver, these cytokines may be highly expressed in IR-resistant animals. Although inhibitory to IR-induced TNF-α and/or IL-1β when administered exogenously, endogenous IL-4, IL-10, and IL-13 may not consistently exert immune-regulatory functions. While IL-13 KO mice show exacerbated liver IRI compared with IL-13 proficient counterparts, IR-induced TNF-α and CXCL8 (MIP-2) production in IL-13 deficient and wild-type (WT) mice was comparable. Although the cellular sources of IL-4 and IL-13 in the liver itself have not been defined, their most significant effect seems to be on the direct protection of hepatocytes from ROS-induced cell death. A role for IL-10 as a key immune regulatory cytokine in IRI has been suggested. In most experimental systems, IL-10 neutralization is both necessary and sufficient to recreate a pro-inflammatory phenotype in IRI-resistant organs. Multiple innate immune cell types (DCs, macrophages, and PMNs) can produce IL-10 to exert regulatory functions. Indeed, KCs can prevent organ damage in a liver IRI model through an IL-10 dependent mechanism.

Which types of liver NPCs produce IL-10 in response to IRI? Although KCs may produce IL-10 in response to endotoxin *in vitro*, its relevance to IRI *in vivo* remains unclear. In contrast, stressed liver conventional DCs may exert immune-regulatory functions by producing IL-10 via a TLR9-mediated mechanism (Bamboat et al., 2010b). Thus, liver NPCs, which are responsible for the initiation of IR-inflammation cascade may also be critical to the self-limitation of the response, in a "context dependent" manner. Consistent with this concept, macrophages and DCs can produce pro- and anti-inflammatory mediators in response to the very same TLR ligand.

As IRI activates both pro- and anti-inflammatory gene activation programs, the question arises, as to which are the key mechanisms that determine the final outcome of local inflammatory responses? It is possible that the kinetics of innate immune responses, differences in the cell types involved, and their responsiveness to pro- and anti-inflammatory products may all equally contribute to the eventual outcome of IRI. Alternatively, endogenous ligands generated at different stages of IRI may trigger pro- and anti-inflammatory responses sequentially, possibly via distinct TLR pathways and/or in different cell types. Addressing these key questions should help identify novel targets that can be used to selectively suppress pro-inflammatory injury pathways in transplant recipients.

T cells, NK cells, and NKT cells in IRI

In addition to KCs and DCs, T cells, NK, and NKT cells are also involved in IRI. Although liver IRI occurs in a sterile environment, CD4 T cells are important in IR-triggered pro-inflammatory responses (Zhai et al., 2011; Zwacka et al., 1997) and similarly in kidney. Indeed, livers in CD4-deficient hosts or in WT mice depleted of CD4 T cells are protected from IR damage. In contrast, CD8 T cell depletion or targeted deficiency minimally affects the severity of IRI. The key role of CD4 T cells poses a number of questions regarding their activation and function in an innate immune response. Since naïve T cell activation typically requires activation by specific Ag for their differentiation into functional effectors, it is unlikely that they play a major role in the very acute phase of IRI. However, memory T cells can be activated quickly to secrete cytokines or upregulate cell surface costimulatory molecules to amplify IRI. Consistent with this, in the liver, resident CD4 T cells are enriched with effector memory phenotype, which is defined as CXCR3+CD62L^{low}CD4+ T cells. CD4 blocking Ab to prevent CD4 TCR-mediated activation without concomitant cell depletion has shown that *de novo* CD4 T cell activation is not required for their function. Furthermore, mice sensitized with allo-Ag have enhanced CD4 T cell-mediated IR immune responses, and RAG-deficient TCR transgenic mice with fewer effector T cells have attenuated IRI.

Naïve CD4 T cells can differentiate into multiple T helper cell subsets including Th1, Th2, Th17, or regulatory T cells (Treg). T cell transfer studies indicate a more profound effect of Stat4-dependent Th1 cells in IRI, consistent with the pathogenic role of Th1 cells in IRI. In contrast, the putative role of Th17 or Treg cells, seen in other organ damage models remains to be determined, at least in the liver. Interestingly, a possible role of the CD154-CD40 costimulatory pathway in the activation of macrophages during IRI has been proposed (Shen et al., 2009). Although CD154 blockade in WT mice or in nude mice reconstituted with CD154-deficient CD4 T cells are protected against liver IRI, a CD40 agonist readily induced organ injury in CD4-KO mice. CD40 signaling has also been shown to synergize with various TLR ligands to facilitate pro-inflammatory phenotype in DC and macrophages with the elaboration of functional IL-12p70. Thus, different T cell types may regulate immune activation in IRI.

T cell immunoglobulin mucin (TIM) family of cell surface proteins has attracted much attention as novel regulators of host immunity. TIM-1 is expressed primarily on Th2 cells, and some natural killer (NK) and NKT cells (Figure 7.2). Notably, TIM-1 is also known as KIM-1 expressed by kidney tubular cells where its expression is of great interest in acute kidney injury. The expression of TIM proteins on hepatocytes is less defined. TIM-4, one of the major TIM-1 ligands, is expressed by macrophages and DCs. Hence, TIM-1/TIM-4 costimulation may dictate the nature and intensity of T cell–macrophage interactions. Using a model of liver "warm" IRI, we have documented the importance of TIM-1/TIM-4 pathway in liver IRI, and the ability of anti-TIM-1 mAb to ameliorate the hepatocellular damage and to improve liver function. The beneficial effect of blocking TIM-1 signaling in liver IRI was accompanied by decreased local PMN infiltration/activation, inhibition of T lymphocyte/macrophage sequestration, and diminished homing of TIM-4+ cells in the ischemic livers. The induction of pro-inflammatory cytokine/chemokine programs was also blunted. Figure 7.5 proposes mechanisms by which TIM-1, expressed primarily by activated T cells, can mediate tissue damage through inflammation as well as T cell/macrophage activation. In the "direct" pathway, TIM-1 on activated Th2 cells cross-links TIM-4 to directly activate macrophages. In the "indirect" pathway, TIM-1 on activated Th1 cells triggers IFN-γ that results in macrophage activation. Regardless of the pathway, activated macrophages elaborate cytokine and chemokine programs that facilitate the ultimate organ damage.

Unlike TIM-1–TIM-4 pathway, the interaction between TIM-3, which is expressed mostly on Th1 cells, and its major endogenous ligand, Gal-9 expressed by a wide array of cells including macrophages (Figure 7.2), inhibits Th1 immunity and promotes tolerance in transplant recipients. Interestingly, an intact TIM-3–Gal-9 "negative" costimulation signaling is needed to prevent excessive liver IRI (Uchida et al., 2010). Indeed, TIM-3 blockade worsened IR-hepatocellular damage, increased IFN-γ but depressed IL-10 expression in IR-stressed livers. Interestingly, the function of TIM-3 is dependent on an intact TLR4 axis, as

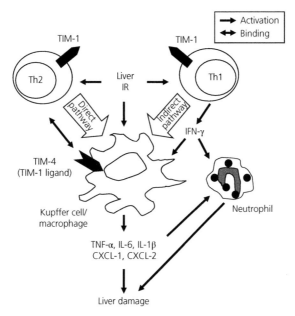

Figure 7.5 TIM-1–TIM-4 "positive" costimulation in hepatic IRI. Th1 and Th2 cells express TIM-1, whereas macrophages express TIM-4, the TIM-1 ligand. Liver IR activates Th1, Th2 and macrophages. TIM-1 on Th2 cells cross-links TIM-4 to directly activate macrophages (*direct pathway*), whereas TIM-1 on Th1 cells triggers IFN-γ that may also activate macrophages (*indirect pathway*). Consequently, activated macrophages produce cytokine/chemokine programs that facilitate ultimate organ damage.

α-TIM-3 mAb failed to affect IRI in TLR4 KO mice. Figure 7.6 depicts the potential mechanisms by which TIM-3–Gal-9 pathway controls IRI. TIM-3 blockade on activated Th1 cells increases their production of IFN-γ, which in turn enhances the activation of KCs, macrophages, and neutrophils, and upregulates TLR4 expression. Activated macrophages elaborate cytokine/chemokine programs through TLR4 pathway to promote organ damage that can be negatively modulated via TIM-3 signaling. We currently favor the notion that TIM-3 pathway may exert "protective" function by depressing IFN-γ production, thereby sparing the liver from IR-mediated damage in a TLR4-dependent manner. However, although the blockade of "positive" TIM-1/TIM-4 or enhancement of "negative" TIM-3/Gal-9 costimulation might be essential, further studies are needed to accurately assess their therapeutic potential given the opposing effects of TIM-1 and TIM-3 signaling in liver IRI. As PD-1–PD-L1 pathway has also been shown to promote liver cytoprotection, harnessing the mechanisms of negative costimulation pathways should prove instrumental in protecting organ damage in IRI.

In addition to T cells, NK and NKT cells also play important roles in IRI (Figure 7.2). Although depletion of NK1.1 cells (NK and NKT) largely fails to affect the severity of IRI at early time-points, it significantly reduces the hepatocellular damage in a later phase. In contrast, NK cells contribute to kidney IRI

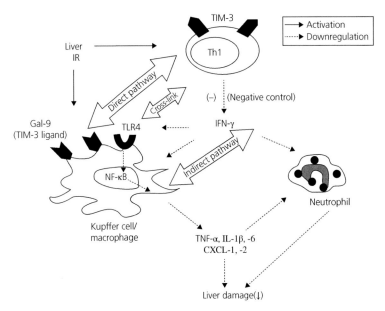

Figure 7.6 TIM-3–Gal-9 "negative" costimulation in hepatic IRI. IR triggers activation TIM-3 expression by activated macrophages and Th1 cells. TIM-3 signaling negatively regulates Th1 cells by suppressing TLR4-NF-κB pathway via IFN-γ, which in turn stimulates Gal-9 and mitigates macrophage activation. Diminished pro-inflammatory cytokine/chemokine programs ameliorate the hepatocellular damage and promote liver homeostasis.

through the interaction of NKG2D receptors with Rae-1 expression by tubular cells. The infiltration of kidney by NK cells can be blocked by the removal of osteopontin expression locally within the kidney. Removal of NK participation in genetically altered deficient mice abrogates renal IRI, which can be restored by the adaptive transfer of NK cells. Collectively, there is a large body of evidence supporting a key role for NK cells in kidney IRI. In the liver, suppression of NKT cells are clearly important. Activation of NKT cells (which comprise almost 50% of liver T cells) is mediated by CD1d, a molecule that is expressed by most liver cells and which presents glycolipid antigens released by necrotic cells, to NKT cell invariant TCRs. NKT cells are heterogeneous, and, similar to T cells, NKT cell subsets play distinctive roles *in vivo*. Indeed, type II NKT cells have been shown to prevent liver IRI when activated by specific glycolipid ligand sulfatide. IR-triggered NK cell activation is dependent on CD39 to hydrolyze ADP to AMP. Indeed, CD39-deficient livers were resistant to IRI, and IFN-γ production by their NK cells was diminished, possibly due to P2 receptor activation (Beldi et al., 2010). This might be a cell-type or organ-specific effect, as CD39 expression on endothelial cells was protective in kidney and cardiac IRI models. Thus, T cells, NKT cells, and NK cells are all involved, possibly at different stages of IRI, by providing costimulatory signaling via direct cell–cell interactions or cytokine modulation.

Conclusions

IRI remains a major issue in clinical transplantation. Inflammation is the common pathway in tissue damage during IRI and this involves the activation of both innate and adaptive immune cells. IRI promotes graft rejection and limits long-term graft survival. There is considerable cross-talk between various cell types and molecular pathways in IRI, which are only now being appreciated in transplantation. While clinical transplantation is primarily focused on inhibiting recipient immune responses, there is much to be gained by inhibiting IRI in the transplanted organs, by targeting the organ itself. Along with conventional immunosuppression in transplant recipients, reducing local production of inflammatory mediators and tissue injury in transplanted organs prior to implantation can attenuate rejection responses and ultimately improve long-term transplant survival.

References

Bamboat ZM, Balachandran VP, Ocuin LM, Obaid H, Plitas G, DeMatteo RP. Toll-like receptor 9 inhibition confers protection from liver ischemia-reperfusion injury. Hepatology 2010;51: 621–632.

Bamboat ZM, Ocuin LM, Balachandran VP, Obaid H, Plitas G, DeMatteo RP. Conventional DCs reduce liver ischemia/reperfusion injury in mice via IL-10 secretion. The Journal of Clinical Investigation 2010;120:559–569.

Beldi G, Banz Y, Kroemer A, Sun X, Wu Y, Graubardt N, Rellstab A, et al. Deletion of CD39 on natural killer cells attenuates hepatic ischemia/reperfusion injury in mice. Hepatology 2010;51:1702–1711.

Ikeda T, Yanaga K, Kishikawa K, Kakizoe S, Shimada M, Sugimachi K. Ischemic injury in liver transplantation: Difference in injury sites between warm and cold ischemia in rats. Hepatology 1992;16:454–461.

Shen X, Wang Y, Gao F, Ren F, Busuttil RW, Kupiec-Weglinski JW, Zhai Y. CD4 T cells promote tissue inflammation via CD40 signaling without de novo activation in a murine model of liver ischemia/reperfusion injury. Hepatology 2009;50:1537–1546.

Tsung A, Sahai R, Tanaka H, Nakao A, Fink MP, Lotze MT, Yang H, et al. The nuclear factor HMGB1 mediates hepatic injury after murine liver ischemia-reperfusion. The Journal of Experimental Medicine 2005;201:1135–1143.

Uchida Y, Ke B, Freitas MC, Yagita H, Akiba H, Busuttil RW, Najafian N, et al. T-cell immunoglobulin mucin-3 determines severity of liver ischemia/reperfusion injury in mice in a TLR4-dependent manner. Gastroenterology 2010;139:2195–2206.

Zhai Y, Shen XD, O'Connell R, Gao F, Lassman C, Busuttil RW, Cheng G, et al. Cutting edge: TLR4 activation mediates liver ischemia/reperfusion inflammatory response via IFN regulatory factor 3-dependent MyD88-independent pathway. Journal of Immunology 2004;173:7115–7119.

Zhai Y, Busuttil RW, Kupiec-Weglinski JW. New insights into mechanisms of innate–adaptive immune-mediated tissue inflammation. American Journal of Transplantation 2011; 11:1563–1569.

Zhu P, Duan L, Chen J, Xiong A, Xu Q, Zhang H, Zheng F, et al. Gene Silencing of NALP3 protects against liver ischemia-reperfusion injury in mice. Human Gene Therapy 2011; 22:853–864.

Zwacka RM, Zhang Y, Halldorson J, Schlossberg H, Dudus L, Engelhardt JF. CD4(+) T-lymphocytes mediate ischemia/reperfusion-induced inflammatory responses in mouse liver. The Journal of Clinical Investigation 1997;100:279–289.

CHAPTER 8

Immune responses to transplants

Denise J. Lo[1] and Allan D. Kirk[1,2]

[1]Department of Surgery, Emory Transplant Center, Emory University School of Medicine, Atlanta, USA
[2]Department of Surgery, Duke University School of Medicine, Durham, USA

CHAPTER OVERVIEW

- The alloimmune response involves adaptive and innate immune systems; T and B cells are the principle mediators of cellular and antibody-mediated rejection.

- Distinct immunologic and histologic differences exist between acute cellular, antibody mediated, and chronic rejection.

- Tolerance strategies include immunoregulation, costimulation blockade, and mixed chimerism; mechanisms of tolerance induction may differ from those that are needed to sustain it.

- Memory T cells are a significant barrier to tolerance induction.

- Understanding the mechanisms behind rejection and tolerance will guide the development of innovative therapies to improve transplant outcomes.

- The identification of biomarkers for rejection and/or tolerance could initiate individualized immune modulation regimens.

Introduction

Organ transplantation is the accepted and indeed the preferred treatment for most forms of end-stage organ failure. However, many challenges remain in the field. Current antirejection therapies are nonspecific, and thus require a careful balance between under- and overimmunosuppression. Unfortunately, there is no clear metric for establishing an individual's therapeutic window for immuno-suppression, and clinical management remains largely empiric. As many immuno-suppressive agents target ubiquitous cellular processes, their use results not only in the intended immune modulation but also in substantial off-target tox-icities. Biologic therapies, such as antibodies and fusion proteins that more

---

Transplant Immunology, First Edition. Edited by Xian Chang Li and Anthony M. Jevnikar.
Companion website: www.wiley.com/go/li/transplantimmunology

specifically target pathways mediating transplant rejection, have the potential to prevent rejection with fewer nonimmune effects, but their chronic use is only now being explored.

In general, improvements in immunosuppression, surgical technique, and organ preservation have resulted in better short-term allograft survival. Unfortunately, this has not translated into an equivalent progress in long-term graft survival. Chronic graft rejection, typically characterized by progressive allograft fibrosis and loss of parenchymal function, arises from the cumulative effects of many immune and nonimmune processes. Preventing chronic graft loss has become the predominant issue facing the transplant community.

The concept of transplant tolerance has been pursued with keen interest since the landmark work of Sir Peter Medawar (Billingham et al., 1953). Considerable resources have been dedicated to elucidating the mechanisms surrounding tolerance and for developing strategies to induce durable allograft acceptance without immunosuppression. This significant undertaking is rendered even more formidable by the fact that the immune system is a dynamic entity; it is constantly being challenged by new antigens and pathogens that can perturb the balance between rejection and tolerance. Strategies to induce tolerance therefore need to be equally adaptive to accommodate the nuances of the immune system as a "moving target."

Tranpslant rejection

The hallmark of the immune system is its capacity to discriminate between physiological variation and threatening disturbances. Many specialized immune mechanisms have evolved to protect the host from harmful pathogens while tolerating self-tissues and benign neo-antigens, thus facilitating protective immunity with remarkably little autoimmunity. While the function of the immune system may be to protect against infection or "danger," the immune system, if not suppressed, also efficiently recognizes an organ transplant from a genetically disparate individual. This initiates an immune response, or an alloresponse, against the transplant. Rejection of organ allografts is the result of numerous innate and adaptive immune cells, and to a large extent is related to the foreign major histocompatibility complex (MHC). Innate immune activation sets the stage for an adaptive response, with T cells evoked as the central mediators of cellular rejection and B cells playing an essential role, typically with the help of T cells, in antibody-mediated rejection (ABMR). Table 8.1 highlights the key features of innate and adaptive immunity in immune responses, including allograft rejection. These responses can happen acutely as well as insidiously over a lengthy period of allograft function.

Table 8.1 Features of innate versus adaptive immunity.

Characteristic	Innate	Adaptive
Function	Immunity against bacterial, viral, and fungal infections	Cellular immunity, antibody production
Components	NK cells, macrophages, dendritic cells, granulocytes, complement	T and B lymphocytes
Receptors	Pattern recognition receptors	T cell receptor, B cell receptor
Antigen specificity	No	Yes
Requirements for activation	Receptor recognition of pathogen- or danger-associated molecular patterns (PAMPs and DAMPS)	Receptor engagement by antigen bound to self-MHC, costimulation
Clonal distribution	No	Yes
Effector functions	Phagorcytosis, direct cytotoxicity, inflammatory chemokine and cytokine secretion	Cytokine secretion, direct cytotoxicity, antibody production
Role in rejection	Not well understood	Cellular and humoral rejection

Clinical manifestations of rejection
Hyperacute rejection
Hyperacute rejection is the most dramatic form of rejection. It results when high titers of preformed antibodies against donor polymorphic MHC antigens cause a severe, complement-dependent rejection that can occur within minutes to hours of reperfusion. Antibodies bind antigens on allograft endothelium and initiate complement-mediated lysis, endothelial damage, and clotting cascades that result in immediate graft thrombosis and failure. Though untreatable, hyperacute rejection related to alloantibodies is nearly universally preventable when lymphocytotoxic crossmatching is performed accurately to detect preformed donor-specific antibody (DSA).

Acute cellular rejection
Without adequate immunosuppression after transplantation, allograft rejection invariably ensues. Acute T cell-mediated rejection (TCMR) can occur within a few days after transplantation and most commonly occurs within 6 months of transplant. However, it can occur even later in transplants, as in the case of patients that have stopped immunosuppression abruptly. As previously discussed, acute rejection results largely from direct allorecognition mediated by hyperphysiological numbers of T cells activated by donor MHC. Unlike hyperacute or chronic rejection (CR), TCMR episodes can be treated with intensified immunosuppression, and expeditious resolution of acute rejection is necessary to limit tissue damage and preserve graft function. TCMR results in a very stereotypical histopathologic pattern characterized by inflammatory changes

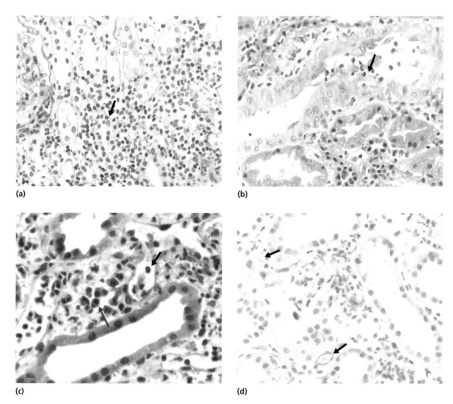

Figure 8.1 Acute cellular- and humoral-mediated rejection. Acute cellular rejection in a renal allograft showing typical (a) tubulitis with dense lymphocytic infiltrates and (b) arteritis. Acute humoral rejection in a renal allograft demonstrating (c) peritubular capillaritis (black arrow) and infiltrating plasma cells (red arrow) and (d) C4d deposition (all images 40× magnification).

and interstitial lymphocytic infiltrates with or without vasculitis (Cornell et al., 2008) (Figure 8.1a and b). Lymphocytic infiltrates are predominantly composed of T cells with accompanying macrophages. Only a minority of the graft infiltrating T cells in rejection are likely to be antigen-specific. Strong inflammatory, cytokine, and chemokine signals recruit non-antigen-specific effectors into the graft. In particular, effector T cell-derived IFN-γ drives the inflammatory and cellular response during acute cellular rejection (ACR). IFN-γ induces expression of several important genes in donor allograft cells as well as in recipient mononuclear cells. Chemokines such as CXCL9, CXCL10, CXCL11, and CCL5 are upregulated and foster additional cellular recruitment. Donor cells upregulate MHC molecules resulting in an increased potential for allorecognition.

Antibody-mediated rejection

Antibody-mediated rejection, or "humoral" rejection, represents a distinct entity that is T cell-dependent, but may or may not be accompanied by a T cell infiltrate and associated TCMR. For humoral immunity, T cell help is essential for the generation of long-lived plasma cells and memory B cells that are responsible for the production of DSAs (Figure 8.2). Patients that have been previously sensitized to donor antigen and have preformed DSA are at the highest risk. ABMR may be a result of high titers of *de novo* DSA or a resurgence of preformed DSA, which were at low levels and below the detection limits of the clinical crossmatch. Alternatively, resting alloreactive memory B cells may be stimulated to produce DSA soon after transplantation. The clinical course of ABMR may be indistinguishable from TCMR and requires a biopsy for diagnosis. ABMR is associated with accumulation of neutrophils and monocytes; microvascular thrombosis; and often but not always, deposition of C4d, a degradation product of the activated complement factor C4b (Figure 8.1c and d). C4d staining can be highly correlated with neutrophil infiltration, fibrinoid necrosis, and circulating DSA (Djamali et al., 2014).

Complement fixation ability greatly enhances an antibody's potency to promote rejection. Antibody isotypes have varying degrees of classical complement cascade activation (IgG3 >IgG1 >IgG2 > IgG4). Kidney transplant patients with ABMR have been found to have increased IgG3 levels, whereas those with stable allografts only exhibited a rise in IgG4. Blockade of the classical complement pathway was shown to protect against ABMR in animal models. Additionally, in kidney transplantation, DSAs that bind the C1q fraction of complement have been associated with poor outcomes compared to DSAs that do not bind C1q.

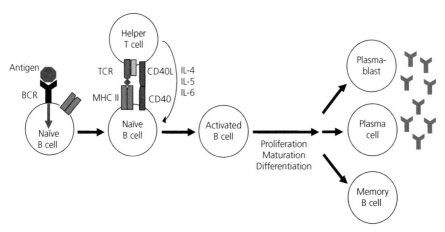

Figure 8.2 Generation of antibody-producing plasma cells and memory B cells. B cell activation begins when the B cell receptor (BCR) recognizes, binds, and internalizes foreign antigens. These antigens are processed and presented on the B cell surface by major histocompatibility complex (MHC) class II molecules. Antigen-specific helper T cells recognize antigen bound by MHC, express costimulatory molecules including CD40L, and secrete cytokines that trigger full B cell activation and proliferation. With this T cell help activated B cells are enabled to mature and differentiate to become antibody-secreting plasmablasts and plasma cells or long-lived memory B cells.

Chronic rejection

Chronic rejection is a broad classification that has been used to describe late deterioration of allograft function that occurs over time in most patients. Descriptive nomenclature for CR varies by organ, and includes chronic allograft nephropathy or interstitial fibrosis/tubular atrophy (IF/TA) in kidneys, chronic coronary vasculopathy in heart, bronchiolitis obliterans in lungs, and vanishing bile duct syndrome in liver. Though clinical manifestations of CR are organ-specific, many organs undergoing CR exhibit unifying histolopathologic features. Proliferative vascular lesions including intimal hyperplasia and neointimal proliferation of smooth muscle cells result in chronic allograft vasculopathy. Additionally, epithelial and fibroblast proliferation and collagen deposition contribute to the fibrous replacement that is synonymous with CR. Cumulative allograft damage results in ischemia, extensive fibrosis, and progressive graft dysfunction.

Compared to acute rejection, the mechanisms of CR are less well understood, largely because CR is not a single entity, but rather a stereotypic response to sublethal cellular injury. Ischemia reperfusion and other non-antigen-specific injuries likely contribute, as these have been associated with increased vasculopathy and CR. Both CD4 T_H1 and CD8 effector T cells also play a role in CR, perhaps most explicitly through the production of IFN-γ. Additionally, chronic allograft injury is often associated with alloantibody formation, implicating B cells as major culprits in CR. Alloantibody complement fixation is likely to be of critical importance in executing damage, as previously described.

Unsolved issues

Despite recent advances, there are still many gaps in our understanding of rejection. A critical dilemma in transplantation is how to achieve precision targeting of effector populations while leaving regulatory cells unharmed. Although commonly used therapies such as calcineurin inhibitors (CNIs) and interleukin-2 (IL-2) receptor blockers are very effective at preventing rejection, they also target mechanisms that Treg cells rely on for activation and proliferation. Newer modalities such as costimulation blockade also may adversely affect Treg cells, which are dependent on costimulation for homeostasis and function. It will be important to identify additional pathways to target effector T cells while sparing regulatory populations; thus tipping the balance in favor of regulation.

Importantly, CR is a multifactorial process and the relative impact of immune and nonimmune insults underlying late allograft failure needs to be further elucidated. There is a lack of highly effective therapeutic options for chronically failing allografts, attesting to the complexity of the problem. The significant contribution of antibody responses in patients with late allograft failure highlights the need for therapeutic modalities that better prevent allosensitization in addition to improved treatments for already sensitized patients. Finally, additional non-T and B effector cells that are not controlled by current immunosuppression will need to be considered.

Key areas of research
Noninvasive tests for rejection

One major area of research in transplantation is the search for noninvasive tests, or biomarkers, to detect—or even predict—rejection episodes prior to organ damage and adverse clinical sequelae. For example, in kidney transplantation there has been considerable interest in developing urinary markers as noninvasive detection of rejection. In a multicenter study from the consortium of clinical trials in organ transplantation (CTOT) , detection of discreet urinary mRNA profiles composed of cytokines and T cell-related markers, including perforin, CXCL9,CXCL10, CXCR3, CD3, and granzyme B, were correlated with acute rejection. Similar efforts are being applied to bronchoalveolar lavage fluids from lung transplants and peripheral blood correlates for all organs. The development of a noninvasive test that would be able to reliably and accurately predict rejection episodes would be an invaluable clinical metric. However, caution must be used in developing such screening or diagnostic tests, taking into consideration cost-effectiveness, sensitivity, and specificity. For example, one particular challenge in developing reliable urinary biomarkers in kidney transplantation is distinguishing rejection from other immune-related events, such as the presence of the BK virus. Confusion between a pathogen-associated immune response versus rejection could misguide "preemptive" immunosuppression adjustments, potentially doing more harm than good.

Therapeutics for antibody-mediated rejection

Antibody-mediated rejection has only recently gained due respect for its significant prevalence and morbidity in transplantation. Most current therapies are T cell-centric, but with heightened insight into the mechanisms of ABMR, B cell-specific therapies are surfacing and may show promise in the treatment of ABMR (Djamali et al., 2014).Two TNF family ligands important for B cells survival, activation, and differentiation are B-lymphocyte stimulator (BlyS, also known as BAFF) and APRIL. The cognate B cell receptors (BCRs) for these factors include BMCA, TACI, and BAFF-R (BAFF-R binds BlyS alone). Belimumab, a humanized mAb to BlyS, was shown to be effective in treating SLE and is in preliminary trials as a desensitization agent. Atacicept (TACI-Ig) is a fusion protein of the extracellular binding domain of TACI bound to the Fc portion of IgG1, and prevents B cell stimulation by inhibiting BlyS and APRIL. In preliminary studies, atacicept was shown to cause a dose-dependent decrease in circulating immunoglobulin levels and B cell counts, and represents a potential desensitization agent and/or treatment for ABMR.

Rituximab, a chimeric anti-CD20 mAb that causes B cell depletion through antibody- and complement-dependent cytotoxicity has been used as part of desensitization protocols in renal transplantation. Newer biologic therapies include proteosome inhibitors, which induce apoptosis in rapidly dividing and metabolically active cells, and anticomplement antibodies. Bortezomib, an inhibitor of the 26s proteosome, was approved for the treatment of multiple myeloma, and there are reports of both successful reversal of ABMR and desensitization with bortezomib. Treatment with eculizumab, a humanized anti-C5 monoclonal antibody currently approved for the treatment of complement-associated disorders, has been shown to decrease the incidence of ABMR in highly sensitized individuals. Its use in treating refractory ABMR remains limited due to its cost and paucity of randomized studies.

Transplant tolerance

Transplant tolerance is a state of lasting antigen-specific, immunologic unresponsiveness in the absence of chronic immunosuppression. Sir Peter Medawar's description of acquired tolerance in mice proved that a sentinel event could modulate the immune system sufficiently to lead to a sustained acceptance of an allograft (Billingham et al., 1953). This landmark work also showed that a spectrum of tolerance exists, and a high degree of variability can be expected for any given manipulation. Though tolerance has been induced in multiple, immunologically naïve experimental animal models (Larsen et al., 1996), the achievement of consistent and robust donor-specific tolerance unfortunately remains elusive in clinical transplantation. This difficulty is due to a large extent to the enormous diversity of immunologic exposure experienced by human patients. Thus, the "road to tolerance" requires a comprehensive understanding of the immune processes of tolerance as well as the mechanisms that exist to thwart it.

Mechanisms of central tolerance

A fundamental feature of the immune system is "self from non-self" discrimination. The immune system has developed overlapping selection mechanisms to purge self-reactive lymphocytes and protect from inappropriate self-recognition. This selection process, known as central tolerance, begins in the primary lymphoid organs where immature lymphocytes differentiate from lymphoid progenitors. B cell precursors develop in the bone marrow, while T cell precursors migrate to the thymus for selection and maturation.

T cells

Immature CD8/CD4 double-positive thymocytes undergo T cell receptor (TCR)-β and α gene locus rearrangement, generating a broad TCR repertoire. The fate of each immature thymocyte depends on the ability of its new TCR to recognize self-peptides bound to MHC. The vast majority of cells are unable to recognize a self-peptide-MHC complex with any avidity and undergo the default program of apoptosis. Additionally, cells that recognize thymic stromal antigens also avidly undergo induced cell death. This process of clonal deletion, or negative selection, eliminates strongly self-reactive lymphocytes and is critical in preventing autoimmunity. Cells with TCRs that weakly recognize self-MHC molecules receive a "rescue signal," or are positively selected, producing a population of thymocytes that are self-MHC restricted. These cells undergo further differentiation to become CD8 or CD4 single-positive T cells (Griesemer et al., 2010).

B cells

B cells precursors remain in the bone marrow where they undergo stochastic V(D)J receptor gene rearrangement, yielding an enormously diverse repertoire of receptors. In fact, this random process generates a significant proportion of B cells (up to 45%) that do not undergo a successful recombination event, and these pro-B cells are lost at this stage. Immature B cells that have unacceptable, strongly autoreactive BCRs undergo clonal deletion. Immature B cells also retain expression of RAG1 and RAG2, the genes primarily responsible for V(D)J recombination, and are able to undergo further recombination in a process known as receptor editing. In this manner, immature B cells can attempt additional recombination events to generate useful, non-self-recognizing BCRs (Kirk et al., 2010) (Figure 8.3).

Mechanisms of peripheral tolerance

The vast majority of self-reactive lymphocytes are eliminated through central tolerance mechanisms. However, self-reactive cells can escape deletion in the central lymphoid organs and require control in the periphery. As well, maintenance of tolerance to "self" requires nonthymic mechanisms in later life,

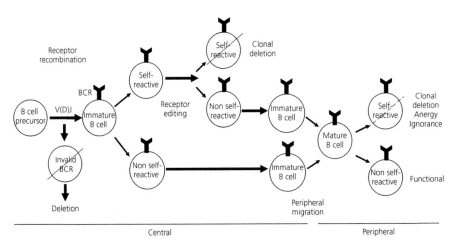

Figure 8.3 B cell central and peripheral tolerance. B cell precursors reside in the bone marrow where each cell begins development by undergoing V(D)J gene receptor rearrangement to generate a unique BCR. Cells that produce a nonfunctional BCR are lost at this stage. Immature B cells are tested for autoreactivity before exiting the bone marrow, a process known as central tolerance. B cells that are self-reactive are deleted or can undergo further receptor rearrangement (receptor editing) prior to deletion in an attempt to rescue the cell. Non-self-reactive B cells are released into the periphery where additional peripheral mechanisms to control escaped self-reactive B cells include clonal deletion, anergy, and ignorance.

as the thymus involutes in adults. Therefore, multiple redundant mechanisms exist to control self-reactive cells that encounter *de novo* self-antigen in the periphery, and these include regulation, deletion, anergy or ignorance. Tolerance of mature lymphocytes generated outside the central lymphoid organs is known as peripheral tolerance.

T cells

As in the thymus, T cells that strongly cross-link peripheral antigen are programmed to undergo deletion. Further peripheral control of mature, self-reactive T cells relies heavily on a naïve T cell's costimulatory (signal 2) requirement for activation. Under conditions of infection, inflammation or tissue injury, the innate immune system provides signals that upregulate costimulatory molecules on APCs, facilitating T cell activation. In contrast, naïve T cells that recognize and bind antigen presented by APCs in the absence of costimulation, as in the case of self-antigen recognition, receive an inactivating signal that renders these cells unresponsive, or anergic, to that specific antigen. T cells also may be temporarily activated, but without sustained support this activation is followed by apoptosis in a process known as activation-induced cell death (AICD).

B cells

Self-reactive B cells that have evaded both clonal deletion and receptor editing in the bone marrow can be controlled in the periphery by further clonal deletion, anergy, or immunologic ignorance (Kirk et al., 2010). Mature B cells that bind strongly to peripheral antigen will also undergo apoptosis or clonal deletion. Cells that encounter an abundance of soluble antigen can become anergized by modulating their antigen responsiveness via desensitization to BCR signaling. Weakly reactive B cells can also bypass other mechanisms of tolerance and simply exist in a state of immunological ignorance to their cognate antigen. Multiple extrinsic mechanisms exist that allow B cells to persist in a state of ignorance. Engagement of the BCR may be so weak that no intracellular signal is generated, and B cells additionally may be limited by a lack of T cell help.

Tolerance induction strategies
Immune regulation

In contrast to deletional mechanisms of tolerance, immunoregulation is an active process whereby a population of suppressor cells control or regulate the activity of another cell population. Some regulatory populations include CD4$^+$ IL-10-secreting T_R1 cells, TGF-β-secreting T_H3 cells, CD4$^-$CD8$^-$ 'double-negative T cells", and CD8$^+$CD28$^-$ T cells. However, the most efficient and critical regulators of immunity are CD4$^+$FoxP3$^+$ regulatory T (Treg) cells (Wood et al., 2012). The importance of Treg cells in maintaining self-tolerance was realized when it was observed that thymectomized neonatal mice and adult rats both develop autoimmune disease, but adoptive transfer of CD4$^+$ T cells from healthy animals prevented this autoimmunity. Additionally, both *scurfy* mice and human patients deficient in FoxP3 gene expression, now known to be a master transcription factor for Treg development and function, developed a severe constellation of autoimmune and allergic sequelae (Hori et al., 2003).

Treg cells make up about 5–10% of the circulating CD4 T cell population in healthy humans. Natural Treg (nTreg) cells mature in the thymus while induced Treg (iTreg) cells have been converted from conventional effector T cells into a regulatory population. *In vitro* studies have shown that TCR stimulation is required to activate Treg cells, which subsequently control other cells in a contact-dependent manner. Treg cells also can exert their suppressive functions via soluble mediators including TGF-β, IL-10, and IL-35. They have been shown to control effector populations by inhibiting cytokine production and secretion, downregulating costimulatory molecules, and inhibiting proliferation, and anergy or apoptosis. Once activated by their cognate antigen, Treg cells can suppress T cell responses irrespective of antigen specificity. This phenomenon of linked suppression may be the result of a Treg-induced functional modification or "decommissioning" of APCs (Figure 8.4). Treg cells constitutively express CTLA-4 and can inhibit B7 molecules on APCs, thereby limiting

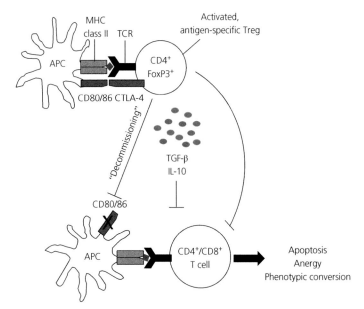

Figure 8.4 Regulatory T cells induce linked unresponsiveness. Activated CD4+CD25+FoxP3+ regulatory T (Treg) cells can suppress both APCs as well as other T cells that possess the same antigen specificity. Treg cells recognize donor antigen that has been processed and presented by MHC class II molecules on APCs via the indirect pathway. After engagement, Treg cells can functionally modify, or "decommission," APCs and suppress antigen-specific T cells through contact-dependent (CTLA-4; Fas-FasL pathway) and contact-independent (IL-10, TGF-β) mechanisms. CTLA-4, cytotoxic T-lymphocyte antigen 4; IL-10, IL-10; TGF-β, transforming growth factor-β.

alloreactive T cell activation. Treg cells also can downregulate costimulatory and MHC molecule expression on immature APCs, and induce mature APCs to undergo apoptosis. Therefore, linked suppression is a powerful way for a small number of allo-specific Treg cells to balance a much larger effector T cell population.

Costimulation blockade

Costimulation blockade is a T cell-targeted therapy designed to foster anergy or AICD of alloreactive cells, specifically by permitting alloantigen recognition and TCR signaling (signal 1) in the absence of costimulation (signal 2) (Figure 8.5). Costimulation blockade most effectively targets naïve T cells that require strong costimulatory signals for full activation. Additionally, costimulation blockade has been shown to prevent alloantibody formation in preclinical and clinical studies, presumably by blocking activated CD4 T cell help to B cells.

Two of the best-characterized costimulatory pathways are the CD28-B7 and CD40-CD40L pathways, and multiple mAbs have been developed to block these interactions. Anti-CD40L mAbs targeting CD40L on T cells have been convincingly effective in experimental animal models (Larsen et al., 1996). However, their use in clinical trials was halted after unexpected thromboembolic events occurred, with CD40L expression on activated platelets being implicated. Despite these results the efficacy of CD40-CD40L pathway blockade was so compelling

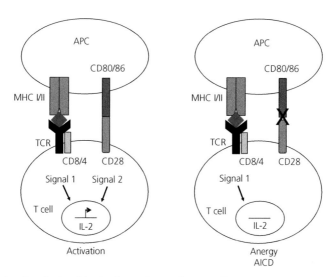

Figure 8.5 Costimulation blockade. Both signals 1 (T cell receptor (TCR) engagement) and 2 (costimulatory signal) are required for full naïve T cell activation. When the TCR is engaged in the absence of signal 2, T cells are rendered anergic and become unable to respond. T cells may also temporarily be activated but are unable to sustain activation without additional costimulatory support and undergo apoptosis, known as activation-induced cell death.

in preclinical studies that interest in this pathway has persisted. Several antibodies targeting CD40 are currently in development and have shown efficacy in preclinical models. CD40 is not highly expressed on platelets and therefore is not expected to cause the same thrombotic complications as does the CD40L blockade.

The CD28-B7 costimulation pathway has been intensely pursued in clinical costimulation blockade development. Abatacept (CTLA4-Ig) and belatacept (LEA29Y) are two CTLA-4 analog fusion proteins that bind to B7 (CD80 and CD86) molecules on APCs, preventing CD28-B7 costimulation. Belatacept, a second-generation, high-affinity variant of abatacept, was investigated in the large-scale, multicentered BENEFIT trial (Vincenti et al., 2010).Three-year results showed that belatacept treatment resulted in superior renal function and similar allograft survival compared to the CNI cyclosporine. Belatacept patients had a higher rate of early acute rejection, indicating that costimulation blockade-resistant populations were able to mediate rejection. Many adjuvant therapies to control these populations are under preclinical or clinical testing. Nevertheless, costimulation blockade is a promising immunomodulatory therapy in that it may spare the nephrotoxic side effects of CNIs, block alloantibody formation, and promote tolerance by facilitating anergy or AICD of alloreactive cells. More recently, anti-CD28 domain antibodies have been developed and are under preclinical testing. Follow-up is needed to determine the long-term efficacy of costimulation blockade-based therapies and their effects on regulatory cells and protective immunity.

Donor-specific transfusion

It has long been appreciated that alloantigen exposure can result in sensitization and generation of alloreactive cells that can foster rejection. However, a number of preclinical and clinical studies on donor-specific transfusion (DST) in the form of transfused donor bone marrow or splenocytes have shown DST to be pro-tolerant in specific circumstances, particularly when paired with costimulation blockade. DST differs from mixed chimerism induction by bone marrow transplantation in that transfused cells are eliminated with no attempts to induce donor cell engraftment or macrochimerism. When paired with costimulation blockade, this modality delivers a bolus of donor antigen while simultaneously inhibiting the costimulatory signals necessary for full T cell activation. Therefore, DST may be used as a potent adjunct to costimulation blockade, whose tolerogenic potential is dependent on the presence of donor antigen, to promote anergy or AICD. Historically, whole blood was transfused in kidney patients pre-transplant, for immunomodulation. While this may have benefited some patients, it also resulted in sensitization in others. As the effect was modest, and was completely lost using leukodepleted blood, the practice was abandoned in favor of more robust strategies to induce tolerance.

Mixed chimerism

Another strategy to achieve tolerance is through the induction of mixed chimerism, a process by which preconditioned recipients receive a donor hematopoetic stem cell (HSC) transplant to achieve a coexistent state of donor and recipient hematopoetic cells in primary lymphoid organs (Pilat & Wekerle, 2010). Recipients are preconditioned using a variety of therapies that include chemotherapy, myeloablation, thymic irradiation, costimulation blockade, T cell depletion and standard immunosuppression to prepare the recipient for donor bone marrow engraftment. The mixed chimeric state differs from full chimerism where donor hematopoetic stem cells comprise 100% of the recipient's bone marrow, substantially increasing the risk for graft-versus-host disease (GVHD).

Tolerance protocols that rely completely on peripheral mechanisms such as clonal deletion can potentially be overwhelmed by the continuous thymic output of alloreactive T cells. In contrast, the establishment of mixed chimerism leads to a continuous, self-renewing source of donor-derived APCs that can be used to educate the recipient to the "new-self" via central mechanisms. Several groups have reported their clinical experience with combined bone marrow and solid organ transplantation tolerance induction trials. Kawai and colleagues (Kawai et al., 2008) reported a trial of five patients who underwent combined HSC and kidney transplantation. The nonmyeloablative conditioning regimen included cyclophosphamide, thymic irradiation, T cell depletion with anti-CD2 antibodies, and cyclosporine, and maintenance immunosuppression was weaned after one year. All patients achieved transient chimerism with no cases of GVHD. Four patients were withdrawn from all immunosuppression and maintained stable renal allograft function for the duration of the reported follow-up period (5.3 years). One patient lost the graft secondary to refractory ABMR, and rituximab and steroids subsequently were added to the regimen. These results show that operational tolerance through mixed chimerism is feasible in clinical transplantation, though a rigorous induction regimen is required. Several versions of strategies exist currently for chimerism and operational tolerance, with various effectiveness and morbidity related to partial myeloablation.

Mechanisms of tolerance resistance
Memory T cells

Memory T cells are well-recognized obstacles to tolerance induction, particularly in clinical transplantation. These cells can develop after direct exposure to alloantigen, during pregnancy, blood transfusions, and prior transplants, and possess unique features that are very different from that of naïve T cells (Table 8.2). However, viral pathogen exposures also generate a repertoire of memory T cells, some of which are cross-reactive to alloantigen, a phenomenon known as heterologous immunity. This was shown by Adams and colleagues (Adams et al., 2003) who demonstrated that in contrast to naïve mice, mice that were exposed to multiple previous viral infections were refractory to

Table 8.2 Characteristics of naïve and memory T cells.

Characteristic	Naïve	Memory
Frequency (antigen specific)	Extremely low (1:10,000)	Readily detectable (1-20 per 1000 cells)
Costimulation	Required	Reduced
Adhesion molecules	Low LFA-1, CD2	Increased LFA-1, CD2, VLA-4
Antigen sensitivity	Requires high titers	Responds to low frequency
Antigen presenting cells	Professional (dendritic cells)	Non professional
Homing	Lymphoid tissues	Lymphoid and non-lymphoid tissues
Effector functions	None	Cytokine production, cytotoxicity
Kinetics of action	Slow (days)	Rapid (hours)
Lifespan	Normal	Indefinite

costimulation blockade-based tolerance induction. In fact, in humans, up to 45% of heterologously derived memory T cells were shown to have alloreactive potential, indicating that alloreactive memory T cells are relevant, even in "naïve" recipients that have not been sensitized through traditional pathways. Alloreactive memory T cells are mediators of costimulation blockade resistance and a barrier to the establishment of stable mixed chimerism. Some mixed chimerism strategies have employed profound T cell depletion to eliminate mature T cells, but this approach leaves patients at increased risk for serious infectious complications.

Homeostatic repopulation

Lymphocyte depletional induction agents are now more commonly used in clinical transplantation. Depletional agents include polyclonal anti-T lymphocyte/thymocyte preparations (Thymoglobulin®, ATGAM®) and monoclonal antibodies against lymphocyte markers including CD3 (OKT3) and CD52 (alemtuzumab). Depletional strategies have the advantage of reducing alloreactive T cell precursor frequencies during the time of surgical trauma, reperfusion injury, and inflammatory immune activation. Moreover, the immune system is given the opportunity to "reset" itself, and careful attention to how the immune system reconstitutes is prudent.

Homeostatic proliferation following profound lymphocyte depletional therapies has been recognized as a barrier to tolerance (Wu et al., 2004). In clinical trials, alemtuzumab monotherapy was shown to induce profound and long-lived T and B cell depletion with moderate monocyte and natural killer (NK) cell depletion. However, patients experienced acute rejection despite profoundly low

T cell counts, and grafts were laden with monocytic infiltrates on histology. This finding suggests that other cell populations can mediate rejection with minimal T cell support. A study by Cherkassky and colleagues found that patients given antithymocyte globulin induction therapy showed decreased donor-specific responsiveness post-transplantation compared to patients that received IL-2 receptor blockade induction. Rather than a selective depletion of alloreactive T cells, this result may reflect the emerging concept that the repopulating T cell repertoire may be shaped by the continual presence of alloantigen in the setting of immunosuppressive therapies. Thus, while experimental studies have shown that depletion-resistant and homeostatic repopulating cells tend to be memory-like cells, they may not be allo-specific.

Non-tolerogenic immunosuppression

Most current immunosuppressants nonspecifically inhibit broad cellular pathways rather than targeting specific immune mechanisms that contribute to rejection. CNIs, such as tacrolimus and cyclosporine, are effective prophylaxis against rejection but have well-known off-target toxicities. Tacrolimus binds to FK506-binding protein, inhibiting the calcineurin-calmodulin pathway and downstream IL-2 synthesis. While tacrolimus is excellent at inhibiting T cell activation and proliferation it also blocks mechanisms of tolerance that depend on TCR signaling, such as anergy, AICD, and promotion of iTreg cells.

Rapamycin (sirolimus) may be an attractive alternative to CNIs in tolerance induction protocols. Rapamycin complexes with FK506-binding protein 12 (FKBP12) and inactivates mammalian target of rapamycin (mTOR), a key mediator of cellular differentiation, proliferation, and other physiologic cellular functions. Rapamycin has been shown to inhibit T cell proliferation, promote T cell anergy induction, inhibit DC maturation, and promote FoxP3 expression in conventional T cells. In the setting of depletional therapy, sirolimus treatment was found to attenuate effector memory T cell generation while relatively preserving Treg cells, creating a more favorable balance between effector and regulatory populations. Therefore, though CNIs are the mainstay of current maintenance regimens, rapamycin is more likely to be compatible with tolerance induction strategies.

Challenges and unresolved issues in tolerance

While many of the mechanisms described here have been used to induce long-term allograft acceptance in animal models, tolerance in clinical transplantation has been extremely difficult to achieve (Newell et al., 2006). True immunologic tolerance requires that virtually all alloreactive cells be eliminated or tolerized. Depletional strategies effectively reduce the alloreactive T cell-precursor frequency, but may be unable to contend with repopulating memory T cells or new alloreactive T cells emerging from the thymus or extra-thymic sites. CNIs are effective at controlling alloreactive naïve and memory T cells, but are not conducive to tolerance. Mixed chimerism strategies require concomitant bone marrow transplantation and preconditioning regimens still remain rigorous, even for the healthiest of patients.

Secondly, the mechanisms that are required to induce tolerance may not be the same mechanisms that are needed to maintain it. Once tolerance is established, regulation is likely to be a major mechanism in sustaining it. Costimulation blockade as maintenance therapy may facilitate ongoing anergy or AICD of peripheral alloreactive lymphocytes and thymic emigrants. However, the ever-changing landscape of the immune system renders tolerance a metastable state. Minor infections in a functionally tolerant patient may generate enough immune activation to ignite a small number of alloreactive cells and overcome the threshold for rejection.

Additionally, each organ has its own unique characteristics, and therefore, differential propensity for tolerance induction. The divergent natures of cell-based transplants, such as hematopoietic stem cells and islet cells, versus vascularized solid organ allografts suggest that these types of transplants will respond differently to various tolerance induction strategies. Within solid organ transplants the liver has remained the organ that is most susceptible to tolerance, likely because of its immune privilege. In contrast, tolerance induction will be significantly more difficult in organs that have a much higher immunogenicity, such as the small bowel.

Acknowledging the great burden and side effects of current immunosuppressive therapy there has been a surge of immunosuppression minimization protocols. A clinical alternative to true immunologic tolerance is the achievement of "prope tolerance," ("near tolerance") with functional allograft acceptance using minimal maintenance immunosuppression. The risk benefit ratio of complete cessation of immunosuppression versus minimal maintenance therapy, immunologic and drug level monitoring, potential physiologic strain during induction, and the individual patient all need to be considered carefully when implementing tolerance strategies. Whether the goal is true immunologic tolerance or prope (i.e., "near") tolerance, it would be reasonable to implement tolerance-promoting strategies as part of immunosuppression minimization protocols to enhance the likelihood of their success.

Key areas of research in tolerance
Regulatory T cells

There are still many unanswered questions regarding Treg cell biology and the optimal approach to harness the tolerogenic potential of Treg cells. The number of alloreactive natural and induced Treg cells is relatively small compared to the number of effectors generated in an alloresponse. One means of tipping the balance in favor of regulation would be to deliberately induce or expand Treg cells. There is keen interest in mechanisms that promote Treg cell survival and induction *in vivo*. Although an ideal approach may be to target and expand alloreactive nTreg cells *in vivo*, there is no way to distinguish alloreactive from non-alloreactive nTreg cells. In contrast, since iTreg cells are derived from effector T cells and possess the same antigen specificity, these may be potent donor-specific suppressors in a transplant setting. *Ex vivo* expansion of donor-specific Treg cells with subsequent infusion is being explored aggressively as a potential tolerance induction mechanism. However, iTreg cells have demonstrated lineage plasticity and have been shown to differentiate into pathologic phenotypes including CD4$^+$CD25$^-$ effectors and T$_H$17 cells in the setting of inflammatory cytokines. The features and conditions that distinguish which cells will remain suppressors from those that will differentiate into other harmful phenotypes remain unknown. The viability and stability of infused Treg cells after lengthy *ex vivo* expansion is uncertain, and these questions will need to be addressed to move Treg-based therapies into the clinic.

Biomarkers

Discovery of molecular signatures of tolerance, or biomarkers, could represent invaluable surrogate data in clinical tolerance protocols, informing clinicians of the opportunity to wean immunosuppression in carefully studied patients (Turka & Lechler, 2009). However, there are many challenges to identifying clinically applicable biomarkers. First, in kidney transplantation, spontaneous tolerance is a rare occurrence. Many spontaneously tolerant patients have discontinued immunosuppression secondary to noncompliance or serious adverse events associated with immunosuppression rather than within carefully controlled studies. Secondly, there may not be a universal tolerance signature for all patients. Tolerance signatures are likely to vary with the organ transplanted, as studies in tolerant liver and kidney patients found very different signatures. Sánchez-Fueyo and colleagues found that tolerant liver transplant patients demonstrated an increase in gene transcripts associated with NK cells and γδ T cells. In contrast, in two separate studies (Newell et al., 2010; Sagoo et al., 2010) in tolerant kidney patients, both reported an increase in peripheral B cells as well as B cell-associated gene transcripts. In addition, tolerance signatures may change with the degree of donor-recipient HLA mismatch, the type of immunosuppression given, and the etiology of organ failure. Thus, considerable work and validation still remains before biomarkers can be widely and reliably applied.

Immune privilege and accommodation

Immune privilege

The concept that certain tissues in the body were exempt or "privileged" from normal immune responses began with the observation that the immune system responded differently to allografts depending on where on the body they were placed. Immune privileged sites that show decreased responses to foreign antigens traditionally include the brain, eyes, testes, and uterus. The immune privilege of the brain and the anterior chamber of the eye were long attributed to the relatively impervious blood–tissue barrier that denies free access to these sites. However, it is now recognized that while anatomic immune sequestration may confer a degree of intrinsic immune privilege, it is one of multiple factors contributing to this phenomenon and many tissues can acquire immune privilege. Distinct from systemic immune tolerance, immune privilege now is thought to be a local, tissue-specific functional status where foreign antigens elicit an unexpectedly weak or absent immune response (Forrester et al., 2008).

Contributions from both active and passive protective mechanisms are hypothesized to determine the relative immune privilege of each tissue. Many sites of privilege demonstrate increased expression of immunomodulating molecules, including Fas ligand, TRAIL, PD-1 (programmed death PD-1), PD-2, TGF-β, IL-10 and a family of molecules that inhibit NK cells, that are likely to contribute to suppression of an immune response. Peripheral DCs that present alloantigen derived from normal homeostatic turnover may have a tolerizing effect by stochastically presenting alloantigen to alloreactive T cells in the absence of costimulation. Small numbers of DCs have a regulatory phenotype and produce indoleamine 2-3 dioxidase (IDO), an important enzyme in tryptophan metabolism. Interestingly, IDO⁺ DCs have been shown to alter T cell responses and induce antigen-specific Treg cells.

In solid organ transplantation, the liver is the organ most prone to tolerance and exhibits a unique form of immune privilege. Liver allografts seem to be relatively unaffected by positive crossmatch, ABO incompatibility, or HLA matching. Transplanted livers have a decreased incidence of hyperacute and CR, and some can spontaneously recover after severe acute rejection. Liver allografts can also protect other extrahepatic grafts derived from the same donor, suggesting that the liver can induce donor-specific hyporesponsiveness. One hypothesis is that the immune privilege of the liver stems from its chronic exposure to LPS endotoxin produced by intestinal flora. Typically, LPS is recognized by TLRs and induces a strong pro-inflammatory response. In contrast, *in vitro* studies have shown that freshly isolated Kupffer cells, which have TLRs that recognize LPS, secreted the anti-inflammatory cytokine IL-10 in response to LPS instead. This altered cytokine milieu may skew the differentiation and function of local immune cells to promote liver tolerance. Recently, there has been increased recognition that the kidney also has the capacity to immunoregulate responses directed at itself and other cotransplanted organs. The mechanisms in kidney immunomodulation are not defined but are likely related to the ability of tubular epithelial cells to engage lymphocytes and express diverse mediators including IL-6, TGFβ, IL-37, and chemokines.

Accommodation

The presence of donor-directed antibodies in the absence of allograft damage is a phenomenon known as accommodation (Lynch & Platt, 2010). This finding was initially described in ABO-incompatible kidney transplantation when recipients treated to clear blood group antibodies prior to transplant were found to have a re-emergence of anti-blood group antibodies after transplantation without apparent allograft damage. Biopsies of ABO-incompatible functioning allografts showed persistent blood group antigens on endothelial surfaces. Similar findings have been demonstrated in patients with pre-existing or *de novo* DSA and evidence of complement deposition on C4d staining. Some of these patients progressed to graft dysfunction whereas others maintained clinical function. Therefore, the coexistence of surface antigen and circulating antibodies without allograft injury suggests that unrecognized interactions between the allograft and recipient could be responsible for this seemingly paradoxical relationship.

Accommodation may phenotypically appear to be identical to classic tolerance, but distinctly differs in that an intact immune response (i.e., antibody production) remains present, whereas in classic tolerance there is an absence of immune response(s). In animal models evidence exists that support allograft resistance to injury and increased control of complement deposition. In xenotransplantation models accommodated grafts were found to have upregulated expression of CD59, a protein regulator of complement that may be important in preventing the formation of the complement membrane attack complex.

Host responses that may facilitate accommodation include changes in the functional quality of antibodies, such as class switching to isotypes that bind complement less efficiently. The type of antibody or antibody titer may also have significance. Some have hypothesized that the presence of low-affinity antibodies (i.e., ABO IgM) or sub-saturating levels of IgG may allow endothelial cells to adapt and mobilize cytoprotective and complement control mechanisms. Despite adequate graft function, accommodated grafts may still be subject to immune toxicities that contribute to poor long-term function.

Summary

While exciting discoveries in immunology have translated into new therapeutics and significant progress in clinical transplantation, the next era will need to focus on ways to extend long-term graft survival and predictably induce robust immunologic tolerance. The recent surge in the development of biologic therapies acknowledges the importance of targeting immune pathways specific to rejection, while leaving protective and homeostatic functions unperturbed. Technical advances in immune monitoring, such as DSA detection, have fostered better recipient-donor matching. Additional pretransplant immune evaluation could be expanded to include flow cytometric characterization of T cell repertoires and detection of donor-specific T cell precursor frequency and functionality. Comprehensive immune profiling may be a critical adjunct to the clinical evaluation of a patient and could more precisely determine a patient's risk for rejection, potential for tolerance, or potential responsiveness to a given therapy. As the armamentarium of therapeutic agents grows and technical innovation enhances our ability to understand and monitor the immune system, these strides forward will ultimately translate into improved patient care and propel us forward to tackle the challenges ahead.

References

Adams AB et al. Heterologous immunity provides a potent barrier to transplantation tolerance. J Clin Invest 2003; 111:1887–1895.

Billingham RE, Brent L, Medawar PB. Actively acquired tolerance of foreign cells. Nature 1953; 172:603–606.

Cornell LD, Smith RN, Colvin RB. Kidney transplantation: mechanisms of rejection and acceptance. Annu Rev Pathol Mech Dis 2008; 3:189–220.

Djamali A et al. Diagnosis and management of antibody-mediated rejection: current status and novel approaches. Am J Transplant 2014; 14:255–271.

Forrester JV, Xu H, Cornall R. Immune privilege or privileged immunity? Mucosal Immunol 2008; 1:382–381.

Griesemer AD, Sorenson EC, Hardy MA. The role of the thymus in tolerance. Transplantation 2010; 90:465–474.

Hori S, Nomura T, Sakaguchi S. Control of regulatory T cell development by the transcription factor FoxP3. Science 2003; 299:1057–1061.

Kawai T et al. HLA-mismatched renal transplantation without maintenance immunosuppression. N Engl J Med 2008; 358:353–361.

Kirk AD, Turgeon N, Iwakoshi N. B cells and transplantation tolerance. Nat Rev Nephrol 2010; 6:584–593.

Larsen CP et al. Long-term acceptance of skin and cardiac allografts after blocking CD40 and CD28 pathways. Nature 1996; 381:434–438.

Lynch RJ, Platt JL. Accommodation in renal transplantation: unanswered questions. Curr Opin Organ Transplant 2010; 15:481–485.

Newell KA, Larsen CP, Kirk AD. Transplant tolerance: converging on a moving target. Transplantation 2006; 81:1–6.

Newell KA et al. Identification of a B cell signature associated with renal transplant tolerance in humans. J Clin Invest 2010; 120(6):1836–1847.

Pilat N, Wekerle T. Transplantation tolerance through mixed chimerism. Nat Rev Nephrol 2010; 6:5994–605.

Sagoo P et al. Development of a cross-platform biomarker signature to detect renal transplant tolerance in humans. J Clin Invest 2010; 120(6):1848–1861.

Turka LA, Lechler RI. Towards the identification of biomarkers of transplantation tolerance. Nat Rev Immunol 2009; 9:521–526.

Vincenti F et al. A phase III study of belatacept-based immunosuppression regimens versus cyclosporine in renal transplant recipients. Am J Transplant 2010; 10:535–546.

Wood KJ, Bushnell A, Hester J. Regulatory immune cells in transplantation. Nat Rev Immunol 2012; 12:417–430.
Wu Z et al. Homeostatic repopulation is a barrier to transplant tolerance. Nat Med 2004; 10:87–92.

Further reading

Afzali B, Lomardi G, Lechler RI. Pathways of major histocompatibility complex allorecognition. Curr Opin Organ Transplant 2008; 13:438–444.
Chalasani G et al. Recall and propagation of allospecific memory T cells independent of secondary lymphoid organs. Proc Natl Acad Sci USA 2002; 9:6175–6180.
Murphy SP, Porrett PM, Turka LA. Innate immunity in transplant tolerance and rejection. Immunol Rev 2011; 241:39–48.

CHAPTER 9

Principles of hematopoietic cell transplantation

Sung Choi and Pavan Reddy

Blood and Marrow Transplantation Program, Department of Internal Medicine, Division of Hematology/Oncology, University of Michigan Comprehensive Cancer Center, Ann Arbor, USA

CHAPTER OVERVIEW

- The indications and process of hematopoietic cell transplantation
- The complications of HCT
- Graft-versus-host disease (GVHD): the role of human leukocyte antigen matching
- Induction and effector phase of GVHD
- Limitations of models and current gaps in GVHD biology

Introduction

Hematopoietic cell transplantation (HCT) allows for the replacement of an abnormal lympho-hematopoietic system with a normal one. It is a definitive therapy for many malignant and nonmalignant diseases (Table 9.1).The development of novel strategies that use donor leukocyte infusions (DLIs), nonmyeloablative conditioning, and umbilical cord blood transplantation (CBT) have expanded the indications for allogeneic HCT over the past several years, especially among older patients. Improvements in the treatment of infection prophylaxis, immunosuppressive medications, supportive care and DNA-based human leukocyte antigen (HLA)-tissue typing have collectively contributed to improved outcomes after allogeneic HCT (Gooley et al., 2010). While the number of allogeneic HCT continues to increase with more than 20,000 allogeneic HCTs performed annually, graft-versus-host disease (GVHD) remains a major complication of allogeneic HCT, limiting its broader application. Depending on the timeframe following allogeneic HCT, GVHD can be either acute or chronic. Acute GVHD is assessed

---

Transplant Immunology, First Edition. Edited by Xian Chang Li and Anthony M. Jevnikar.
© 2016 John Wiley & Sons, Ltd. Published 2016 by John Wiley & Sons, Ltd.
Copyright ® American Society of Transplantation 2016.
Companion website: www.wiley.com/go/li/transplantimmunology

Table 9.1 Indications for allogeneic hematopoietic cell transplantation.

1. Hematologic malignancies
   a. Acute and chronic leukemias
   b. Myeloproliferative disorders
2. Solid tumors
   a. Hodgkin's lymphoma
   b. Non-Hodgkin's lymphoma
3. Bone marrow failure sndromes (BMFS)
   a. Aplastic anemia
   b. Myelodysplastic syndrome
   c. Inherited BMFS (e.g., Diamond–Blackfan anemia, Dyskeratosis congenital, Fanconi anemia,
      Severe congenital anemia, Schwachmann–Diamond syndrome, Diamond–Blackfan anemia)
4. Immunologic disorders
   a. Severe congenital immunodeficiency disorder
   b. Wiscott–Aldrich syndrome
5. Other blood or metabolic disorders
   a. Sickle cell anemia
   b. Thalassemia
   c. Gaucher disease

according to the modified Glucksberg criteria (Table 9.2) (Przepiorka et al., 1995). It is responsible for 15–40% of transplant-related mortality and remains the major cause of morbidity after allogeneic HCT, while chronic GVHD occurs in up to 50% of patients who survive beyond the first 3 months after HCT (Weiden et al., 1979).

Three requirements for the development of GVHD were formulated by Billingham (Billingham, 1966). First, the bone marrow graft must contain mature T cells. In both experimental and clinical allogeneic HCT, the severity of GVHD correlates with the number of donor T cells transfused. Second, the recipient must be incapable of rejecting the transplanted cells, that is, an immuno-compromised host. A patient with a normal immune system will usually reject cells from a foreign donor, while in an allogeneic transplant setting the recipient is prevented from doing so by immunosuppression prior to the hematopoietic cell infusion. Third, the recipient must express tissue antigens that are not present in the donor. Over the years, we have gained considerable insights into the biology of this complex disease process. Herein, we will summarize the current understanding of the pathophysiology of acute GVHD in the context of Billingham's principles, followed by a discussion on potential therapeutic strategies.

Principles of HCT

The hematopoietic stem cell (HSC) is phenotypically and clinically defined as $CD34^+$ marrow cells lacking known myeloid or lymphoid lineage markers (Korngold & Sprent, 1987). The features of HSC that make clinical transplantation

Table 9.2 Staging and grading of acute graft-versus-host disease (GVHD).

Stage	Skin	Liver (bilirubin)	Gut (stool output/day)
0	No GVHD rash	<2 mg/dl	Adult: <500 ml/day
1	Maculopapular rash<25% BSA	2–3	Adult: 500–999 ml/day or persistent nausea, vomiting, or anorexia, with a positive upper GI biopsy
2	Maculopapular rash 25–50% BSA	3.1–6	Adult: 1000–1500 ml/day
3	Maculopapular rash>50% BSA	6.1–15	Adult: >1500 ml/day
4	Generalized erythoderma plus bullous formation and desquamation>5% BSA	>15	Severe abdominal pain with or without ileus, or grossly bloody stool (regardless of stool volume)

- For GI staging: the "adult" stool output values should be used for patients greater than or equal to 50 kg in weight
- Three day averages for GI staging based on stool output. If stool and urine are mixed, stool output is estimated to be 50% of total stool/urine mix.
- For stage 4 GI: the term "severe abdominal pain" will be defined as:
- Pain control requiring institution of opioid use, or an increase in on-going opioid use. PLUS
  (a) Pain that significantly impacts performance status, as determined by the treating physician.
  (b) If colon or rectal biopsy is positive, but stool output is <500 ml/day (<10 ml/kg·day), then consider as GI stage 0.
- There is no modification of liver staging for other causes of hyperbilirubinemia.

Source: Przepiorka et al. (1995).
Overall Clinical Grade:
  Grade 0 No stage 1–4 of any organ.
  Grade 1: Stage 1–2 rash and no liver or gut involvement.
  Grade 2: Stage 3 rash, or Stage 1 liver involvement, or Stage 1 GI.
  Grade 3: Stage 0–3 skin, with Stage 2–3 liver, or Stage 2–3 GI.
  Grade 4: Stage 4 skin, liver or GI involvement.

feasible are their regenerative capacity, ability to home to the marrow space after intravenous infusion, and capacity to survive cryopreservation. These characteristics facilitate complete and sustained replacement of the patient's lympho-hematopoietic system, including red cells, platelets, white cells, and tissue-resident moncyte/macrophages, such as pulmonary alveolar macrophages, Kupffer cells of the liver, osteoclasts, and Langerhans cells of the skin. Following intravenous infusion, a significant percentage of HSCs are retained in the marrow through interactions between integrins expressed on the surface of these cells and the adhesion molecules on vascular endothelial cells in the marrow.

HSCs for transplantation are described according to the relationship between the donor and recipient and according to their anatomic source. When the donor is identical to the recipient, the HCT is called syngeneic (identical). In allogeneic HCT, HSCs are provided by a nonidentical donor. The donors can be members either related or unrelated to the patients. Regardless, with this type of HCT, there is a risk of both graft rejection, such as in solid organ transplants and GVHD. Thus, HCTs are almost always performed with immunosuppressive drugs. Depending on whether the donors are matched for major histocompatibility complex (MHC) antigens, the HCT can be further characterized as MHC-matched or MHC-mismatched allogeneic HCT.

The primary sources of HSCs are typically from the bone marrow or peripheral blood. The HSCs from the peripheral blood are harvested by apheresis following the administration of hematopoietic growth factors such as granulocyte colony-stimulating factor (G-CSF) or granulocyte/macrophage colony-stimulating factor (GM-CSF). Most centers aim to infuse a HSC dose of 5.0×10^6 CD34$^+$ cells per kilogram of body weight. In patients who do not have matched related or unrelated donors, cord blood (CB) is being increasingly used as the source of HSCs (a total nucleated cell dose of $2.5 \times 10^7 \mathrm{kg}^{-1}$ or $2.0 \times 10^5 \mathrm{kg}^{-1}$ CD34$^+$ cells). HSCs are often infused without depleting other immune cells, in which the T cells are responsible for the immune reconstitution and GVH responses.

Prior to HSC infusion, a conditioning regimen is administered to the patient in order to eradicate the patient's disease and, in the case of allogeneic transplantation, to also provide adequate immunosuppression to prevent rejection of the graft (Figure 9.1: phase 1). The appropriate regimen for any particular patient is determined according to the nature of the disease, the source of stem cells, and the patient's overall health. For example, a conditioning regimen may not be required in the treatment of Severe Combined Immune Deficiency (SCID) using matched sibling marrow. Generally, there are no abnormal cells to eliminate, and the primary immunodeficiency of the patient prevents rejection of the graft cells. In contrast, in patients with hematologic malignancies, the type and intensity of the conditioning regimens are designed based on the presumed sensitivity of the particular malignancy. Although more aggressive regimens have typically been used in transplants for malignancies, the observation that much of the antitumor/leukemic effect of transplantation derives from allogeneic graft-versus-leukemia (GVL) effect (Weiden et al., 1979) has led to the development of less intensive or nonablative regimens that are as effective and more tolerable. This innovation has allowed for increased application of allogeneic HCT to the elderly and to those who have decreased performance status.

Following HCT, with proper preparation and matching, the donor HSCs engraft, which is clinically reflected by the peripheral blood counts. The neutrophils are the first to engraft and they typically begin to increase within 10–14 days after transplantation (Figure 9.1: phases 2–3). If bone marrow is the source of stem cells, the granulocyte count reaches 100 mm^{-3} by days 14–16 and 1000 mm^{-3} by about day 23–28. Platelet recovery occurs slightly after granulocytes. The use of methotrexate as part of GVHD prophylaxis may delay

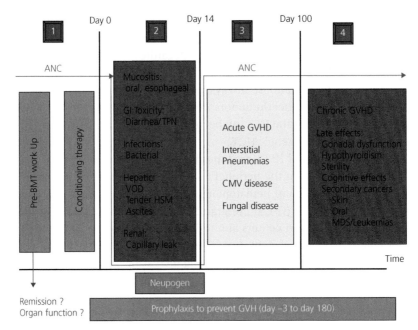

Figure 9.1 Four phases of allogeneic hematopoietic cell transplantation (HCT). The
average length of hospital stay for patients undergoing allogeneic HCT is approximately 28–35
days, characterized by four phases: (1) the conditioning regimen, (2) myelosuppression, (3)
deconditioning, and (4) cell count recovery. The conditioning regimen administered during
Phase 1 leads to a decline in counts of white blood cells, hemoglobin, and platelets
(myelosuppression), increasing the risk of painful mucositis, bleeding complications, organ
toxicities, and life-threatening infections (Phase 2). It is not uncommon for HCT patients to
require intravenous narcotics and total parenteral nutrition for effective pain and nutrition
management, respectively. The risk of acute GVHD and infectious complications increase during
Phase 3, which is then followed by risk of chronic GVHD and other late effects in Phase 4.

engraftment by a few days, whereas the use of a myeloid growth factor (G-CSF
or CM-CSF) may accelerate engraftment. Allogeneic HCT is commonly performed under the cover of immunosuppression, primarily with calcineurin
inhibitors (CNIs) such as cyclosporine or tacrolimus to prevent rejection and
GVHD. CNIs are often combined with either methotrexate or mycophenolate
mofetil or rapamycin early after HCT.

Complications of HCT:

(a) **Conditioning regimen-related complications:** The immediate toxicities
vary according to the specific agents used, but usually include nausea, vom-
iting, rash, and diarrhea. The patients are at risk for potentially serious complications as a result of pancytopenia (infection and bleeding) before
engraftment is complete. Most patients also develop oral mucositis during
the neutropenic phase and alopecia (Figure 9.1: phase 2). Certain complications result from the specific agent used, for example, hemorrhagic cystitis

from the use of high-dose cytoxan. In addition, two specific complications occur in patients that receive myeloablative regimens, namely, veno-occlusive disease (VOD) of the liver and idiopathic pneumonia syndrome (IPS). VOD of the liver occurs within 1–4 weeks after transplant in approximately 10% of patients and presents as a syndrome of ascites, tender hepatomegaly, and jaundice. VOD is treated with supportive care, although recent studies suggest that defibrotide may be beneficial. IPS is seen in 5–10% of patients between 28 and 90 days after transplant. IPS is also treated supportively and generally has poor outcomes (Figure 9.1: phase 3).

(b) **Infectious complications**: Most patients develop granulocytopenia and fever during the first 2 or 3 weeks post transplant. Positive blood cultures (mostly gram positive) are found in about one-third of patients (Figure 9.1: phase 2). In most centers, prophylactic antibiotics are used to treat febrile granulocytopenic patients. Following engraftment, most centers use prophylaxis, including fluconazole, against invasive fungal infections, sulfa-based drugs for Pneumocystis carinii, and acyclovir for herpes zoster. The most significant infections that occur in the interval between successful engraftment and day 100 include aspergillus, cytomegalovirus (CMV), and respiratory syncytial virus (RSV) disease (Figure 9.1: phase 3). Approximately 75% of patients with detectable antibody to CMV pre-transplant have some evidence of CMV activation post-transplant. Ganciclovir is administered pre-emptively or for the treatment of clinical disease. Prolonged immunosuppression from GVHD and its treatment enhances the risk substantially for CMV, for fungal as well as bacterial infections.

(c) **Immune-related complications:** The primary immune-related complications are rejection of the donor graft by the host immune system (graft failure) or GVHD with attack of the host by the engrafted donor immune system (Figure 9.1: phase 3–4). The risk of rejection is relatively low (<5%) with current preparative regimens and immunosuppression, along with adequate infusions of HSCs. Risk of graft failure increases substantially when insufficient HSC numbers are infused, as in the case of CBT.

GVHD: Principles

Genetic basis of GVHD

Billingham's third postulate stipulates that the GVH reaction occurs when donor immune cells recognize disparate host antigens. These differences are governed by the genetic polymorphisms of HLA and non-HLA systems.

(a) **HLA matching:** Alloreactive T-cell activation in the setting of HSC can occur whether the presenting MHC molecule is matched or mismatched. Although covered elsewhere in greater detail, briefly, human MHC is composed of HLA antigens encoded by the MHC gene complex on the short arm of chromosome 6 and are broadly divided into class I, II and III regions by their products. Class I antigens (HLA-A, B, and C) are expressed on almost all cells of the body, while class II antigens (DR, DQ, and DP) are primarily expressed on hematopoietic cells, although their expression can be induced on other cell types following inflammation. In contrast to solid organ transplants in which matching may have less immediate impact, the incidence of acute GVHD in HCT is directly related to the degree of MHC mismatching (Flomenberg et al., 2004). The role of HLA mismatching in CBT is more difficult to analyze compared to unrelated donor HCT, as allele typing of CB units for HLA-A, B, C, DRB1, and DQB1 is not routinely performed. Nonetheless, the total number of HLA disparities between the recipient and the CB unit has been shown to correlate with risk of acute GVHD as the frequency of acute GVHD is lower in patients transplanted with HLA-matched (6/6) CB units (Flomenberg et al., 2004).

(b) **Minor histocompatibility antigens:** In MHC-matched allogeneic transplants, which represent the usual situation clinically, donor-derived T cells can recognize MHC-bound peptides derived from the protein products of polymorphic genes (minor histocompatibility antigens or MiHAs) that are present in the host, but not in the donor (Goulmy et al., 1996). A significant number (40%) of patients will develop acute GVHD despite receiving HLA-identical grafts as well as optimal immune suppression. MiHAs are widely expressed, but can differ in their tissue expression. This might be one of the reasons for the unique target organ involvement in GVHD. A preponderance of MiHAs, such as HA-1 and HA-2, are expressed on hematopoietic cells, which might account for making the host immune system a primary target for the GVH response and may also account for the critical role of direct presentation by recipient antigen-presenting cells (APCs) in causing anti-tumor and GVHD responses. By contrast, other MiHAs, such as H-Y and HA-3, are ubiquitously expressed. MiHAs are not equal in their ability to induce lethal GVHD and instead show hierarchical dominance. Furthermore, the difference in single immuno-dominant MiHAs alone is not insufficient for causing GVHD in murine models, although T cells targeting single MiHAs can induce tissue damage in a skin explant model (Fontaine et al., 2001). The role of specific and immuno-dominant MiHAs that are relevant in clinical GVHD has not been systematically evaluated in large groups of patients.

(c) **Other non-HLA genes:** Genetic polymorphisms in several non-HLA genes such as in killer-cell immunoglobulin-like receptors (KIRs), cytokines, and nucleotide-binding oligomerization-domain containing 2 (NOD2) genes have recently been shown to modulate the severity and incidence of GVHD.

KIRs on natural killer (NK) cells that bind to the HLA class I gene products are encoded on chromosome 19. Polymorphisms in the trans-membrane and cytoplasmic domains of KIRs govern whether the receptor has inhibitory (i.e., KIR2DL1, -2DL2, -2DL3, and 3DL1) or activating potential. Two competing models have been proposed for HLA-KIR allo-recognition by donor NK cells following allogeneic HCT: "missing self" and the "missing ligand" models. Both models are supported by several clinical observations (Ruggeri et al., 2002).

Pro-inflammatory cytokines, involved in the classical "cytokine storm" of GVHD (discussed later), cause pathologic damage to target organs, typically the skin, liver, and gastrointestinal (GI) tract. Several cytokine gene polymorphisms, in recipients and donors, have been implicated. Specifically, tumor necrosis factor (TNF) polymorphisms (TNFd3/d3 in the recipient, TNF-863 and -857 in donors and/or recipients and TNFd4, TNF-α-1031C and TNFRII-196R- in the donors) have been associated with an increased risk of acute GVHD (Antin & Ferrara, 1992). The three common haplotypes of the interleukin-10 (IL-10) gene promoter region in recipients, representing high, intermediate, and low production of IL-10, have been associated with severity of acute GVHD following HLA-matched sibling donor allogeneic HCT. By contrast, smaller studies have found neither IL-10 nor TNF-α polymorphisms to be associated with GVHD following HLA-mismatched CBT. Interferon-gamma (IFN-γ) polymorphisms of the 2/2 genotype (high IFN-γ production) and 3/3 genotype (low IFN-γ) have been associated with decreased and increased acute GVHD, respectively (Lin et al., 2003).

NOD-2 and caspase-activating recruitment domain 15 (CARD15) gene polymorphisms in both the donors and recipients were recently shown to have a striking association between GI GVHD and overall mortality following related and unrelated donor allogeneic HCT. Taken together, it is likely that non-HLA gene polymorphisms play different roles in GVHD depending on the donor source (related vs. unrelated), HLA disparity (matched vs. mismatched), graft source (CB vs. BM vs. peripheral blood stem cells), and the intensity of the conditioning (Paczesny et al., 2010).

Immunobiology of acute GVHD

GVHD can be considered as a complex immune process that consists of: (a) triggers, (b) sensors, (c) mediators, and (d) effectors (Figure 9.2).

Triggers for GVHD

Like all immune responses, certain triggers are critical for the induction of acute GVHD. These include:

1. **Genetic disparities that include HLA** and the non-HLA factors, which have been discussed and outlined earlier.
2. **Nongenetic factors,** which are related to damage induced by conditioning regimens and underlying diseases.

Under most circumstances, the initiation of adaptive immune responses is triggered or augmented by early innate immune responses, which are triggered by exogenous and endogenous molecules in the context of sterile or nonsterile

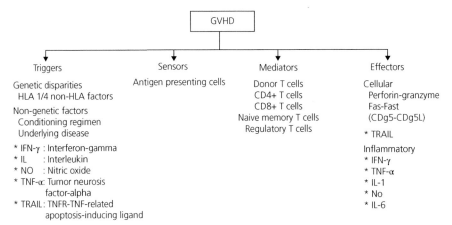

Figure 9.2 Immunobiology of acute GVHD. Acute graft-versus-host disease (GVHD) can be understood by triggers that are critical for its induction, APCs that sense allodisparity, donor T cells that mediate its pathogenesis, and cellular and inflammatory effectors that amplify GVHD, leading to target organ injury of the skin, liver, and/or gastrointestinal tract.

tissue injury and inflammation. This is likely the case in the induction of acute GVHD. Pathogen-associated molecular patterns (PAMPs) from the endogenous microflora initiate cell signaling pathways that activate cytokine secretion. PAMPs, such as lipopolysaccharide (LPS), muramyl dipeptides (MDP), and other Toll-like receptor (TLR) and nucleotide-binding oligomerization domain (NOD)-like agonists are released during the chemo- and radio-therapeutic conditioning regimens. In this way, the conditioning regimens amplify the secretion of pro-inflammatory cytokines, such as IL-1, TNFα, and IL-6, described as a "cytokine storm" (Hill et al., 1997).

NOD2 recognizes MDP, which is an important structure of bacterial pepti-doglycan. Single nucleotide polymorphisms in the NOD2 gene locus have been associated with increased risk of Crohn's disease and also of GVHD, both conditions characterized by intestinal inflammation. Therefore, the role of NOD2 was recently examined in experimental models of GVHD. While NOD2 deficiency of donor T cells or bone marrow did not impact GVHD, NOD2 deficiency in recipients increased GVHD through enhanced alloreactive T cell responses by host APCs (Penack et al., 2009). Intestinal stem cells (ISCs) have been described as targets of GVHD, damaged by direct insult from the pre-HCT conditioning regimen. Given the role of Wnt signaling in intestinal epithelial cell proliferation, R-spondin1 (R-Spo1) was tested in allogeneic BMT. R-Spo1, an activator of the Wnt pathway, stimulated ISC proliferation and protected against conditioning-induced gastrointestinal damage (Takashima et al., 2011). These findings demonstrated a critical role of ISCs in GVHD. Investigators have also studied the role of inflammation (GVHD) on the intestinal microbiota after allogeneic HCT. Prior to onset of GVHD, flora diversity was similar to controls.

This was lost, however, after GVHD. Additionally, there were increases in *Lactobacillales* and decreases in *Clostridiale*, but these changes were not observed in the absence of GVHD.

IL-22 has recently been reported to regulate inflammatory conditions, given its protective effects in the intestinal epithelium. In allogeneic HCT, recipient mice deficient in IL-22 had significantly increased apoptosis in crypts, damage to the intestinal stem cell compartment, and loss of epithelial integrity. Consistent with studies in inflammatory bowel disease and colitis, IL-22 demonstrated cyto-protective effects during GVHD (Hanash et al., 2012). In another study exploring the role of intestinal microbiota in GVHD, the investigators focused on Paneth cells, which are located within the crypts of ISCs (Eriguchi et al., 2012). Paneth cells secrete α-defensins, providing antimicrobial properties. During GVHD, Paneth cells were damaged, α-defense in expression was decreased, and E. coli levels were elevated, leading to systemic infection and increased gastrointestinal pathology (Eriguchi et al., 2012). This study extends the important role of ISCs and intestinal flora change in GVHD. More recently, neutrophil infiltration within the mouse GI tract (ileum) was analyzed after allogeneic HCT by myelop-eroxidase imaging. Tissue damage by neutrophils appeared to be associated with reactive oxygen species production. Interestingly, neutrophils lacking TLR2, 3, 4, 7, and 9 had decreased GVHD, suggesting its potential contribution to GVHD (Schwab et al., 2014).

In addition to the exogenous microbial-associated molecules, endogenous triggers as a consequence of damage, known as damage-associated molecular patterns (DAMPs), might also play a critical role in GVHD. In fact, the pro-inflammatory cytokines themselves might serve as DAMPs. As such, the type of damage (apoptosis *vs* necrosis) and the specific DAMPs will be relevant, but remain poorly understood. ATP has been described as an endogenous danger signal in the activation of $P2X_7R$, contributing to GVHD pathogenesis. It has been shown that ATP binding to $P2X_7R$ can cause the assembly and activation of the protein 3 (Nlrp3)-inflammasone. The activation of this inflammasone by uric acid (DAMP) increased GVHD severity by mediating IL-1β production (Jankovic et al., 2013). By contrast, sialic acid-binding immunoglobulin-like lectins (Siglecs) mediate inhibitory signals as an antagonist of DAMPs. Recent work showed that expression of Siglec-G was downregulated by tissue damage, increasing its impact by DAMPs. However, this was attenuated through the Siglec-G-CD24 axis with a CD24 fusion protein, thereby interfering with DAMP effects and decreasing GVHD (Toubai et al., 2014).

Sensors of GVHD
APCs might be considered the sensors for acute GVHD. The APCs sense DAMPs, present the MHC-disparate or miHA-disparate protein, and provide the critical secondary (costimulatory) and tertiary (cytokine) signals for activation of the alloreactive T cells, the mediators of acute GVHD (Figure 9.3).

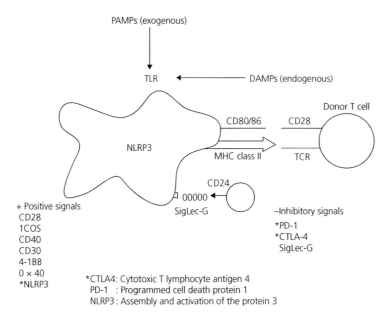

Figure 9.3 Sensors of GVHD. Antigen presenting cells sense pathogen-associated molecular patterns (PAMPs or exogenous microbial associated molecules) and damage-associated molecular patterns (DAMPs or endogenous triggers, such as protelytic products, ATP, ions, uric acid, HMGB1, S100 protein family, and oxidized lipoprotein). The interaction between the MHC complex on APCs and the T-cell receptor (TCR) on T cells and other co-stimulatory molecules and their ligands on APCs lead to T cell activation, proliferation, differentiation, and survival. These interactions are regulated positively or negatively by numerous cytokines, chemokines, and other immune cell subsets.

Pathways of antigen presentation: APCs allow sensing of allo-disparity through MHC and peptide complexes. Dendritic cells (DCs) are the most potent APCs and primary "sensors" of allo-disparity. Recipient DCs that have been primed by the conditioning regimen can process and present MHC and peptide complexes to donor T cells at the time of transplant (Shlomchik et al., 1999). At later time points, donor DCs may take over this role (Reddy et al., 2005). Donor APC-derived IL-23 has recently been shown to play an important role in the pathophysiology of GVHD. Langerhans cells (LCs) may also be sufficient for the induction of skin GVHD. However, when other types of host APCs were intact, GVHD was similar in LC-deficient and LC-sufficient recipients, suggesting that LCs may be conditional in GVHD (Paczesny et al., 2010).

Different modes of antigen presentation have also been described. In allogeneic HCT, recipient DCs present endogenous and exogenous antigens to donor CD8+ and CD4+T cells, respectively (direct antigen presentation). Exogenous antigens are also presented to donor CD8+ T cells by MHC class I or donor CD4+ T cells by MHC class II expressed by donor DCs via an indirect pathway. Traditionally, the MHC class I and class II pathways were thought to be independent, but recent studies suggest that endogenous antigens released by lysosomal ruptures through a mechanism known as autophagy can be presented to CD4+ T-cells via the class II pathway. We now know that there is no predilection for allo-peptides to be recognized by either CD4+ or CD8+ mediated presentation. Interestingly, recipient B cells were recently examined, which were not found to have a major impact on GVHD induced by CD4+ or CD8+ T cells (Paczesny et al., 2010).

Both subsets of dermal DCs (CD1a⁺ and CD14⁺) in recipients have been shown to be rapidly depleted and replaced by donor cells. They induce cytokine expression in memoryCD4⁺ T cells as well as in the activation and proliferation of CD8⁺ T cells, suggesting that they contribute to GVHD by sustaining the alloreactive responses of previously activated T cells. However, kinetics of the switch from recipient to donor APCs, contributions of different APCs subsets, importance of direct alloantigen presentation, and magnitude of indirect alloantigen presentation in GVHD remain to be determined. Recently, plasmacytoid dendritic cells (pDCs) have received interest because of their tolerogenic role. However, the impact of pDCs in acute GVHD remains unclear and additional studies are needed. A novel molecular pathway, the Ikaros-Notch axis, was investigated and found to have importance in DC biology and be critical in host hematopoietic-derived APCs for modulating GVHD responses (Paczesny et al., 2010).

Costimulation: As noted, APC provide critical costimulation signals for "turning on" the acute GVHD process. The interaction between the MHC-allopeptide complex on APCs and the T cell receptor (TCR) of donor T cells is insufficient to induce T cell activation. A second signal via T cell costimulatory molecules and their ligands on APCs is required to achieve T cell activation, proliferation, differentiation, and survival. *In vivo* blockade of positive costimulatory molecules reduces acute GVHD, (Blazar et al., 1994) while blockade of inhibitory signals exacerbates acute GVHD in murine models (Table 9.3).

Modulation of APC functions in GVHD: In addition to inflammatory cytokines and DAMP ligands that influence GVHD, other factors can modulate APC functions. Exposure to granulocyte colony-stimulating factor (G-CSF) shortly after allogeneic HCT, in combination with a total body irradiation (TBI) regimen, was recently shown to significantly worsen GVHD in mice. TBI rendered host DCs responsive to G-CSF by upregulating the expression of the G-CSF receptor. Stimulation of host DCs by G-CSF subsequently activated a cascade of events characterized by donor NKT cell activation, IFN-γ secretion and amplification of donor cytotoxic T lymphocyte (CTL) function during the effector phase of GVHD. These data may explain the increased incidence of GVHD seen in patients receiving prophylactic G-CSF (Paczesny et al., 2010).

Table 9.3 Constimulatory pathways.

	T cell	**APC**
Adhesion	ICAMs	LFA-I
	LFA-1	ICAMs
	CD2 (LFA-2)	LFA-3
Recognition	TCR/CD4	NIIIC hi
	TCR/CD8	Mi-Icc I
Costimulation	CD28	CD80/86
	CD152 (CTLA-4	CD80/86
	ICOS	B7H/B7RP-1
	PD-1	PD-L1, PD-L2
	Unknown	B7-H3
	CD154 (CD40L)	CD40
	OX40	OX4OL
	4-1BB	4-1BBL
	HVEM	LIGHT
	CD24	Siglec-G

HVEM HSV glycoprotein D for herpes virus entry mediator; LIGHT, homologous to lymphotoxins, shows inducible expression, and competes with herpes simplex virus glycoprotein D for herpes virus entry mediator (HVEM), a receptor expressed by I lymphocytes.

Indoleamine 2,3-dioxygenase (IDO) plays an important role in tryptophan catabolism and has been shown to be critical for immune tolerance. Histone deacetylase inhibitors, such as suberonylanilide hydroxamic acid (SAHA; vorinostat), have been shown to reduce GVHD in murine models through the induction of IDO in a STAT-3-dependent manner (Figure 9.4). Vorinostat was recently tested in a Phase 1/2 clinical trial, which showed that reduction in grade 2–4 acute GVHD following related donor, reduced the intensity of the conditioning allogeneic HCT (Choi et al., 2014).

Recent studies have also shown that several innate and adaptive immune cell subsets negatively affect the functions of APCs. For example, (i) host gamma-delta (γδ) T cells, which are cells commonly found in the GI tract and skin, are associated with reduced APC activation and suppressed GVHD in MHC-mismatched mouse models; (ii) NK cells, which are inhibited by the recognition of class I alleles on target cells via KIRs, downregulate APC-mediated activation of T cells by directly killing APCs. NK cells have been shown to mitigate GVHD and retain GVL responses by inhibiting alloreactive T cells; (iii) NKT cells: Host NKT cells can negatively regulate APCs' interactions with donor T cells in a Th2-dependent manner. In contrast, donor NKT cells activate this response. Interestingly, low doses of adoptively transferred donor NKT cells have been shown to suppress GVHD by decreasing the production of IFN- γ and TNF-α in an IL-4-dependent mechanism; and (iv) B cells: The role of B cells in acute GVHD is currently under investigation, particularly regarding their possible role in attenuating GVHD.

Mediators of GVHD

Donor T cells are the critical mediators of acute GVHD regardless of the type of antigen severity. The alloantigen composition of the host determines which donor T cells subsets differentiate and proliferate to become effector cells.

CD4+ and CD8+ T cells: CD4 and CD8 are the coreceptors for MHC class II and class I receptors, respectively. As mentioned previously, in the majority of HLA-matched allogeneic HCTs, acute GVHD may be induced by either or both CD4+ and CD8+ subsets. The repertoire and immuno-dominance of the GVHD-associated peptides presented by MHC class I and class II molecules have not been clearly defined. One approach to retaining the beneficial GVL effects while eliminating the negative effects of GVHD is to selectively deplete subsets of donor alloreactive T cells in the hematopoietic cell inoculums using a TCR Vß repertoire analysis with CDR3-size spectra typing. It has been shown that GVL in allogeneic recipients could be restored without GVHD induction when the adoptive transfer of TCR-transduced allogeneic CD8+ T cells was given in combination with PD-L1 blockade (Paczesny et al., 2010).

Naïve and memory T cells: T cells in murine models can be categorized into naïve (CD62L+CD44-), central memory (CD62L+CD44+), and effector effector memory (CD62L-CD44+) subsets. Donor naïve CD62L+ T cells are the primary alloreactive T cells that drive the GVHD reaction while the donor effector memory CD62L-T cells do not (Anderson et al., 2003). It is possible to modulate the alloreactivity of naïve T cells by inducing anergy with costimulation blockade, deletion via cytokine modulation, or mixed chimerism. Donor effector memory T cells that are nonalloreactive do not induce GVHD, and yet are able to transfer functional memory (Anderson et al., 2003) and mediate GVL. In addition, lymphopenia-induced proliferation gives rise to cells that are memory-like T cells and enhance the GVL effect after DLI. In contrast, memory T cells that are alloreactive and donor specific can cause severe GVHD. However, it has been demonstrated that enhancing the alloreactivity of effector memory T cells can cause GVHD, which is much less severe and possibly more transient in nature (Paczesny et al., 2010). These findings may be better understood with further analyses that define tracking of alloantigen-specific T cells (naïve,

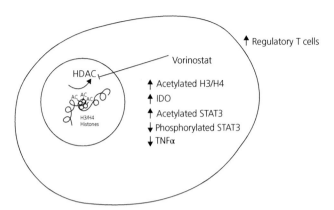

Figure 9.4 Histone deacetylase inhibition and GVHD. Vorinostat combined with standard GVHD prophylaxis in the related donor reduced intensity conditioning setting has been shown to reduce the incidence of grade 2–4 acute GVHD by day 100 post-HCT. This correlated with significantly increased acetylated H3/H4 histones, indoleamine-2,3-dioxygenase (IDO), signal transducer and activator of transcription 3 (STAT-3), decreased phosphorylated STAT-3, increased regulatory T cells, and increased plasma levels of tumor necrosis factor-alpha (TNF-α).

central memory, and effector memory subsets) in experimental GVHD and GVL models with defined TCR repertoires.

Regulatory T cells (Tregs): Distinct subsets of regulatory T cells exist: the naturally occurring CD4+CD25+ Tregs that express the Forkhead Protein P3 (FOXP3), CD4+CD25-IL10+ Tr cells, γδ T cells, double negative (DN) T cells, and NKT cells. In mice, naturally occurring Tregs develop in the thymus, prevent autoimmunity, and suppress pathology inflicted by uncontrolled immune responses. Naturally occurring donor-derived Tregs suppress the proliferation of conventional T cells, prevent GVHD, and preserve GVL effects depending upon the ratio of effector T cells to Tregs (Edinger et al., 2003; Taylor et al., 2002). Furthermore, viral immunity is preserved in the presence of Tregs after allogeneic HCT. The mechanisms for suppression in the context of GVHD remain completely unknown. The influence between host NKT cells and host IL-4 on the accumulation of donor Tregs has been shown to protect against GVHD. Importantly, clinical trials exploiting the properties of Tregs for the suppression of GVHD are ongoing, but isolation and expansion of human Tregs remain challenging and labor-intensive. The stability of Foxp3 expression limits the ability of adoptively transfused Tregs to attenuate GVHD. A novel approach to prevent acute GVHD in the allogeneic HCT setting would be to manipulate the immune system to take advantage of important T cell interactions, specifically involving NKT cells and Tregs. Advances in Treg biology may provide therapies that favorably impact the overall outcome of allogeneic HCT. CD4+ DLI combined with low-dose recombinant IL-2 has recently been shown to expand Tregs *in vivo* following allogeneic HCT. Adaptive IL-10-secreting Tr1 also promoted tolerance in GVHD via IL-10 or TGFß release, or possibly contact-mediated inhibition of cell growth. Although IL-10 and IDO have been implicated in Treg-mediated responses, alloantigen expression by host APCs has been shown to be sufficient and necessary for GVHD suppression by donor Tregs, independent of IL-10 or IDO production by host APCs (Paczesny et al., 2010).

Th subsets: Based on the dominant cytokines that are produced upon activation, CD4+ T cells can be characterized by various subsets namely Th1, Th2, and Th17 cells. The Th1 cytokines (IFN-γ, IL-2 and TNF-α) have been implicated in the pathophysiology of acute GVHD. IL-2 production by donor T cells remains the main target of many current clinical therapeutic and prophylactic approaches. Emerging data indicate an important role for IL-2 in the generation and maintenance of $CD4^+CD25^+$ Foxp3+ Tregs, suggesting that prolonged interference with IL-2 may have an unintended consequence in the prevention of the development of long-term tolerance after allogeneic HCT. Furthermore, the role of Th1 cytokines is complex. For example, exogenous administration of IFN-γ or T cells from IFN-γ deficient donors demonstrated a reduction and enhancement of GVHD, respectively. Accordingly, IFN- γ might play a differential role in the severity of distinct GVHD target organs. Thus, whether Th1 cytokines act as regulators or inducers of GVHD severity may be contextual. These data support earlier work showing that both Th1 and Th2 cells contribute to acute GVHD, with each subset causing injury to specific tissues (Paczesny et al., 2010).

Several different cytokines that polarize donor CD4+ T cells to Th2, such as IL-4, IL-11, and IL-18, as well as G-CSF and rapamycin, have been associated with reduced acute GVHD. In addition, donor T cells lacking the ability to secrete Th2 cytokines have increased GVHD severity. Furthermore, STAT-5 overexpression in CD4+ T cells regulated Th2 cytokine production, thereby reducing GVHD while retaining GVL (Paczesny et al., 2010). The role of IL-17-producing CD4+ T cells (Th17) in GVHD remains unclear. Several other cytokines are currently being examined (Paczesny et al., 2010).

T cell trafficking into target organs: Donor T cells migrate to secondary lymphoid organs where they recognize allo-antigens on either recipient or donor APCs, and become activated. They then exit the lymphoid tissues and traffic to the target organs where they cause tissue damage. Although almost all tissues express alloantigens, the three main clinical target organs of acute GVHD are the skin, liver, and GI tract. The thymus is also a GVHD target organ (Weinberg et al., 2001). The lung, although a major target of chronic GVHD, is a less common target of acute GVHD. The reasons for such selectivity of target organs are largely unknown. The spatiotemporal expression of cytokine and chemokine gradients might provide one explanation. Indeed, the trafficking of donor T cells into the GVHD target organs is chemokine-dependent. Chemokines, including CCL2-5, CXCL2, CXCL9-11, CCL17, and CCL27, are overexpressed by the liver, spleen, skin, and lungs during acute GVHD. T cells expressing the CXCR3 and CCR5 receptors cause acute GVHD in the liver and GI tract. Integrins and their ligands are also implicated in donor T cell trafficking into target organs. The integrin α4ß7 and its ligand MadCAM-1 are essential for homing of donor T cells to the Peyer's patches and the induction of intestinal GVHD. It is unlikely that a single chemokine or integrin accounts for the majority of GVHD as their roles are redundant. In addition, the trafficking of donor T cells has been shown to depend on other factors, such as the conditioning regimen as well as cytokine release.

Effectors and amplifiers of GVHD

The effector phase that leads to GVHD target organ damage is a complex cascade that involves cytolytic cellular effectors, such as CD8+ CTLs, CD4+ T cells, NK cells, and inflammatory molecules, such as TNFα, IFN-γ, and reactive oxygen species.

Cellular effectors: Cellular effectors usually require cell-cell contact to kill the cells of the target tissues using perforin-granzyme, Fas–FasL (CD95-CD95L), or TNFR-TNF-related apoptosis-inducing ligand (TRAIL) pathways (Kagi et al., 1994). CD8+CTLs are the major effectors of GVHD. Perforin and granzyme are stored in the cytotoxic granules of CTLs, secreted upon the recognition of target cells, and induce lysis by the perforation of target cell membranes. Fas clustering on the surface of target cells are induced by binding to FasL on CD8+ T cells, resulting in the formation of a death-inducing signal complex and the triggering of apoptosis on target cells. Other CTL killing mechanisms involve TNF death ligand receptor–triggered apoptosis by the activation of the TNF/TNFR, TRAIL, TNF-related weak inducer of apoptosis (TWEAK), and lymphotoxin ß (LTß)/ LIGHT pathway. The CD4+ effector T cells act mainly through the Fas–FasL and secondarily through the granzyme pathway.

Inflammatory effectors: Inflammatory pathways do not require cell-cell contact to kill target cells. Cellular damage is amplified by inflammatory mediators, including IFN-γ produced by T cells, TNFα and IL-1 produced by T cells and monocytes/macrophages, and nitric oxide (NO) produced by monocytes/macrophages. IL-6 has also been identified as a critical cytokine that promotes a pro-inflammatory response during GVHD and inhibits the reconstitution of Tregs. While an important role for IL-6 in GVHD has been shown, the findings were independent of T effector cell expansion or donor Treg responses. It is possible that reduction in GVHD is a consequence of direct reduction in IL-6 induced inflammation and cytopathic damage of the target tissues (Paczesny et al., 2010). Building on preclinical observations, early blockade of IL-6 after allogeneic HCT is currently being tested in a clinical trial of GVHD prevention.

The role of several effector molecules that cause GVHD is increasingly being better understood. However, the effector pathways that are employed for negatively regulating GVHD remain largely unknown.

Limitations of models and current gaps in GVHD biology

The biology of acute GVHD summarized in step-wise models remain as the predominant models for the current understanding of the biology of acute GVHD (Figure 9.1). While they elegantly summarize the complex biology of GVHD, they are limited by reductionist approaches. Indeed the observations derived from a collection of two-dimensional data points give an impression that GVHD is a linear, step-wise cascade that occurs in discrete stages. Thus, while useful for the purpose of this discussion, they do not account for the three-dimensional aspects and the critical role of milieu, space, and time. Clearly, the biology of GVHD is complex and involves multiple cells and pathways that play distinct, overlapping, or antagonistic roles in a feed-back or feed-forward manner, and all of these are context-dependent. For example, recent experimental data on various cellular subsets and cytokines and their interactions, when put together, leads to a complex network of interactions that would be difficult to categorize into distinct stages. As such, an additional explanation must be sought to complement these models. One such approach would be to understand the biology of GVHD from a system-based multiscale model. Rather than dividing the complex biology of GVHD into its components and stages, it may be more instructive to take an integrative systems biology approach that combines computational and mathematical modeling with direct experimentation to link spatial and temporal scales. Such a model would be interactive and dynamic and the properties of a single cell would be appropriately contingent on its relationship with other cells as well as the activities of many other molecules within the network. The data that are available to date on the biology of GVHD can potentially be incorporated into a multiscale model that spans from single cells to target organ systems. We anticipate that such a model would be a combination of an agent-based model (single cells) to ordinary differential equations (ODEs) for the organ system. The generation of one such model is currently under development by our group. We believe that the development of such an integrative approach is imperative to providing a mechanistic explanation of GVHD that is both robust and contextual.

Acknowledgments

S.C. is recipient of St. Baldrick's Foundation Scholar Award and is supported by National Institutes of Health grant AI091623-01.

P.R. is recipient of Leukemia Lymphoma Society Clinical Scholar Award and Basic Science Award from American Society of Transplantation. P.R. is supported by National Institutes of Health grants AI-075284, HL-090775 and CA-143379 to P.R.

References

Anderson, B.E., et al., Memory CD4+ T cells do not induce graft-versus-host disease. *J Clin Invest*, 2003. **112**(1): pp. 101–8.

Antin, J.H. and J.L. Ferrara, Cytokine dysregulation and acute graft-versus-host disease. *Blood*, 1992. **80**(12): pp. 2964–8.

Billingham, R.E., The biology of graft-versus-host reactions. *Harvey Lect*, 1966. **62**: pp. 21–78.

Blazar, B.R., et al., In vivo blockade of CD28/CTLA4: B7/BB1 interaction with CTLA4-Ig reduces lethal murine graft-versus-host disease across the major histocompatibility complex barrier in mice. *Blood*, 1994. **83**(12): pp. 3815–25.

Choi, S.W., et al., Vorinostat plus tacrolimus and mycophenolate to prevent graft-versus-host disease after related-donor reduced-intensity conditioning allogeneic haemopoietic stem-cell transplantation: a phase 1/2 trial. *Lancet Oncol*, 2014. **15**(1): pp. 87–95.

Edinger, M., et al., CD4+CD25+ regulatory T cells preserve graft-versus-tumor activity while inhibiting graft-versus-host disease after bone marrow transplantation. *Nat Med*, 2003. **9**(9): pp. 1144–50.

Eriguchi, Y., et al., Graft-versus-host disease disrupts intestinal microbial ecology by inhibiting Paneth cell production of alpha-defensins. *Blood*, 2012. **120**(1): pp. 223–31.

Flomenberg, N., et al., Impact of HLA class I and class II high-resolution matching on outcomes of unrelated donor bone marrow transplantation: HLA-C mismatching is associated with a strong adverse effect on transplantation outcome. *Blood*, 2004. **104**(7): pp. 1923–30.

Fontaine, P., et al., Adoptive transfer of minor histocompatibility antigen-specific T lymphocytes eradicates leukemia cells without causing graft-versus-host disease. *Nat Med*, 2001. **7**(7): pp. 789–94.

Gooley, T.A., et al., Reduced mortality after allogeneic hematopoietic-cell transplantation. *N Engl J Med*, 2010. **363**(22): pp. 2091–101.

Goulmy, E., et al., Mismatches of minor histocompatibility antigens between HLA-identical donors and recipients and the development of graft-versus-host disease after bone marrow transplantation. *N Engl J Med*, 1996. **334**(5): pp. 281–5.

Hanash, A.M., et al., Interleukin-22 protects intestinal stem cells from immune-mediated tissue damage and regulates sensitivity to graft versus host disease. *Immunity*, 2012. **37**(2): pp. 339–50.

Hill, G.R., et al., Total body irradiation and acute graft-versus-host disease: the role of gastrointestinal damage and inflammatory cytokines. *Blood*, 1997. **90**(8): pp. 3204–13.

Jankovic, D., et al., The Nlrp3 inflammasome regulates acute graft-versus-host disease. *J Exp Med*, 2013. **210**(10): pp. 1899–910.

Kagi, D., et al., Fas and perforin pathways as major mechanisms of T cell-mediated cytotoxicity. *Science*, 1994. **265**(5171): pp. 528–30.

Korngold, R. and J. Sprent, Purified T cell subsets and lethal graft-versus-host disease in mice, in *Progress in Bone Marrow Transplant*, R.P. Gale and R. Champlin, Editors. 1987, Alan R. Liss, Inc.: New York. pp. 213–8.

Lin, M.T., et al., Relation of an interleukin-10 promoter polymorphism to graft-versus-host disease and survival after hematopoietic-cell transplantation. *N Engl J Med*, 2003. **349**(23): pp. 2201–10.

Paczesny, S., et al., New perspectives on the biology of acute *GVHD*. *Bone Marrow Transplant*, 2010. **45**(1): pp. 1–11.

Penack, O., et al., *NOD2* regulates hematopoietic cell function during graft-versus-host disease. *J Exp Med*, 2009. **206**(10): pp. 2101–10.

Przepiorka D., Weisdorf D., Martin P., Klingemann H.G., Beatty P., Hows J., Thomas E.D. 1994 Consensus Conference on Acute GVHD Grading. *Bone Marrow Transplant*, 1995. **15**(6): pp. 825–8.

Reddy, P., et al., A crucial role for antigen-presenting cells and alloantigen expression in graft-versus-leukemia responses. *Nat Med*, 2005. **11**(11): pp. 1244–9.

Ruggeri, L., et al., Effectiveness of donor natural killer cell alloreactivity in mismatched hematopoietic transplants. *Science*, 2002. **295**(5562): pp. 2097–100.

Schwab, L., et al., Neutrophil granulocytes recruited upon translocation of intestinal bacteria enhance graft-versus-host disease via tissue damage. *Nat Med*, 2014. **20**(6): pp. 648–54.

Shlomchik, W.D., et al., Prevention of graft versus host disease by inactivation of host antigen-presenting cells. *Science*, 1999. **285**(5426): pp. 412–5.

Takashima, S., et al., The Wnt agonist R-spondin1 regulates systemic graft-versus-host disease by protecting intestinal stem cells. *J Exp Med*, 2011. **208**(2): pp. 285–94.

Taylor, P.A., C.J. Lees, and B.R. Blazar, The infusion of ex vivo activated and expanded CD4(+) CD25(+) immune regulatory cells inhibits graft-versus-host disease lethality. *Blood*, 2002. **99**(10): pp. 3493–9.

Toubai, T., et al., Siglec-G-CD24 axis controls the severity of graft-versus-host disease in mice. *Blood*, 2014. **123**(22): pp. 3512–23.

Weiden, P.L., et al., Antileukemic effect of graft-versus-host disease in human recipients of allogeneic-marrow grafts. *N Engl J Med*, 1979. **300**(19): pp. 1068–73.

Weinberg, K., et al., Factors affecting thymic function after allogeneic hematopoietic stem cell transplantation. *Blood*, 2001. **97**(5): pp. 1458–66.

CHAPTER 10

Therapeutic approaches to organ transplantation

Philip F. Halloran[1], Chatchai Kreepala[1], Gunilla Einecke[2], Alexandre Loupy[3,4], and Joana Sellarés[1]

[1] Alberta Transplant Applied Genomics Centre, Department of Medicine, Division of Nephrology and Transplant Immunology, University of Alberta, Edmonton, Canada

[2] Department of Nephrology, Hannover Medical School, Hannover, Germany

[3] Kidney Transplant Department, Necker Hospital APHP, Paris, France

[4] INSERM UMR 970, Epidemiology, PARCC Cardiovascular Research Institute, Paris, France

---

CHAPTER OVERVIEW

- Immunosuppression drugs are required for transplant survival; they act by inhibiting key steps in T cell and B cell responses or by depleting lymphocytes.

- The commonly used immunosuppression drugs include small-molecule drugs and protein biologics.

- Immunosuppression drugs are efficacious in suppressing T cell-mediated acute cellular rejection, but less so in other forms of rejection.

- Antibody-mediated rejection is a major cause of late graft loss, and prevention of donor-specific HLA antibody production and antibody-mediated rejection are increasingly important.

- Development of tolerance-compatible immunosuppression protocols remains an important goal in transplantation.

Introduction

Rejection has always been a key issue in organ transplantation, and, therefore, administration of immunosuppression drugs (ISDs) that inhibit rejection remains a centerpiece in transplant survival. However, rejection exhibits very different forms and features, which can be broadly divided into T cell-mediated rejection (TCMR) and antibody-mediated rejection (ABMR). Rejection is also very dynamic, and the risks of graft rejection change over time. TCMR is mainly a risk in the first 6 months, but becomes very rare after several years, even in nonadherent patients. The risk of ABMR in transplant patients emerges over time, despite the absence of donor-specific antibodies (DSAs) at the time of transplantation, and contributes substantially to late graft loss (Halloran, 2004). Thus, different

---

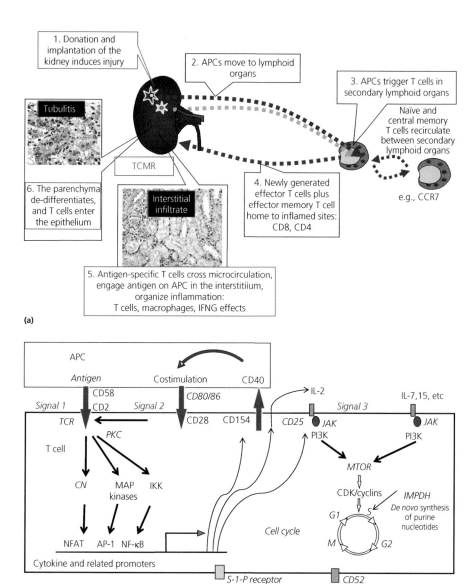

(a)

1. Donation and implantation of the kidney induces injury

2. APCs move to lymphoid organs

3. APCs trigger T cells in secondary lymphoid organs

Naïve and central memory T cells recirculate between secondary lymphoid organs

Tubulitis

TCMR

e.g., CCR7

6. The parenchyma de-differentiates, and T cells enter the epithelium

Interstitial infiltrate

4. Newly generated effector T cells plus effector memory T cell home to inflamed sites: CD8, CD4

5. Antigen-specific T cells cross microcirculation, engage antigen on APC in the interstitiium, organize inflammation: T cells, macrophages, IFNG effects

(b)

APC

Antigen   Costimulation   CD40

IL-2   IL-7,15, etc

Signal 1   CD58   CD80/86   Signal 2   Signal 3

CD2

TCR   CD28   CD154   CD25   JAK   JAK

T cell   PKC   PI3K   PI3K

MTOR

CN   MAP kinases   IKK   CDK/cyclins   IMPDH

G1   S   De novo synthesis of purine nucleotides

NFAT   AP-1   NF-κB   Cell cycle

M   G2

Cytokine and related promoters

S-1-P receptor   CD52

Activation   Proliferation

Homing to inflamed sites

Figure 10.1 (a) Pathogenesis of T cell-mediated rejection (TCMR). Dendritic cells of donor and host origin become activated and migrate from the graft to secondary lymphoid organs, where they present donor antigen to naïve and central memory T cells, which ordinarily recirculate between lymphoid tissues. The encounter with their cognate antigen on dendritic cells causes the T cells to become activated, leading to clonal proliferation and differentiation. Effector T cells and effector memory T cells home to the graft, where they again encounter antigen in interstitial antigen-presenting cells, triggering inflammation and resulting in TCMR lesions, such as interstitial inflammation and tubulitis. **(b) Key events in activation, proliferation and homing of T cells: a simplified three signal model.** Antigen on APCs triggers T-cell receptors (TCRs) (**signal 1**) and synapse formation. CD80 and CD86 on APCs engage CD28 on the T cells to provide **signal 2**. These activate the calcium–CN pathway, the mitogen-activated protein (MAP) kinase pathway, and the protein kinase C (PKC)–IKK pathway, which activate transcription factors such as NFAT, AP-1, and NF-kB, respectively. The result is production of cytokines and expression of cytokine receptor on activated T cells, for example Interleukin-2 (IL-2). IL-2 delivers growth signals (**signal 3**) through the PI-3K and mammalian target-of-rapamycin pathway (mTORpathway), which initiates the cell cycle. Lymphocytes require *de novo* synthesis of purine nucleotides for replication, regulated by inosine monophosphate dehydrogenase (IMPDH).

approaches are needed in the clinic to address the different rejection responses mechanistically (Figures 10.1 and 10.2).

In theory, rejection could be prevented by inducing antigen specific tolerance, but this remains elusive in practice. As a result, rejection must be controlled by the use of ISDs that nonspecifically suppress immune responses. Fortunately, graft survival is facilitated by the natural antigen-specific adaptations of the host immune response to the persistence of alloantigens, which results in a form of partial adaptive tolerance that likely occurs in all successful transplants, but requires ISDs to remain stable. While every ISD has been claimed to produce tolerance at some time or under certain conditions, no ISD or protocol induces transplant tolerance that completely prevents TCMR and ABMR, except for donor stem cell transplantation and induction of chimerism. Thus, ISDs must be continued to maintain this state of graft acceptance. However, this practice also creates a myriad of complications, mostly due to drug toxicities after long-term usage, which adversely affect both patient and graft survival. This chapter outlines how ISDs prevent rejection and why they produce undesired effects, as well as the emerging approaches to eliminate or minimize

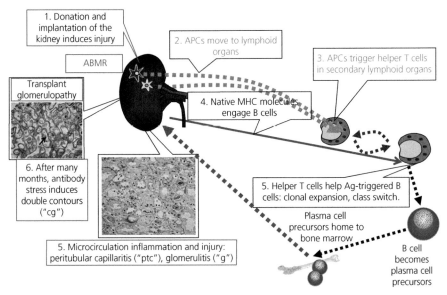

Figure 10.2 Pathogenesis of antibody-mediated rejection (ABMR). Dendritic cells of donor and host origin become activated and migrate from the graft to secondary lymphoid organs, where they present donor antigen to naive and central memory T cells. These T cells recirculate between lymphoid tissues. Naïve B cells become activated through antigen primed T helper cells in the secondary lymphoid organs. They then undergo clonal proliferation, antibody class switching and affinity maturation to become plasma cell precursors and migrate to the bone marrow. They then differentiate into memory B cells or plasma cells that produce alloantibody HLA donor-specific. Donor-specific HLA alloantibody targets the endothelium in the graft producing the typical lesions present in antibody-mediated rejection, such as glomerulitis, peritubular capillaritis, and transplant glomerulopathy.

those effects. This chapter focuses on ISDs that are approved for use in kidney transplantation, but many issues covered here are applicable to other organ transplants as well.

General aspects of ISDs

Immunosuppressive drugs include small-molecule drugs (Tables 10.1 and 10.2) and protein/biologic drugs (Tables 10.3 and 10.4). They are often used in combinations to achieve additive efficacy and to reduce toxicity. Most small-molecule ISDs are derived from microbial products, and the drug targets are usually highly conserved proteins in evolution. At clinically tolerated doses, small-molecule drugs do not saturate their targets. For example, cyclosporine acts by inhibiting calcineurin (CN), but inhibits only partially at the doses used clinically (Budde et al., 2011). Thus, the effects of the drug are proportional to the concentration of the drug, which makes dosing and monitoring critical. Partial saturation also explains why rejection can still occur despite the presence of ISDs, and why combinations of agents are required to control rejection.

Protein biologics can be depleting or nondepleting, and include polyclonal antibodies, monoclonal antibodies, fusion proteins, and intravenous immune globulin (IVIG). Monoclonal antibodies can be murine, chimeric, and humanized or human products. Depleting reagents are antibodies that destroy large numbers of T cells, B cells, or both. They are usually used for induction therapies. Recovery from severe lymphocyte depletion takes years, and may never be complete in older adults. Nondepleting biologics are monoclonal antibodies or fusion proteins that reduce T cell responses without compromising the numbers of lymphocytes. They typically target a cell surface molecule required for T cell activation such as CD25, which is the high affinity interleukin-2 (IL-2) receptor used for proliferation. These drugs have low nonimmune toxicity because they target proteins that are expressed only in immune cells.

Table 10.1 Classification of small-molecule immunosuppressive drugs commonly used in organ transplantation.

- Immunophilin-binding drugs
  - Cyclophilin-binding CN inhibitors: cyclosporine
  - FKBP-binding CN inhibitors: tacrolimus
  - FKBP-binding mTOR inhibitors: sirolimus (rapamycin), everolimus
- Inhibitors of *de novo* purine synthesis: IMPDH inhibitors
  - MPA: mycophenolate mofetil, enteric-coated MPA
- Antimetabolites
  - Azathioprine

CN, calcineurin; FKBP, mTOR, mechanistic target of rapamycin; IMPDH, inosine monophosphate dehydrogenase; MPA, mycophenolic acid.

Table 10.2 The features of small-molecule ISDs.

Drug	Description	Mechanism	Nonimmune toxicity and comments	Monitoring
cyclosporine; voclosporine (aka ISA247)	11-amino-acid cyclic peptide from *Tolypocladium inflatum*	Prodrug: binds to cyclophilin to create cyclosporine: cyclophilin complex; complex inhibits CN phosphatase, which prevents activation of transcription factors needed to transcribe proteins critical to T cell activation; thus prevents T cell activation	Hypertension, hyperlipidemia; post transplantation diabetes mellitus, nephrotoxicity; hemolytic–uremic syndrome, neurotoxicity, gum hyperplasia, skin changes, hirsutism	trough monitoring or checking levels < 2 h after administration required
tacrolimus (FK506)	Macrolide antibiotic from *Streptomyces tsukubaensis*	Prodrug; binds to FKBP to create drug: FKBP complex; complex inhibits CN phosphatase, which prevents activation of transcription factors needed to transcribe proteins critical to T cell activation; thus prevents T cell activation	Effects similar to those of cyclosporine but with a lower incidence of hypertension, hyperlipidemia, skin changes, hirsutism, gum hyperplasia, post-transplant diabetes mellitus, neurotoxicity	trough monitoring required

Drug	Source	Mechanism	Adverse effects	Monitoring
sirolimus (aka rapamycin); everolimus	Triene macrolide antibiotic from S. hygroscopicus from Easter Island (Rapa Nui)	Prodrug; binds to FKBP to create drug: FKBP complex; complex inhibits MTOR and prevents ribosomes from translating growth factor–driven cell cycling; thus inhibits clonal expansion	Hyperlipidemia. Delayed wound healing. Prolongs delayed graft function; increases the toxicity of CN inhibitors; thrombocytopenia, mouth ulcers, pneumonitis, interstitial lung disease	Yes when used as main ISD. Lipid monitoring required.
mycophenolic acid (mycophenolate and enteric-coated mycophenolate	Mycophenolic acid from penicillium molds	Inhibits IMPDH. which is necessary for balancing GMP versus AMP; the imbalance prevents de novo purine synthesis, selectively preventing proliferation of T and B cells	Gastrointestinal symptoms (mainly diarrhea), neutropenia, mild anemia; absorption reduced by cyclosporine	blood-level monitoring not required but may improve efficacy

Continued

Table 10.2 Continued

Azathioprine	Prodrug that releases 6-mercaptopurine	As 6-mercaptopurine incorporated into thioguanine nucleotides that interfere with DNA synthesis; thioguanine derivatives may inhibit *de novo* purine synthesis	Leukopenia, bone marrow depression, macrocytosis, liver toxicity (uncommon); blood-count (monitoring required); pancreatitis	Monitoring not required: Purine analogue allopurinol may greatly increase toxicity and requires *azathioprine* dose reduction.
Sotrastaurin (aka AEB071)	Synthetic small-molecule drug	Inhibits protein-kinase-C, which plays a role in signal 1, and thus blocks early T cell activation	Gastrointestinal, particularly constipation; mild tachycardia	Regimens for use in organ transplantation are being evaluated
Tofacitinib (formerly tasocitinib; aka CP-690,550)	Synthetic small-molecule drug	Inhibits JAK3 (and other JAKs) to impair signaling of a number of cytokines	Anemia; neutropenia; increased cholesterol; increased PTLD at higher doses	Development in organ transplantation is not clear; In trials for rheumatoid arthritis

Fingolimod (aka FTY720)	Sphingosine-like derivative of myrlocin from ascomycete Fungus	Antagonist (superagonist) for sphingosine-1-phosphate receptors on lymphocytes, effectively blocking these receptors and enhancing homing to lymphoid tissues and preventing egress, causing lymphopenia by trapping lymphocytes in gut-associated lymphoid tissues	Reversible first-dose bradycardia, potentiated by general anesthetics and beta-blockers: nausea, vomiting, diarrhea, increased liver-enzyme levels	Trials in transplantation were stopped; Being developed for treatment of multiple sclerosis
Prednisone	Prodrug converted by liver into prednisonolone. synthetic corticosteroid	Many different actions at different dose levels: Acts via steroid receptors to influence transcription of many genes via CRE in DNA: at higher doses has receptor independent action:	Cataracts, hypertension, hyperglycemia, osteoporosis, Cushingoid habitus, impaired growth	Monitor side effects (hypertension, lipids, glucose, bone metabolism)

Table 10.3 Protein-based ISDs in use or recently in trials for organ transplantation.

- Depleting
  - Polyclonal antithymocyte globulin
  - Anti-CD52 (alemtuzumab, Campath-1H)
- Nondepleting/partially depleting
  - Anti-CD25 (basiliximab)
  - CTLA4Ig (belatacept)
  - Anti-CD2 (alefacept)
  - Anti-LFA3 (efalizumab) (withdrawn)
  - Anti-CD40
- For managing/preventing ABMR, see below

All ISDs exhibit the following features:

1. Therapeutic effects: Suppression of rejection can be achieved by depleting lymphocytes, diverting lymphocyte traffic, or blocking lymphocyte activation pathways (Figure 10.3).
2. Off-target effects on the immune system: Immunosuppression leads to increased episodes of infection as well as cancers, such as nonmelanoma skin cancers and post-transplantation lymphoproliferative disease (PTLD). These effects are related to the duration and intensity of immunosuppression, and in some cases the specific ISD used.
3. Nonimmune toxic effects: These effects are more common with small-molecule drugs and are related to the mechanism of action of the drug, because of effects of the drug on targets molecules with physiologic roles in nonimmune tissues. For example, nephrotoxicity of CN inhibitors may reflect the role of CN within the renal resistance in arteries and arterioles.

Small-molecule drugs

Mycophenolic acid
Mycophenolic acid (MPA) interestingly, is a product of penicillium molds that were first isolated more than 100 years ago and as a crystalline material was noted to inhibit the growth of bacilli. Although it was found to be immunosuppressive in the 1960s, its potential as a small-molecule ISD was only realized in the 1990s. It is available in two forms: mycophenolate mofetil (MMF, a synthetic ethyl ester of MPA) and enteric coated MPA.

Mechanism of action
MPA acts by inhibiting the enzyme inosine monophosphate dehydrogenase (IMPDH), which is crucial for *de novo* purine synthesis in lymphocytes (Figure 10.4). Purines can be synthesized either *de novo* or can be recycled by salvage pathways. Lymphocytes require *de novo* synthesis, while other cell types

Table 10.4 Details of Protein ISDs.

Drug	Description	Mechanism	Nonimmune toxicity and comments	Monitoring
Antithymocyte globulin (ATG) (rabbit/equine)	Rabbit immunoglobulin, horse immunoglobulin	Cytotoxic antibodies directed against antigens expressed on T-cells mediate T-cell effects via inhibition of proliferative responses.	Severe cytokine-release syndrome, pulmonary edema, acute renal failure, GI disturbances, changes in CNS system. Long-term use of this agent has been associated with increased risk of post-transplant lymphoproliferative disease.	Monitoring of symptoms of cytokine release
Muromonab-CD3 (OKT3) (no longer available)	Mouse monoclonal antibody against the to the CD3 structure that transduces signals for the T cell receptor	Binding of muromonab-CD3 to T-cells results in early activation, which leads to cytokine release, followed by blocking T-cell functions.	Cytokine release syndrome including gastrointestinal symptoms, headache, acute renal failure or pulmonary edema as a result of capillary leak, and rarely, severe CNS manifestations such as cerebral edema or cortical blindness. Pre-medication required.	Monitoring of symptoms of cytokine release; now rarely used in clinical transplantation
Basiliximab (daclizumab is no longer available)	Chimeric monoclonal antibody against CD25 component of the IL-2 receptor.	Selective blockade of IL-2 receptors on activated T-lymphocytes blockage, therefore prevention of IL-2-induced T cell activation	GI disturbances, uncommon hypersensitivity reactions	No monitoring required

Continued

Table 10.4 Continued

Alemtuzumab	Humanized monoclonal antibody against CD52	Binds to CD52, an antigen present on all B and T lymphocytes and the majority of monocytes, macrophages and NK cells. The potential actions include internalization, blockade, or lysis of the receptor-bearing cells	Mild cytokine-release syndrome, neutropenia, anemia, idiosyncratic pancytopenia, autoimmune thrombocytopenia, thyroid disease	immunodeficiency complications (infections and cancer)
Belatacept	Fusion protein combining CTLA-4 with the Fc portion of IgG	Binds to the CD80 and CD86 surface molecules on antigen-presenting cells, preventing them from triggering the CD28 receptor on T-cells, and thus blocking costimulation	Increased risk of graft and CNS PTLD; should not be used in EBV-negative recipients. Increased risk of early TCMR and of late progressive multifocal leukoencephalopathy (PML), and of M tuberculosis infection in endemic areas	given intravenously every 4–8 weeks; no monitoring required

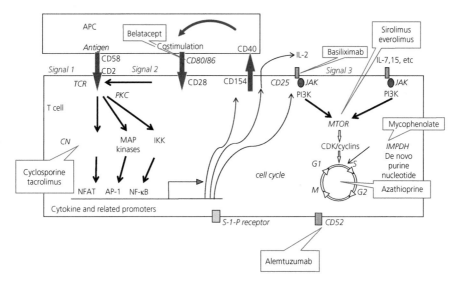

Figure 10.3 Sites of action of ISDs in relationship to key T cell events.

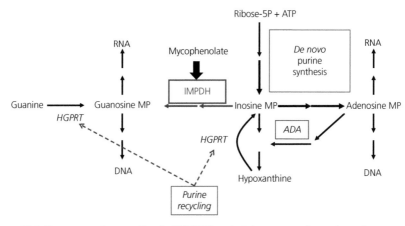

Figure 10.4 *De novo* purine synthesis: IMPDH maintains guanosine–adenosine nucleotide balance, and is the target of mycophenolate. Lymphocytes require *de novo* purine synthesis to proliferate, and IMPDH is a key enzyme for this process. Inosine monophosphate is the precursor of adenosine monophosphate and guanosine monophosphate, and the balance between these proteins requires IMPDH. The inhibition of IMPDH by mycophenolate causes depletion of guanosineMP, creating an imbalance in purine nucleotide levels, which inhibits *de novo* purine synthesis.

such as neurons use salvage pathways. The inhibition of IMPDH by MPA causes depletion of guanosine monophosphate (GMP), which creates a relative excess of adenosine monophosphate (AMP). The imbalance between purine nucleotide levels inhibits *de novo* purine synthesis, thus arresting replicating lymphocytes in S phase. Inhibition of the cell cycle in lymphocytes is the principal mechanism by which MPA confers immunosuppression. MPA diminishes the clonal expansion of B and T cells, decreases generation of effector T cells, and suppresses primary antibody responses.

Efficacy
Mycophenolate was developed as a replacement for azathioprine. Several clinical trials established the efficacy of mycophenolate along with cyclosporine and corticosteroids in the prevention of renal allograft rejection, compared with treatment with azathioprine. Mycophenolate and MPA are now widely used in most tacrolimus-based regimens.

Adverse effects and drug interactions
The main toxic effects are leucopenia, anemia, and gastrointestinal symptoms particularly diarrhea. Marked gastrointestinal adverse effects are handled by reducing the dose, by switching to another formulation, or by stopping the drug. Mycophenolate has no direct renal toxicity and does not confer cardiovascular risk, but may increase cytomegalovirus disease. It has been associated with some protection against *Pneumocystis jiroveci* pneumonia. Mycophenolate may not be well absorbed in patients who are concurrently receiving antacids, cholestyramine, or ferrous sulfate. There is a growing awareness as well of teratogenic effects and it should be avoided in pregnancy.

Azathioprine
Azathioprine, developed by Elion and Hitchings (Nobel Prize in medicine, 1988), was the first ISD to achieve widespread use in organ transplantation.

Mechanism of action
Azathioprine acts by releasing 6-mercaptopurine (6-MP), a purine analog that is incorporated into DNA as a purine. It interferes with cell division, thus functioning as an antiproliferative agent. Intracellular metabolism by hypoxanthine-guanine phosphoribosyltransferase converts 6-MP to thioinosinic acid and thioguanylic acid. Thioguanylic acid is incorporated into developing strands of DNA, interfering with DNA synthesis. This is unlike MPA, which is not a nucleotide and cannot be incorporated into DNA. Thioinosinic acid suppresses intracellular synthesis of guanylic and adenylic acids from inosinic acid and interferes with purine synthesis. This suppresses proliferation of activated B and T lymphocytes, as well as other cell types such as red cell precursors. Azathioprine also reduces the number of circulating monocytes by blocking the cell cycle of promyelocytes in the bone marrow. Effects on erythyrocyte precursors interfere with cell division and cause macrocytosis.

Adverse effects and drug interactions
The major side effect is dose-dependent bone marrow suppression: anemia, leucopenia, and thrombocytopenia, and occasionally pancreas and liver toxicity. These effects respond to a reduction or transient discontinuation of the drug.

Azathioprine can cause gastrointestinal problems such as anorexia or nausea. Other adverse effects include hair loss. The principal drug interaction with azathioprine is with allopurinol, which slows the elimination of 6-MP by inhibiting xanthine oxidase. The dose of azathioprine should be reduced by 66–75% when used with allopurinol; but given the risk of complete bone marrow suppression and failure, the combination should be avoided if possible.

CN inhibitors

Two classes of ISDs inhibit the phosphatase CN: cyclosporine, a cyclic fungal peptide with 11 amino acid residues; and tacrolimus, a macrolide antibiotic. Voclosporin (ISA247) is a semi-synthetic analog of cyclosporine currently under investigation (phase 3 Trials), and its mechanism is presumably the same as that of cyclosporine.

Mechanism of action

Both cyclosporine and tacrolimus are "prodrugs" that bind to intracellular immunophilins to create the complexes that are the true active drugs. Thus, cyclosporine binds cyclophilin, and tacrolimus binds FKBP, and the drug-receptor complexes inhibit CN.

CN is activated by the engagement of T cell receptors (TCRs), activation of tyrosine kinases and of phoshpolipase C-γ1 (PLC- γ1), releasing calcium stored in the endoplasmic reticulum, and opening membrane calcium-release-activated calcium channels (CRACs). The calcium influx or current through the CRAC provides a crucial step for the activation of CN (Figure 10.5). The activated CN dephosphorylates the inactive cytosolic form of the transcription factors of the NF/AT family, leading to the transcriptional activation of many genes associated with T cell activation, such as IL-2, tumor necrosis factor alpha, interferon-gamma, and CD40L. Thus, cyclosporine or tacrolimus prevents TCR engagement from delivering signal 1, thereby preventing or reducing expression of T cell activation proteins such as cytokines and CD40L, which prevents cell proliferation and expression of effector functions.

Efficacy

Trials of cyclosporine versus tacrolimus have found similar efficacy, depending on the dose. The largest trial, the Symphony study in *de novo* renal transplants, showed superior renal function and control of rejection in patients that were on tacrolimus and mycophenolate compared to three ISD combinations involving cyclosporine or sirolimus. Conversion to tacrolimus has been used as a rescue therapy for refractory rejection in patients taking cyclosporine.

Adverse effects and drug interactions

Cyclosporine and tacrolimus have similar toxicity profiles, related to the concentration of the drug. Both cause varying degrees of nephrotoxicity, hyperlipidemia, diabetes, hyperkalemia, hypomagnesemia, and neurotoxicity (mainly

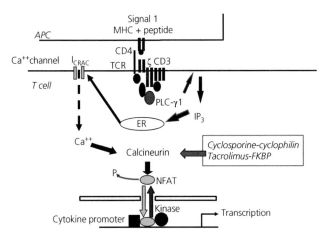

Figure 10.5 Calcineurin inhibitors prevent activation of nuclear factor of activated T cells (NFATs). Engagement of T cell receptors (TCRs) activates the calcium-CN pathway, through activation of tyrosine kinases and phospholipase C-γ1 (PLC-γ1), releasing calcium stored in the endoplasmic reticulum, and opening membrane calcium-release-activated calcium channels. The calcium current through the CRAC increases the cytoplasmic level of calcium, which becomes essential for activating CN. The activated CN dephosphorylates the inactive cytosolic form of the transcription factor NFAT, which leads to its translocation to the nucleus where it activates the transcription of many genes associated with T cell activation.

tremor). Gingival hyperplasia, hirsutism, hypertension, and hyperlipidemia are more frequently observed with cyclosporine. Tacrolimus induces more tremor and post-transplantation diabetes mellitus. Both can induce hemolytic–uremic syndrome, often associated with elevated drug levels.

The main concern with CN inhibitors is dose-dependent nephrotoxicity, which is primarily due to renal vasoconstriction. Prolonged vasospasm may explain the hyalinosis of the glomerular afferent arterioles. However, hyalinosis can occur in other settings (e.g., hypertension, diabetes mellitus, and pre-existing donor lesions) and is not specific to CN inhibitor nephrotoxicity. The exact mechanism of vasoconstriction is unclear, but correlates with the immunosuppressive ability, and thus, is probably mediated by CN inhibition. Chronic nephrotoxicity induces nephron loss with interstitial fibrosis and tubular atrophy. The use of cyclosporine and tacrolimus is associated with mild-to-moderate permanent impairment in renal function over time, but this seldom progresses to end-stage renal disease in well-managed kidney transplants.

There are many drugs that can increase cyclosporine and tacrolimus levels, for example, diltiazem, fluconazole, ketoconazole, clarithromycin, and erythromycin. Grapefruit juice contains furanocoumarins, which inhibit the cytochrome P450 system and increase blood levels of cyclosporine and tacrolimus. mTOR inhibitors also increase CN inhibitor exposure (see following text). Some drugs can decrease cyclosporine levels, for example, rifampicin, isoniazid, carbamazepine, phenobarbital, and phenytoin.

Choosing which CN inhibitor to use

Tacrolimus is now the primary CN inhibitor used in solid organ transplantation, but cyclosporine remains widely used in many long-term patients or those intolerant to tacrolimus. Most transplantation programs exploit the strengths of both tacrolimus and cyclosporine, depending on the risks in individual patients. Hypertension, hyperlipidemia, and rejection risk support the use of tacrolimus, whereas a high risk of diabetes (e.g., older age, obesity, and family history) argues for cyclosporine.

Inhibitors of mammalian target of rapamycin (mTOR)

Sirolimus (or rapamycin) is a macrocyclic lactone isolated from *Streptomyces hygroscopycus*. Everolimus is a derivative of sirolimus and has similar effectiveness and side-effects.

Mechanism of action

Sirolimus and everolimus are pro-drugs that engage FKBP to create complexes that engage and inhibit mammalian target of rapamycin (mTOR), but cannot inhibit CN. mTOR is a kinase that regulates 4E-BP1 and the enzyme p70 S6 kinase. Both proteins control the translation of the mRNAs for certain proteins needed for progression from the G1 to the S phase of DNA synthesis. Thus, cytokines and growth factors must activate these steps to trigger G1 to S progression (Figure 10.6). Inhibition of mTOR by the drug—FKBP complex blocks signal 3, preventing cytokine and growth factor receptors from activating the cell cycle. Thus, mTOR inhibitors result in cell cycle arrest in the G1–S phase.

Efficacy

mTOR inhibitors were initially evaluated in combination with cyclosporine, but this combination increases nephrotoxicity, hemolytic–uremic syndrome and hypertension. The use of mTOR inhibitors with tacrolimus has been successful in some centers, but also produces concerns about toxicity. Withdrawing the CN inhibitor in stable patients who are also on mTOR inhibitor reduces renal dysfunction and hypertension, although with a small increase in TCMR episodes.

Adverse effects and drug interactions

The principal nonimmune toxic effects of mTOR inhibitors include hyperlipidemia, thrombocytopenia, and impaired wound healing. Other effects include delayed recovery from acute tubular necrosis in kidney transplants, reduced testosterone concentrations, aggravation of glomerular damage and proteinuria, mouth ulcers, skin lesions, and pneumonitis. However, mTOR inhibitors may reduce cytomegalovirus disease.

Sirolimus and everolimus have antitumor effects and arterial protective effects. Since these agents slow the growth of established experimental tumors, they have potential applications in oncology. mTOR inhibitors may be able to

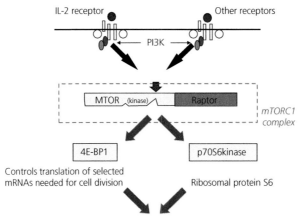

Figure 10.6 mTORkinase (as part of the mTORC1 complex) has many effects on ribosomes, protein translation, and cell replication. The activation of mammalian target of rapamycin (mTOR) requires the formation of the mTORC1 complex, which is composed of mTOR kinase with regulatory proteins such as Raptor. The mTORC1 complex regulates signaling pathways that act in parallel to control events needed for mRNA translation, including phosphorylation of 4E-BP1 (factor-4E-binding protein-1) and activation of ribosomal protein p70 S6 kinase. These events are needed for progression from the G1 to S phase of DNA synthesis.

reduce risks in some cancers, including skin cancer, and have been used in managing Kaposi's sarcoma. Many programs consider the conversion of antirejection drugs to the use of mTOR inhibitors, particularly with cessation of CN. While this is a reasonable strategy, particularly in those patients in which reduction of other drugs has not been effective, or in those where prevention of rejection remains a priority, too aggressive a conversion is often associated with adverse effects. These may be severe enough for patients to discontinue the drug. More gradual reduction of CN and more gradual increase in mTOR drugs may be better tolerated.

The possibility that sirolimus and everolimus can protect arteries is suggested by two observations: mTOR inhibitors incorporated into coronary stents inhibit restenosis, and mTOR inhibitors plus CN inhibitors reduce the incidence of graft coronary artery narrowing in heart transplants. Potential arterial protective effects of sirolimus and everolimus must be weighed against hyperlipidemia.

Sirolimus levels are modified through interaction with some of the drugs that also affect CN inhibitors, for example, when increased with diltiazem and ketoconazole and decreased with rifampicin and some anticonvulsants.

Tofacitinib (Tasocitinib, CP-690550)
Mechanism of action
Tofacitinib inhibits Janus-associated kinases (JAKs). JAKs phosphorylate tyrosines in their downstream transcription-regulation proteins, called signal transducers and activators of transcription (STATs), thus mediating ligand-specific

signal transduction between cell membrane receptors and the nucleus. JAK3, a tyrosine kinase associated with the cytokine receptor gamma chain, participates in the signaling of many cytokine receptors (interleukin- 2, 4, 7, 9, 15, and 21). By inhibiting JAK3 and other JAKs, tofacitinib blocks the signal, the proliferative signals for T and B cells.

Efficacy
The use of tofacitinib in organ transplantation is being evaluated in combination with basiliximab induction, MPA, and steroids to replace CN inhibitors. Patients treated with tofacitinib had acceptable acute rejection rates. By reducing CN inhibitor use, protocols with tofacitinib reduce the prevalence of interstitial fibrosis and tubular atrophy, with improved renal function.

Adverse effects
In trials to date, patients treated with tofacitinib have similar lipid profiles and lower rates of new onset diabetes and hypertension compared to patients treated with CN inhibitors. The incidence of serious infections and bone marrow suppression (anemia and neutropenia) was higher in the tofacitinib groups. Further analyses are ongoing to identify the optimal tofacitinib dose regimen required to balance immunosuppression versus immunodeficiency.

Current status
Tofacitinib has been released for the treatment of rheumatoid arthritis, and is not being developed in organ transplantation.

Prednisone
Corticosteroids continue to be used in kidney transplantation for induction and maintenance immunosuppression and for treatment of rejection. The usual corticosteroids administered are prednisone (oral) and methylprednisolone (intravenous). High-dose intravenous corticosteroids are administered pre-transplantation as part of the induction therapy. This is then followed by oral steroids, which is gradually tapered to a maintenance dose of 5 mg daily on alternate days. The first-line treatment for TCMR is usually a high dose of intravenous methylprednisolone, for example, a bolus of 250–500 mg/day during 3–4 days.

Mechanism of action
Corticosteroids have anti-inflammatory effects and immunosuppressive effects. In low doses, they act by binding with a cytoplasmatic corticosteroid receptor, as part of the glucocorticosteroid hormone mechanism. This complex migrates to the nucleus and binds to specific DNA elements and adjacent proteins, which causes either induction or suppression of gene transcription. They also regulate transcription factors such as activator protein-1 and NFκB. At high doses they have receptor-independent effects such as membrane stabilization. Many of

their effects are on monocytes and macrophages as well as lymphocytes. They also increased leukocyte blood counts by inhibiting margination. The problem with discussing steroid actions is that the many different effects of corticosteroids and the wide range of doses make it difficult to identify the therapeutic action.

Adverse effects

Adverse effects of corticosteroids are common and responsible for significant morbidity, including Cushingoid features, acne, weight gain and excessive appetite, diabetes mellitus, cataracts, osteoporosis, avascular necrosis of the femoral heads, and increased susceptibility to infections, particularly when high doses are administered. Owing to their interaction with the glucocorticoid responsive elements (GREs) of many genes, steroids may display unpredicted effects such as increased hepatitis B viral transcription.

Protein drugs and biologics

Depleting antibodies
Polyclonal antithymocyte globulin

Polyclonal antithymocyte globulin is produced by immunizing horses or rabbits with human (thymic) lymphoid cells, harvesting the IgG, and absorbing out nondesired antibodies (e.g., those against platelets and erythrocytes) (Table 10.5). As an induction agent, polyclonal antithymocyte globulin that has been used for 3–10 days produces profound and durable lymphopenia that slowly recovers over many months. A number of dosing strategies are used including fixed daily dosing versus adjusted on total cell counts. In addition to immunodeficiency complications, toxic effects of polyclonal antithymocyte globulin include thrombocytopenia, cytokinerelease with fever and chills, and occasional serum sickness or allergic reactions. Rabbit preparations of polyclonal antithymocyte globulin

Table 10.5 Drugs and strategies to suppress donor-specific antibodies and prevent or treat antibody-mediated rejection.

- Optimize maintenance agents, correct nonadherence
- Intravenous immunoglobulin (IVIG)
  - low dose
  - high dose
- Plasmapheresis
- Splenectomy
- Immunoabsorption
- Rituximab
- Bortezomib
- Eculizumab
- Emerging B-cell-directed therapies

are favored over horse polyclonal antithymocyte globulin because of greater potency.

Alemtuzumab

Alemtuzumab (referred to in the past as Campath 1H) is a humanized monoclonal antibody against CD52 that massively depletes lymphocyte populations. It is approved for use in treating refractory chronic B cell lymphocytic leukemia, but is used off-label for induction therapy in organ transplantation, primarily in kidney recipients. It has recently been shown to reduce early TCMR in renal transplants, but with no effects on survival to date (Einecke et al., 2009). The pharmaceutical company owning alemtuzumab is developing it for multiple sclerosis, and its future in transplantation is uncertain.

Efficacy

Alemtuzumab is a powerful lymphocyte depleting agent, inducing long-lasting lymphopenia and low rates of TCMR when used in combination with CN inhibitors. Because of the lack of regulatory approval in kidney transplantation, the use of alemtuzumab varies widely. Induction with alemtuzumab is in combination with CN inhibitors and results in very low rates of TCMR.

Alemtuzumab has been used in "tolerogenic" strategies, but this was not successful. Some claims that mTOR inhibitors plus alemtuzumab would induce tolerance have also not been confirmed.

Adverse effects

Adverse effects of alemtuzumab include first-dose reactions, neutropenia, anemia, and rarely pancytopenia and autoimmunity (e.g., hemolytic anemia, thrombocytopenia, and hyperthyroidism). The relative risks of immunodeficiency complications (infections and cancer) with alemtuzumab protocols compared to other protocols are unknown because large phase 3 trials have not been performed.

Nondepleting antibodies and fusion proteins
Basiliximab

Basiliximab is a recombinant chimeric murine/human IgG monoclonal anti-CD25 antibody that is widely used in transplantation for induction. Daclizimab, a humanized form of anti-CD25 antibody, is no longer available.

Mechanism of action

Basiliximab selectively binds to CD25, the α-subunit of high-affinity IL-2 receptors on the surface of activated T lymphocytes. Because expression of CD25 is confined to activated T cells, anti-CD25 antibody causes little general depletion of T cells.

Efficacy
Basiliximab is moderately effective, reducing rejection by about one-third when used with CN inhibitors.

Adverse effects
Basiliximab is largely free from nonimmune toxicity. There is also little evidence of increased risk of infections, malignancies or PTLDs, probably reflecting its limited potency. This is an advantage of basiliximab induction: moderate efficacy with very little toxicity or immunodeficiency complications.

Belatacept
Belatacept is a fusion protein, the product of combining the genes for cytotoxic-T-lymphocyte–associated antigen 4 (CTLA-4) (which engages CD80 and CD86 on antigen-presenting cells) with the hinge region and Fc portion of IgG. Belatacept was approved for use in kidney transplantation in June 2011. It is administered by periodic intravenous injection (5 mg/kg every 4 weeks in the maintenance phase).

Mechanism of action
Binding to the costimulatory ligands CD80 and CD86 disrupts the interaction of antigen-presenting cells with the CD28 receptor on naïve T cells and blocks the costimulatory signaling required for successful activation. This mechanism may be advantageous for controlling T cell help for antibody formation and thus reduce ABMR, although this has not been proven. However, this mechanism may be less effective than other ISDs at controlling memory T cells.

Efficacy
Results of phase 2 and 3 trials demonstrated the efficacy of belatacept in renal transplant recipients with average immunological risk. Belatacept in combination with MMF, glucocorticoids, and anti-CD25 antibody controlled TCMR less well than cyclosporine, but resulted in better renal function and improved cardiovascular side-effect profile, with lower lipids and better blood pressure control. (The excess of early TCMR could reflect memory T cells). Belatacept establishes the concept of long-term use of nondepleting protein ISDs to reduce reliance on CN inhibitors, thus reducing drug-related toxicity. It is also possible (but not proven) that administration of a parenteral drug such as belatacept will reduce nonadherence.

Adverse effects
Belatacept must not be used in patients who are EBV-negative because of the increased risk of PTLD, predominantly in the central nervous system. Progressive multifocal leukoencephalopathy (PML) has been reported in patients receiving belatacept.

Immunosuppression protocols

The common maintenance ISD protocol at present is a CN inhibitor as first line and a mycophenolate as second line, with either low-dose steroid or no steroid. The use of protein induction varies widely: depleting antibodies, basiliximab, or no protein drug induction are all in common use. The newest option of belatacept as first line plus mycophenolate, with low-dose steroid, will probably find increasing use. The first trials of belatacept used anti-CD25 induction. With the release of the drug for general use, other options will be explored, as in steroid withdrawal.

However, hundreds of potential combinations exist, and many new protocols have emerged, most of them including reduced reliance on steroids and CN inhibitors. Developing evidence-based approaches to this confusing choice of protocols presents a challenge.

"Minimization" strategies: pros and cons
New protein ISDs with long-lasting effects on induction therapy increased interest in CN inhibitors and steroid minimization protocols. There was also a period of intense interest in minimization based on the belief that many patients were effectively tolerant. In fact, many of these minimization approaches have not worked as intended. At the same time, there is increasing awareness that much of late graft loss likely reflects under immunosuppression with the emergence of late effector pathways. Thus the late consequences of some minimization protocols have been perhaps lower CN toxicity, but a high incidence of rejection.

Steroid minimization regimen
Steroid minimization protocols aim to reduce or eliminate steroid-related metabolic adverse effects without increasing the rate of acute rejection or allograft loss. Three main strategies have been used: late steroid discontinuation ($\geq$3 months post transplantation), early steroid discontinuation ($\leq$7 days post-transplantation), and complete steroid avoidance. These approaches are probably not equivalent. The main concerns include an increase in TCMR episodes and a possible increase in atrophy-fibrosis.

Late steroid discontinuation ($\geq$3 months post transplantation)
After the introduction of mycophenolate, several trials on late steroid discontinuation were performed in select patients under either cyclosporine or tacrolimus with mycophenolate. Most studies showed a higher rate of acute rejection episodes in the steroid withdrawal group, but no differences in patient survival, graft failure, or function between the steroid withdrawal and steroid maintenance groups were found. Patients on the steroid withdrawal arm usually have less hypertension and lower mean of LDL-cholesterol values.

Steroid avoidance or rapid steroid discontinuation (≤7 days post transplantation)

A trial of this protocol found no differences in patient survival, graft loss, or allograft function, but patients with early withdrawal experienced more mild acute rejection. Moreover, patients in the steroid withdrawal arm had more atrophyscarring. Patients with early withdrawal experienced better serum triglycerides and less weight gain, but no differences were observed regarding cholesterol levels, blood pressure or new-onset diabetes. The FREEDOM trial compared steroid avoidance versus early steroid withdrawal versus standard maintenance, in patients receiving induction with anti-CD25 antibody and maintenance with cyclosporine and mycophenolate. The incidence of acute rejection was higher in the steroid-free and withdrawal groups compared to the standard maintenance group, with the highest rate of acute rejection in the steroid avoidance arm. Moreover, many patients on the two steroid-free groups were back on steroids within 1 year. No major metabolic benefits were detected.

Thus, the randomized controlled trials showed that rapid steroid withdrawal is associated with an increased risk of acute rejection without an increased risk of graft failure. Also, most of the rejection episodes were steroid-sensitive, and no differences in terms of graft function were found. However, the long-term impact of these strategies could not be assessed at this time.

Trials of steroid avoidance strategies in kidney transplantation always force the question "compared to what?" With such a wide range of steroid dosage in common use, many extremely low, it is impossible to determine the net benefit of steroid elimination. The advantage of steroid withdrawal is its potential metabolic benefit, which may reduce cardiovascular risk and improve patient survival. Thus, steroid-free strategies are favorable for patients with metabolic or cardiovascular risk factors. These protocols may not be suitable for higher-risk recipients. In addition, current maintenance dosages of steroids are much lower than before, and the evidence of benefits of withdrawing steroids are often based on controls maintained on higher doses of steroids. The current doses of steroids for maintenance (2.5–5 mg/day or equivalent on alternate days) are less toxic than the higher dosage used previously (e.g., 10 mg/day or 15 mg every second day).

CN inhibitor minimization

CN inhibitors, which have become the fundamental ISDs for preventing rejection, are nephrotoxic and have detrimental metabolic adverse effects. Three main strategies have been used to avoid the adverse effects of CN inhibitors: reduction, substitution or conversion, and avoidance.

CN inhibitor reduction

The choice of a CN inhibitor, and its dose was examined in the Elite–Symphony trial. Four immunosuppressive regimens were compared: standard dose of cyclosporine, MMF and corticosteroids, induction with daclizumab followed by MMF and corticosteroids in combination with low-dose tacrolimus, low-dose cyclosporine, or low-dose-sirolimus. At 12 months post transplant, the regimen with low-dose tacrolimus showed better renal function, lower episodes of acute rejection, and better survival compared to the other regimens. However, the overall results in the reduced-dose cyclosporine were favorable. Patients under sirolimus did not have good results. It is important to note that the levels of CN in various centers are measured by immunoassays, and by mass spectroscopy which measure the parent compounds and do not measure the metabolites.

CN inhibitor substitution/withdrawal

Studies with CN inhibitor conversion to an mTOR have shown variable results. Early cyclosporine conversion (at 3 months post transplantation) to mTOR inhibitors improves renal function, but does not have a major impact on survival. The efficacy and safety of converting maintenance renal transplant recipients from CN inhibitors to sirolimus was evaluated in a prospective, randomized, clinical trial (the CONVERT study). Importantly, the evidence of a renal function (GFR < 40 ml/min) as well as a UPr/Cr ratio greater than 0.11 was not associated with a benefit of the conversion from CN inhibition- to sirolimus-based immunosuppression. Therefore, while being a promising approach for reducing CN inhibitor exposure and toxicity, a switch to sirolimus may not be applicable in all cases and should be avoided in high immunological risk kidney recipients, and those with low function or large proteinuria.

CN inhibitor avoidance

CN inhibitor avoidance strategies have generally been associated with higher rates of acute rejection. The Symphony trial confirms that mTOR inhibitors are less effective than CN inhibitors for the prevention of TCMR, and their early use was associated with high rates of discontinuation and adverse events. The trials with belatacept found that acute rejection was more frequent and severe in the belatacept group (belatacept, MMF, steroids). However, patients treated with belatacept achieved better renal function and had less chronic changes in the biopsy at 12 months than patients treated with cyclosporine, MMF, and steroids.

Managing antibody-mediated rejection and the positive crossmatch patient

Therapies to suppress donor-specific antibodies and treat antibody-mediated rejection

The drugs commonly used for the suppression of DSA or for the prevention and treatment of ABMR are listed in Tables 10.5 and 10.6.

Table 10.6 Details of drugs for prevention and treatment of antibody-mediated rejection.

Drug	Description	Mechanism	Nonimmune toxicity and comments	Monitoring
Intravenous immunoglobulins (IVIG)	Immunoglobulins derived from pooled human plasma from thousands of donors; used In low-dose and high-dose protocols	interactions of IVIG with several components of the immune system via the F (ab') 2 fragment or the Fc fragment; reduction of alloantibodies through inhibition of antibody production and increased catabolism of circulating antibodies	infusion-related complications (aseptic meningitis, thrombotic events, bronchospasm) and hemolytic anemia	No monitoring required
Rituximab	Chimeric (murine/human) monoclonal antibody directed against the CD20 antigen on the surface of B-cells	Depletion of CD20+ B cells	Infusion reactions, uncommon hypersensitivity reactions, infections	CD20+ B cell counts
Bortezomib	Proteasome inhibitor	Reduction of alloantibodies through proteasome inhibition and apoptosis of plasma cells	In treatment of myeloma adverse effects include peripheral neuropathy, sometimes painful; myelosuppression (neutropenia, thrombocytopenia) and zoster	No monitoring required
Eculizumab	humanized monoclonal antibody with high affinity for C5	Blockade of the activation of terminal complement cascade	Infections with Neisseria meningitidis	No monitoring required

Intravenous immunoglobulin (IVIG)

Intravenous immunoglobulin products are derived from human plasma pooled from thousands of donors.

Mechanism of action

The mode of action of IVIG in suppressing ABMR is complex and poorly understood. Proposed mechanisms include reduction of alloantibody levels through inhibition of antibody production and increased catabolism of circulating antibodies, and inhibition of effector mechanisms such as complement or Fc receptors on NK cells and inflammatory cells.

Efficacy

Intravenous immunoglobulin is a component of most desensitization protocols, for prevention of ABMR in transplanting sensitized patients with DSA, or in treating patients who develop ABMR. It is usually used in combination with other treatments for DSA or ABMR. The dosage of IVIG can be low or high. Low-dose IVIG (100 mg/kg) is usually used supplementing plasmapheresis for the treatment of ABMR and is administered after each session of plasmapheresis to add to Fc receptor inhibition of antibody-producing plasma cells. High-dose IVIG (2 g/kg) is also administered either for desensitization or for treatment of ABMR, alone or in combination with other drugs, or is prescribed at monthly intervals if more than one dose is required. Many protocols use IVIG in combination with maintenance ISDs, plasmapheresis, and rituximab. One recent study comparing treatments for ABMR in the first 3 months post-transplant found that graft survival was improved in patients treated with plasmapheresis/IVIG/anti-CD20 compared to high-dose IVIG alone.

Adverse effects

While the tolerability and safety of IVIG is good, complications of IVIG treatment include infusion-related complications (fever, allergic reactions, aseptic meningitis, thrombotic events, and bronchospasm), and hemolytic anemia.

Rituximab

Rituximab, a chimeric anti-CD20 monoclonal antibody, eliminates most B cells and is approved for use in treating refractory non-Hodgkin's B-cell lymphomas, including some PTLDs in organ-transplant recipients. Rituximab is used off-label in combination with maintenance ISDs, plasmapheresis, and IVIG to suppress DSA and to treat both type 1 and type 2 ABMR.

Pharmacokinetics

Rituximab is administered intravenously. Although the standard dosage in lymphomas is a four-cycle treatment of 375 mg/m^2, studies have reported successful results for the treatment of ABMR resistant to standard therapy using a single low-fixed dose (375 or 500 mg). B cell depletion persists for 3–6 months following treatment, and levels return to normal by approximately 12 months.

Mechanism of action

Although most antibodies are made by plasma cells, which are usually CD20-negative, some plasma cells are short-lived and must be replaced by CD20-positive precursors. Thus, depletion of CD20-positive cells reduces some antibody responses. CD20-positive B cells can act as secondary antigen-presenting cells, thus explaining why rituximab may ameliorate long-standing T cell responses. For example, this may be the reason why it suppresses rheumatoid arthritis.

Efficacy

Off-label applications for rituximab include treatment of ABMR, prophylaxis against ABMR, and suppression of preformed HLA antibody. Rituximab in combination with IVIG and plasmapheresis is superior to high-dose IVIG alone for the treatment of ABMR.

Adverse effects

Rituximab is well tolerated, but cases of progressive multifocal leukoencephalopathy have been reported in patients being treated with rituximab in lymphomas.

Bortezomib

Bortezomib is a proteasome inhibitor approved for use in the treatment of multiple myeloma. Proteasome inhibition causes apoptosis of some plasma cells because pro-apoptotic factors must be degraded by proteasomes to avoid apoptosis in plasma cells. In organ transplantation, proteasome inhibitor treatment provides a potential approach to reduce HLA antibodies. Initial limited experience with bortezomib suggests that proteasome inhibitor therapy for ABMR in kidney transplant recipients may have some effect as primary or rescue therapy. In late ABMR (i.e., 6 months or later, post transplant), it is not yet clear whether treatment with proteasome inhibitors results in reduction of antibodies, and whether long-lived plasma cells in the bone marrow are susceptible to bortezomib. Proteasome inhibitor therapy is associated with low rates of opportunistic infection, and does not substantially reduce antibody titers from childhood vaccinations.

Adverse effects

Bortezomib has induced peripheral neuropathy in many patients treated for myeloma, and can induce usually mild bone marrow suppression.

Eculizumab

Eculizumab is a humanized monoclonal antibody against complement factor C5, preventing C5 from activating the terminal complement pathway. Eculizumab is approved for use in the treatment of paroxysmal nocturnal hemoglobinuria (PNH). The rationale for using eculizumab in ABMR is based on the evidence of complement activation (as demonstrated by C4d staining of the peritubular capillaries). Successful prevention and treatment of early ABMR using eculizumab has been reported. Initial experiences with eculizumab treatment at the time of transplantation showed that blockade of terminal complement activation prevented the development of type 1 ABMR in patients with high levels of DSA, despite the persistence of the DSA. Thus, blockade of terminal complement activation is an attractive approach to the prevention of type 1 ABMR. Whether it can prevent the late development of transplant glomerulopathy is still unclear, since this may involve other mechanisms such as NK cell-mediated damage. Experience in paroxysmal nocturnal hemoglobinuria has shown that eculizumab is generally safe and well tolerated. Because susceptibility to infection with *Neisseria meningitides* is increased by complement deficiency, all patients require meningococcal vaccination prior to receiving eculizumab. To date, there is little evidence that complement inhibition with eculizumab suppresses the usual type of ABMR that emerges late after organ transplantation.

Emerging B cell-directed therapies

Several B cell-directed therapies in development for the treatment of B cell malignancies and autoimmune diseases have potential applications for modification of alloantibody responses in transplantation. CD19 is an antigen expressed on all B cells (and follicular dendritic cells), but is also present in early stages of B cell ontogeny and at lower levels on plasma cells. CD22 is expressed on naïve and transitional B cells. An antibody targeted against CD22, epratuzumab, depletes approximately 35% of the total B cell population. This drug is currently in clinical trials in patients with systemic lupus. The B cell activating factor (BAFF) is a member of the tumor necrosis factor cytokine family that is secreted by dendritic cells, macrophages, and neutrophils and contributes to B cell differentiation and activation. Recently, a human monoclonal antibody (belimumab) directed against BAFF was approved for use in the treatment of mild systemic lupus.

Strategies for desensitization and management of the positive crossmatch patient

Desensitization protocols emerged in the late 1990s as approaches to deal with the increasing numbers of sensitized wait-listed patients. Pre-existing sensitization against HLA antigens with DSA constitutes a serious hurdle to transplantation, leading to protracted waiting times for kidney transplant recipients and increased risk of type 1 ABMR, post transplant. Over the past decade, advancements in HLA antibody detection techniques, better diagnosis of ABMR, and the availability of effective regimens have permitted successful kidney transplantation across the HLA barrier. If no donor with a negative crossmatch is available, there are two main approaches:

1. Pre-transplant desensitization to achieve a negative crossmatch.
2. Transplantation across a weak positive crossmatch with heavy treatment to prevent ABMR.

Desensitization

This strategy of eliminating or decreasing pre-existing HLA alloantibody, aiming to reach a negative crossmatch and thus permit kidney transplantation, is mainly applicable to live donors, where transplantation can be performed as soon as the reduction in antibody level has been achieved. The goal of these strategies is to prevent ABMR and its devastating impact on graft outcome. We briefly mention some desensitization strategies.

Desensitization protocols consist of conditioning regimens using IVIG, and/ or anti CD20, and IVIG in combination with plasma exchange. One protocol developed for desensitization consists of high-dose IVIG courses of 2 g/kg every 3 weeks repeated three or four times. A modified protocol is two courses IVIG with the addition of a single 1 g dose of rituximab given between the IVIG courses.

Another choice is plasmapheresis with low-dose IVIG. In the case of deceased donor programs, where the waiting time for a suitable donor is uncertain, high-dose IVIG, alone or in combination with rituximab, is preferred since it provides a more sustained decrease in antibody level.

The real mechanism of IVIG in the setting of desensitization remains to be determined. IVIG possesses immunomodulatory, immunoregulatory, anti-inflammatory, and anti-complement properties, and occupies Fc receptors on effector cells. The use of the proteasome inhibitor bortezomib may be beneficial in the setting of desensitization as this may increase the metabolic activity of plasma cells and increase their susceptibility.

Protocol approaches to inhibit ABMR

The tools currently include anti-CD20, IVIG, and plasmapheresis, at the time of transplantation rather than some time before. Such protocols are more suitable with deceased donors as the timing is brief and constitutes a strategy of voluntary, but controlled risk-taking. Terminal complement blockade post-transplantation is a promising strategy, but needs to be evaluated in the long term. Clinical studies of desensitization using multiple agents indicate that they can permit many sensitized patients to be transplanted (Table 10.7). The use of other single agents as sole agents in desensitization (i.e., rituximab or borte-zomib) has not given consistently successful results. Patient and graft outcomes in patients receiving desensitization protocols are acceptable at least in the short-term period, post transplant. However, a high prevalence of ABMR is still

Table 10.7 Managing risks over time in transplant patients.

- Pre-adaptation
  - ○ Avoid ABMR: PRA, crossmatching
    - ○ Novel kidney sharing strategies to manage sensitized patients
    - ○ Major unmet need: transplant sensitized patients
    - ○ Desensitization: high risk for ABMR, late failure
  - ○ Avoid TCMR
    - ○ TCMR is relatively benign: no chronic rejection
  - ○ Avoid/manage nonspecific injury to the graft
  - ○ Manage infectious risks: CMV, EBV, BK, HCV, PCP
  - ○ Avoid post-transplant diabetes mellitus
- Post-adaptation:
- Vigilance for the three major causes of late graft loss
  - ○ ABMR due to anti-HLA (esp. DSA class II). Monitor DSA status before making decisions
  - ○ Nonadherence, ultimately leading to ABMR
  - ○ Recurrent disease
- "Enough" ISD to stabilize adaptation, prevent DSA: avoid dangerous minimization
- Little evidence for superiority of individual protocols post-adaptation
- Manage mechanism-related toxicities
- Vigilance for immunodeficiency toxicity e.g., PTLD, skin cancer

ABMR, antibody-mediated rejection; DSA, donor-specific antibody; PRA, panel reactive antibody; TCMR, T cell-mediated rejection.

observed and graft survival remains significantly lower than in nonsensitized patients, long-term outcome data are awaited. A recent FDA symposium on desensitization and treatment of AMR focused on the rapid advancements that have occurred in the field of desensitization and some of the issues and concerns desensitization has created. A major concern is the lack of standardization of solid phase assays for DSAs. In addition, despite promising studies, there are still no FDA approved drugs for desensitization (or treatment of ABMR). Despite these concerns, recent reports have summarized what is considered "best practices" for this immunologically disadvantaged group with focuses on the use of IVIG, plasma exchange, and rituximab in various combinations.

The inferior graft outcome as compared to nonsensitized patients has always raised the question of whether highly sensitized patients would be better served by waiting for a compatible organ. A study from the Johns Hopkins group suggests that desensitization strategy may provide a significant survival benefit as compared to waiting for a compatible organ. These findings offer an argument for a broader implementation of desensitization protocols. Such programs necessitate close clinical and immunological monitoring using recent techniques as well as screening biopsies. The alternatives of specific allocation protocols such as paired donor exchange programs must be optimized before these high-risk, resource-intensive programs are considered.

Tolerance induction strategies

Tolerance is often defined as a state in which transplant recipients fail to mount a pathologic injurious response to donor antigens, while responses to other antigens including microbial pathogens are not altered in the absence of continued immunosuppression. Thus, some use the term "operational tolerance," which defines a stable functioning graft and no signs of rejection in the absence of or minimal immunosuppression for an arbitrary period of time, with no apparent compromise in host defense. This is most commonly achieved in liver transplant recipients, particularly those more than 10 years post transplantation. This phenomenon is perhaps due to both the unique features of the liver (mass and ability to regenerate) and induction of T cell clonal exhaustion.

The strategies that are used to achieve tolerance in kidney transplantation include the following:

1. T cell depletion protocols pre-transplantation: These protocols are based on the hypothesis that tolerance can be achieved by inducing severe T cell deletion by thymoglobulin or alemtuzumab. The results have been disappointing in terms of long-term freedom from all ISDs.
2. HLA identical stem cell transplant (SCT) and induction of chimerism: Tolerance has been described in cases of HLA-identical SCT followed by renal transplantation from the same donors, when complete replacement of the recipient's bone marrow with donor hematopoietic cells has been achieved. Performance of SCT and kidney transplantation simultaneously has been used as a tolerogenic strategy in patients with hematologic malignancies and end-stage kidney disease. Also, graft losses due to rejection in these settings are reported. Stem cell transplantation has potential lethal complications and is justified only in cases where it is required to treat a life-threatening hematological malignancy.
3. HLA identical stem cell transplant (SCT) plus "facilitator cells" and induction of chimerism: This experimental protocol has achieved success in highly selected living donor recipients and continues to be evaluated (Ekberg et al., 2007).
4. Late withdrawal of ISDs: Spontaneous tolerance in kidney allograft has been reported in sporadic cases in which immunosuppression was discontinued due to nonadherence or under professional supervision due to life-threatening complications. However, most of these cases eventually develop rejection after ISD withdrawal, months or years after stopping the drugs, probably reflecting the decay of the nonspecific changes in the lymphoid organs. Thus, reported cases with long-term follow-up, normal renal function, and no rejection episodes are rare. Two cohorts of kidney tolerant transplant recipients have been recently reported; these studies showed that tolerant patients had immunologic abnormalities, displaying increased expression of several B-related genes, particularly those involved in B cell differentiation. In liver

transplantation, some patients can be withdrawn from ISDs successfully, particularly if they are many years post transplant, but clinicians remain divided on the risks and benefits of this strategy (El Zoghby et al., 2009). The unique aspects of the liver allograft include its mass and its regenerative capacity, suggesting that it may simply exhaust the antigen-specific T cell (and B cell?) clones.

In summary, no clinical strategy has demonstrated consistent success in achieving tolerance in kidney transplant recipients other than HLA-identical stem-cell transplantation. Thus, the adaptation that exists in a stable organ transplant recipient usually depends on ISDs. At some point, most immunosuppressive agents are billed as tolerogenic, an assertion typically followed by the realization that the state is not durable. Drug-free tolerogenic strategies in kidney or other organ transplants will require large-scale clinical trials.

References

Budde K, Becker T, Arns W, Sommerer C, Reinke P, Eisenberger U, et al. Everolimus-based, calcineurin-inhibitor-free regimen in recipients of de-novo kidney transplants: an open-label, randomised, controlled trial. Lancet 2011;377(9768):837–47.

Einecke G, Sis B, Reeve J, Mengel M, Campbell PM, Hidalgo LG, et al. Antibody-mediated microcirculation injury is the major cause of late kidney transplant failure. Am J Transplant 2009;9(11):2520–31.

Ekberg H, Tedesco-Silva H, Demirbas A, Vitko S, Nashan B, Gurkan A, et al. Reduced exposure to CN inhibitors in renal transplantation. N Engl J Med 2007;357(25):2562–75.

El Zoghby ZM, Stegall MD, Lager DJ, Kremers WK, Amer H, Gloor JM, et al. Identifying specific causes of kidney allograft loss. Am J Transplant 2009;9(3):527–35.

Halloran PF. Immunosuppressive drugs for kidney transplantation. N Engl J Med 2004;351(26):2715–29.

Further reading

Ferguson R, Grinyo J, Vincenti F, Kaufman DB, Woodle ES, Marder BA, et al. Immunosuppression with belatacept-based, corticosteroid-avoiding regimens in de novo kidney transplant recipients. Am J Transplant 2011;11(1):66–76.

Friman S, Arns W, Nashan B, Vincenti F, Banas B, Budde K, et al. Sotrastaurin, a novel small molecule inhibiting protein-kinase C: Randomized phase II Study in renal transplant recipients. Am J Transplant 2011;11(7):1444–55.

Halloran PF, de Freitas DG, Einecke G, Famulski KS, Hidalgo LG, Mengel M, et al. An integrated view of molecular changes, histopathology, and outcomes in kidney transplants. Am J Transplant 2010;10(10):2223–30.

Halloran PF, de Freitas DG, Einecke G, Famulski KS, Hidalgo LG, Mengel M, et al. The molecular phenotype of kidney transplants. Am J Transplant 2010;10(10):2215–22.

Hanaway MJ, Woodle ES, Mulgaonkar S, Peddi VR, Kaufman DB, First MR, et al. Alemtuzumab induction in renal transplantation. N Engl J Med 2011;364(20):1909–19.

Jordan SC, Tyan D, Stablein D, McIntosh M, Rose S, Vo A, et al. Evaluation of intravenous immunoglobulin as an agent to lower allosensitization and improve transplantation in highly sensitized adult patients with end-stage renal disease: report of the NIH IG02 trial. J Am Soc Nephrol 2004;15(12):3256–62.

Montgomery RA, Lonze BE, King KE, Kraus ES, Kucirka LM, Locke JE, et al. Desensitization in HLA-incompatible kidney recipients and survival. N Engl J Med 2011;365(4):318–26.

Newell KA, Asare A, Kirk AD, Gisler TD, Bourcier K, Suthanthiran M, et al. Identification of a B cell signature associated with renal transplant tolerance in humans. J Clin Invest 2010;120(6):1836–47.

Sellares J, De Freitas D, Mengel M, Reeve J, Einecke G, Sis B, et al. Understanding the causes of kidney transplant failure: the dominant role of antibody-mediated rejection and non-adherence. Am J Transplant 2011;12(2):388–99.

Stegall MD, Diwan T, Raghavaiah S, Cornell LD, Burns J, Dean PG, et al. Terminal complement inhibition decreases antibody-mediated rejection in sensitized renal transplant recipients. Am J Transplant 2011;11(11):2405–13.

Stegall MD, Gloor J, Winters JL, Moore SB, Degoey S. A comparison of plasmapheresis versus high-dose IVIG desensitization in renal allograft recipients with high levels of donor specific alloantibody. Am J Transplant 2006;6(2):346–51.

Vincenti F, Charpentier B, Vanrenterghem Y, Rostaing L, Bresnahan B, Darji P, et al. A phase III study of belatacept-based immunosuppression regimens versus cyclosporine in renal transplant recipients (BENEFIT study). Am J Transplant 2010;10(3):535–46.

Vincenti F, Friman S, Scheuermann E, Rostaing L, Jenssen T, Campistol JM, et al. Results of an international, randomized trial comparing glucose metabolism disorders and outcome with cyclosporine versus tacrolimus. Am J Transplant 2007;7(6):1506–14.

Vo AA, Lukovsky M, Toyoda M, Wang J, Reinsmoen NL, Lai CH, et al. Rituximab and intravenous immune globulin for desensitization during renal transplantation. N Engl J Med 2008;359(3):242–51.

CHAPTER 11

Organ-specific features in clinical transplantation

Roslyn B. Mannon

Division of Nephrology, Department of Medicine, University of Alabama at Birmingham, Birmingham, USA

CHAPTER OVERVIEW

- Transplant outcomes are outstanding and continue to improve in the short term; long-term patient and graft survivals are less so and remain a major concern.

- Immunosuppressive therapy is required for transplant survival and is complicated by infection and malignancy. There are no specific tests that can predict the adequacy of immunosuppression.

- Immunosuppressive therapies are remarkably effective against cellular rejection, but are less effective against antibody-mediated injury.

- Viral infections such as hepatitis C in the liver and BK polyoma virus in the kidney remain critical cause of late allograft failure.

- Continued investigation of the immune system should provide insights into donor-specific tolerance.

- The inadequate supply of transplantable organs underlies a current dilemma and has resulted in long-wait lists and continued mortality.

Introduction

Solid organ transplantation has evolved from an experimental procedure to an accepted treatment of organ failures. The success of transplantation has been attributed to the improvements in surgical techniques, in-depth understanding of the alloimmune response, and the development of effective therapies to suppress those responses. In rodent models, different transplanted organs provoke rejection responses that vary in intensity as well as in sensitivity to tolerance induction. For example, rejection of skin allograft is more vigorous than that of other transplants, while liver allografts are often spontaneously accepted in the

---

Transplant Immunology, First Edition. Edited by Xian Chang Li and Anthony M. Jevnikar.
© 2016 John Wiley & Sons, Ltd. Published 2016 by John Wiley & Sons, Ltd.
Companion website: www.wiley.com/go/li/transplantimmunology

absence of any immunosuppression. Similarly, in humans, recipient responses are affected by organ type, with liver being the least immunogenic and small bowel, the most immunogenic. Moreover, the multiplicity of organs transplanted simultaneously is more commonplace now, resulting in a further increase in potential immunologic activation. Thus, when managing an organ graft recipient, the organ-specific features necessitate specific considerations based on the type of organ transplanted, and the complexity of immune risks assessed in the recipient. In this chapter, we will review the current state of organ transplants, identifying the key outcomes, management strategies, and clinical challenges in various types of transplants. We will also address pathways and potential opportunities for further investigation.

Kidney

Current status of kidney transplantation

In 2013, nearly 17,000 kidney transplants were performed in the United States, which includes 5,700 from living donors. However, the waiting list continues to grow in a dramatic fashion. At present, nearly 100,000 individuals are wait-listed for deceased donor kidney transplant in the United States (OPTN/SRTR 2013 annual data report, 2015). It has become obvious that the supply of donor kidneys is terribly insufficient to meet the current demand. This has led to a number of proposed policy strategies to optimize the deceased donor pool. Expanding the deceased organ pool would mean including extended criteria donors (ECD), defined as donors older than 60 years as well as donors older than 50 years with any two of the following criteria: (i) hypertension, (ii) cerebrovascular cause of brain death, or (iii) pre-retrieval serum creatinine (SCr) level >1.5 mg/dl (130 μmol/l).The short-term outcome of such donor kidneys is similar to that of standard criteria donors, although 3- and 5-year survival and function are more problematic. Recipients of these kidneys are generally provided with improved survival compared to matched patients treated with dialysis, although there may be survival risks with the most marginal ECD organs. The engagement of a new allocation system should provide clinicians with the survival benefit estimates of a given kidney.

Along these lines are the recent use of donation after circulatory determination of death (DCDD), which refers to the donor who does not meet the criteria for brain death, but in whom cardiac standstill or cessation of cardiac function occurred before the organs were procured. Similar to brain death donors, DCDD kidneys enjoy similar graft and recipient survival with greater risk of delayed graft function, and no difference in acute rejection rates. Over the past 10 years, the use of ECD and DCDD kidneys has grown by 55 and 794%, respectively. These donors represent opportunities for wait-listed candidates but can be challenging in post-transplant management.

Other strategies to expand the donor pool include paired kidney exchange, in which incompatible living donors are "swapped" with their respective recipients to create acceptable pairs based on both blood types as well as to avoid preformed donor-specific antibodies (Gentry et al., 2011). These strategies are illustrated in Figure 11.1, and demonstrate the potent opportunity to use not only living donor kidneys, but of deceased donors as well. This process is enhanced by including the largest number of possible recipients and donors available. Challenges in this area include the imbalance in blood group O donors, the presence of highly sensitized recipients, geographic barriers, and legal issues. The long-term success of these transplants in highly sensitized recipients remains an issue, particularly in the management of ongoing antibody-mediated injury (Marfo et al., 2011). The ability to define antibody specificities in wait-listed patients by solid phase assays along with rapid high-resolution HLA typing

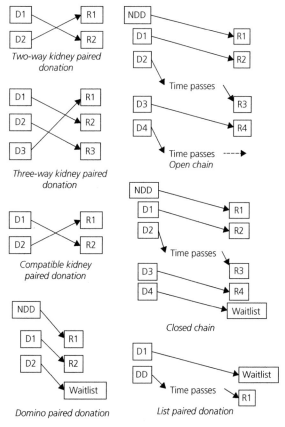

Figure 11.1 Paired kidney donation strategies. Donors (D) and recipients (R) are demonstrated by numbered pairs, and arrows show the route of the donor kidney to the intended recipient. Deceased donors (DDs) and nondirected donors (NDDs) may also participate in enhancing the potential to transplant more recipients. Source: Gentry et al. (2011). Reproduced by permission of Elsevier.

allows for virtual crossmatching across large geographies, looking for "acceptable mismatches" as a way to increase the deceased donor pool. This has been a successful strategy employed in Europe and recently in Canada, to provide kidneys for highly sensitized patients (i.e., cPRA > 95%).

Over the past several decades, both graft and recipient survival have improved dramatically as shown in Table 11.1 due to improved immunosuppression as well as optimized medical care of nonimmune-related issues. Typical antirejection regimens include both induction and maintenance components. Maintenance therapy has long included a combination of three types of agents: corticosteroids, a calcineurin inhibitor (CNI), and an antiproliferative agent. The focus of these therapies is aimed almost exclusively against T cell proliferation and function, rather than B cells or other cells of the innate immune response. In combination with "triple therapy" is the use of induction agents. Typically, in kidney transplantation, this includes both nondepleting monoclonal antibody targeted at CD25 on T cells or lymphocyte depleting strategies such as polyclonal rabbit antithymocyte globulin (ATG) and monoclonal anti-CD52 antibodies. The use of depletional induction has greatly facilitated the development of minimization and avoidance protocols, predominantly aimed at corticosteroids or CNIs. Newer agents for maintenance include mTOR inhibitors, which are substituted for antiproliferative agents, although their significant adverse effects in the early post-operative course have limited their use. The recent approval of belatacept, an inhibitor of the B7-1 and CD28 costimulatory pathway, may herald a new pathway for patient management, which permits complete CNI avoidance.

Patient and graft survival at 1 year has been the focus for many years. With such outstanding early outcomes, clinical trials of new agents would require enormous and costly studies in order to see even minimal improvements in outcomes. It has become clear to the field that new endpoints are needed in designing clinical trials. These may include measures of graft function (i.e., estimated or measured glomerular filtration rate), the extent of allograft fibrosis and tubular atrophy, or other biomarkers of late graft failure. The difficulty in defining these variables has in some ways led to a "failure to progress" period in transplantation, with minimal development of newer agents that may be more specific and less toxic, and the sense that there are available opportunities for early intervention to minimize late graft loss.

Challenges in renal transplantation

Immune monitoring: The need for indefinite immunosuppression is associated with significant complications, such as death due to immunosuppression-related morbidities, and a wide range of drug toxicities. This has led to a critical need in transplantation—the ability to detect sufficient immunosuppression to avoid alloimmune responses while avoiding toxicities of overimmunosuppression. SCr, an insensitive measure of renal function, remains the primary method to monitor acute rejection. However, multiple studies have shown that histologic

Table 11.1 Unadjusted graft and patient survival at 3 months, 1 year, 3 years, 5 years, and 10 years survival (%).

Organ and survival type		Follow-up period				
		3 months Tx 2006–2007 (%)	1 year Tx 2006–2007 (%)	3 years Tx 2004–2007 (%)	5 years Tx 2002–2007 (%)	10 years Tx 1997–2007 (%)
Kidney: deceased donor	Graft survival	95.3	91.0	80.1	69.3	43.3
	Patient survival	98.1	95.6	89.1	81.9	61.2
Kidney: living donor	Graft survival	98.1	96.3	89.6	81.4	59.3
	Patient survival	99.5	98.5	95.3	91.0	77.1
Pancreas alone	Graft survival	85.3	75.5	59.5	51.5	34.7
	Patient survival	98.9	97.8	92.3	88.7	76.1
Pancreas after kidney	Graft survival	87.1	80.0	65.2	53.4	36.9
	Patient survival	98.8	97.0	91.6	84.5	67.5
Kidney–pancreas	Kidney graft survival	96.0	92.5	86.1	78.6	58.3
	Pancreas graft survival	88.7	84.8	79.4	73.4	55.0
	Patient survival	97.9	95.7	91.7	87.2	71.4
Liver: deceased donor	Graft survival	91.2	84.3	74.2	68.4	54.1
	Patient survival	94.3	88.4	79.3	73.8	60.0
Liver: living donor	Graft survival	90.9	86.0	79.0	72.9	62.6
	Patient survival	94.9	91.0	84.9	79.0	69.9
Intestine	Graft survival	90.4	78.9	58.7	39.6	28.9
	Patient survival	96.1	89.3	72.0	57.9	46.4
Heart	Graft survival	92.8	87.9	80.6	73.7	54.2
	Patient survival	93.1	88.3	81.5	74.9	56.0
Lung	Graft survival	91.6	81.6	63.5	51.5	26.2
	Patient survival	92.3	83.3	66.2	54.4	28.6

Continued

Table 11.1 Continued

Heart–lung	Graft survival	85.5	80.5	61.5	43.1	26.2
	Patient survival	85.5	80.6	61.7	44.9	29.0
Kidney–liver	Kidney graft survival	89.8	83.0	71.9	64.4	48.1
	Liver graft survival	90.2	83.7	72.4	66.0	52.7
	Patient survival	93.3	87.4	76.5	71.4	58.9
Kidney–heart	Heart graft survival	94.7	92.6	82.6	76.0	57.5
	Kidney graft survival	90.5	88.2	78.5	72.0	48.7
	Patient survival	97.2	95.8	84.7	77.6	58.8
Liver–intestine	Intestine graft survival	71.4	58.7	55.3	53.0	36.7
	Liver graft survival	71.4	58.7	55.3	53.4	36.7
	Patient survival	73.3	63.3	58.2	58.0	39.0

Data from OPTN/SRTR (http://www.srtr.org) as of May 4, 2009.

features of allograft rejection may be present in the absence of any significant change in SCr. This has led to the performance of allograft biopsies at scheduled periods, the so-called protocol (surveillance) biopsies. However, biopsies are cumbersome, expensive, and are associated with morbidity. Thus, there has been a focus on finding assays that use noninvasively obtained tissue such as serum, urine, and peripheral blood mononuclear cells, to perform genomic, proteomic, and metabolic diagnostic approaches (Mannon & Kirk, 2006). Most of these methods have not been substantiated in larger clinical studies, and the impact of specific induction therapies remains clear. These are discussed further in Chapter 14.

Tolerance treatments and studies: A number of groups are investigating the potential for tolerance induction—that is, creating a milieu that results in donor-specific hypo- or nonresponsiveness. Within the clinical context, a number of centers have reported preliminary data regarding the ability to induce tolerance that is associated with microchimerisms. Insights into the mechanism of tolerance are also being elucidated through cohort studies in both North America and Europe and have suggested a possible role for B cells in a regulatory process. The role of regulatory T cells has long been under study and translational therapies that promote their development and reconstitution are emerging.

Recent studies by Wood et al. suggest that disruption of late allograft failure pathways may be amenable to human Tregs developed *ex vivo* and adoptively transferred. However, it remains an understatement that tolerance has been significantly more difficult to induce in man compared to inbred mouse models and even primates where successes have been identified. Some of the hurdles include heterologous immunity, homeostatic proliferation as a consequence of lymphocyte depletion induction, and the relative resistance of memory T cells found in primates to lymphocyte induction strategies.

Allograft fibrosis: One of the key features of failing kidney allografts is the presence of interstitial fibrosis (IF) and tubular atrophy (TA). Over the past decade, there has been growing appreciation that classifying all allografts as "chronic allograft nephropathy" is inaccurate and unhelpful, as the features of IF/TA frequently accompany most failing kidneys. A concerted effort has been made to identify the etiology of the failing kidney allograft. Indeed, a number of studies now demonstrate that there are identifiable etiologies of late graft failure, some of which have potential therapies (El-Zoghby et al., 2009). Both alloantigen-dependent and -independent events may lead to IF/TA (Figure 11.2). Once injury is initiated, there is an inflammatory process and a proliferative process mediated by chemokines, cytokines, and growth factors such as TGFβ and connective tissue growth factor (CTGF). Ultimately, there is increased extracellular matrix

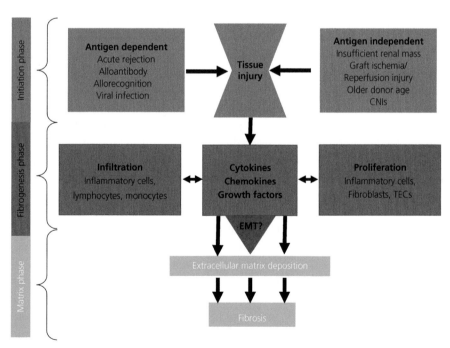

Figure 11.2 A proposed scheme of the events that lead to fibrosis in the failing kidney allograft. Similar mechanisms exist in other solid organs including the heart, lung, and liver.

deposition, either due to overproduction or reduced degradation. The role of epithelial mesenchymal transition remains a controversial but unlikely unifying cause of transplant fibrosis. Moreover, the clinical implications of such a process are also debated. Ultimately, fibrosis of the allograft may simply represent a programmed response to injury and a final common pathway for graft loss. It may however prove to be a useful adjunctive target to other strategies including modification of immunosuppression (Mannon, 2006).

Antibody-mediated injury: Antibody-mediated injury has been a growing focus of study over the past decade, facilitated by our ability to reliably detect even low levels of donor specific antibodies and general agreement on histologic criteria (Racusen et al., 2003). Acute antibody-mediated rejection may occur in the first weeks after transplantation, presenting with acute allograft dysfunction. Appropriate therapy selection has been under significant investigation including the use of rituximab, IVIg, and plasmapheresis (reviewed in Marfo et al., 2011) as well as the proteasome inhibitor bortezomib to inhibit plasma cell function and limiting injury using the C5 complement inhibitor eculizumab.

Late graft failure has become a huge focus for research as well as clinical management as nearly half of graft loss is due to the late and progressive decline in renal function. The participation of antibody in late injury has become even more apparent, although strategies to control remain elusive. Transplant glomerulopathy has been recognized as a key cause of late kidney allograft loss, characterized histologically by the widespread involvement of all glomeruli, enlargement and duplication of the glomerular basement membrane, and endothelial cell activation. Electron microscopy reveals subendothelial accumulation of electron lucent material, duplication of the basement membrane and interposition of mesangial cells into the capillary wall. Glomerular C4d staining may also be seen in this lesion, indicating the participation of antibody-mediated immune responses. Clinically, there is proteinuria, progressive renal dysfunction, and accelerated graft failure. Associated risk factors for development include the presence of anti-HLA antibodies at the time of transplant, late acute rejection and as well as the presence of non-HLA antibodies such as those targeting angiotensin (ATR) receptors. T cell activation and mononuclear cell activation have also been implicated in injury. The use of rituximab, often given along with IVIG, has met with some modest success in uncontrolled studies. The limited effect on an antibody may be due to the limited or absent expression of CD20 on antibody producing cells. Further investigation into the prospective development of glomerulopathy and the contributions of both cellular and antibody-mediated components is clearly needed.

Antibody-mediated injury may also be directed against non-HLA targets, including vascular endothelial cells, tubular basement membrane, and heparan sulfate proteoglycans. Recently, anti-angiotensin II type A receptor antibody has been detected in a subset of kidney transplant recipients with refractory vascular rejection episodes and malignant hypertension, although its role in late graft loss has not been defined. Finally, recent reports link antibodies against major histocompatibility complex (MHC) class I-related chain A (MICA) antigens to worsened graft outcomes.

Late kidney allograft failure: other mechanisms: There are other mechanisms that contribute to late allograft loss. Recurrence of the primary disease that leads to transplant failure is common in kidney transplantation, and the development of effective therapies in transplant is hampered by the lack of therapies effective in the initial disease that led to failure. Another cause of late graft loss is related to CNI-induced nephrotoxicity, which includes both kidney allograft as well as native kidney failure in other solid organ transplants. Also, a substantial number of transplant recipients, especially older adults, die with functioning grafts. The leading causes are cardiovascular disease accounting for approximately 30% of deaths and malignancy for 13% of deaths in the past decade, while, of rate, deaths due to infection are much less common. The rising prevalence of diabetes post-transplant is a significant risk factor. Improved recognition of all risk factors, personalization of drugs and screening for this complication post-transplant will provide for early intervention and a reduction in complication rate.

Infections post-transplant include both common as well as opportunistic microbes (Fishman, 2007). Primary infection with Epstein Barr Virus during immunosuppression may lead to the development of post-transplant lymphoproliferativedisease (PTLD), as there is an unrestricted expansion of EBV-infected B cells. Furthermore, ongoing issues exist for viral infections such as BK polyomavirus. This disorder may be fatal in spite of viral clearance by reduction of immunosuppression. Finally, the invasion of the CNS by the JC virus has been identified as a fatal complication in a number of immunosuppression treatment trials in autoimmune diseases. Such catastrophic outcomes have led to an abrupt abandonment of or reluctance to use some biologic agents in transplantation. Understanding the mechanisms leading to disease, and the appropriate methods to monitor for disease in those at highest risk remain critical questions to answer.

Malignancy remains a common contributor to recipient death. This is in part related to the contribution of viral inducers including EBV in PTLD, Hepatitis B and C in hepatocellular carcinoma, herpes viruses in Kaposi's sarcoma, and human papillomavirus (HPV) in cancers of the female urogenital tract. As well, solid tumors that are more common in the general nontransplant population occur more frequently in transplanted patients (i.e., 2–3x), usually with more severe outcomes. Clearly, limiting transplantation of those recipients at highest risk for cancer development and/or with a past history of cancer may reduce this risk after transplant. Moreover, skin and general cancer screening is a key part of post-transplant care, where the frequency intervals remains controversial in post-transplant kidney recipients.

Liver

Current status of liver transplantation

There are approximately 16,000 candidates on the waiting list for liver transplantation and only 6,200 were transplanted in 2010 (OPTN and SRTR, 2012). The model for end-stage liver disease (MELD) allocation system was instituted in 2002, in an effort to prioritize patients using a numerical score to reflect candidate illness and urgency for life-saving transplantation. Scores range from <9 (less ill; mortality at 3 months 1.9%) to >40 (gravely ill with 71.3% mortality in 3 months), and are ranked based on levels of bilirubin, INR as a reflection of liver synthetic function of coagulation proteins, and SCr. Modifications have also been made to include serum Na, in the attempt to further select recipients (Na-MELD). While there are specific exceptions to MELD scoring including cancers of defined size, these compose a minority of those waiting for a liver transplant. While MELD allocation de-emphasizes wait list times to facilitate transplantation to the sickest patients, wait-listed candidates are challenging to care for with their morbidities. In 2008, about 30% had some level of renal failure, and about 30% with diabetes and/or obesity (Thuluvath et al., 2010).

The limit in available deceased donor livers has led to alternative strategies to find available donors. This includes DCDD, which only accounts for <5% of livers transplanted in 2008 in the United States. The high frequency of nonanastomotic biliary strictures from ischemic cholangiopathy requires the identification of appropriate recipients. Thus, transplantation of the DCDD liver may reduce recipient quality of life after transplant and this must be weighed against the possibility of death on the waiting list. Living organ donors remain a relatively small population of donors (<0.5% per year) overall in the United States. Recent results of the A2ALL study of living liver transplantation has demonstrated survival benefits compared to deceased donor liver transplant in either low- or high-MELD groups and high MELD for those with hepatocellular carcinoma. The benefit in those with low MELD scores is in contrast with past reports of recipients of deceased donor liver transplants, data that provided impetus to change allocation policies.

Patient and graft survival after liver transplant (Table 11.1) have improved over the past decade. At 1 year, adjusted for age, gender, and race, and etiology of liver failure, graft survival in 1998 was 79.5% and up to 85.6% in 2007. Similarly, recipient survival improved from 85.4 to 89.4%, respectively, during those time periods (Thuluvath et al., 2010). A similar trend was seen in recipients of living liver grafts. Age again is a key contributor to outcome, with the worst 5 and 10 year graft survival in those >65 years old. While gender does not impact survival, race has a significant impact on graft survival outcomes in African-Americans being only 60% at 5 years, and falling to 45% at 10 years (Thuluvath et al., 2010). Graft survival is also affected by center and varies across the United States, with the worst outcomes in low volume (<10 transplants/

year), or much higher volumes (>57 transplants/year). Importantly, the presence of metabolic, cholestatic diseases, and biliary atresia were associated with better outcomes than in liver malignancies. Higher MELD scores (>30) had worse outcomes at 1 and 5 years compared to lower MELD scores (11–20). Extremes of donor age (<1 and >65 years) also have a negative impact on survival.

Both clinical and experimental experiences seem to indicate that liver transplants are relatively resistant to transplant rejection. For example, combined organ transplantation with a liver seems to "protect" the other organ from rejection, although the effect may be less apparent or nonexistent in recipients treated with CNI. The role of the antibody has been more subtle in liver than in other organs, likely due to its relatively huge absorptive surface. However long term, antibody does appear to have a worsening effect on graft survival, but not as dramatically as in the kidney. In contrast to other solid organs, HLA matching has no impact on liver transplant outcomes and, currently, is not a consideration in transplant allocation. Finally, there is a growing appreciation of the ability of some recipients to be weaned off immunosuppression in the absence of rejection, many being operationally "tolerant." However, for the most part, immunosuppression remains a requirement for liver transplant recipients.

The selection of immunosuppression depends on its known toxicities, some of which may be specific in certain disease states such as malignancy and hepatitis C. Typical immunosuppression consists of CNI therapy, in spite of its potential nephrotoxicity and profibrotic effects, coupled with corticosteroids and mycophenolate mofetil (MMF). MMF use has been further explored as an avenue for CNI-free treatment with improvement in renal function, but rejection rates are higher when used as a monotherapy compared to CNI. While corticosteroids have been the mainstay in solid organ transplantation, their potential toxicities as well as their ability to induce hepatitis C viral replication are associated with worsened outcomes. The effect of steroids on hepatitis B viral replication is not an issue with effective antibiotics. Consequently, strategies to limit steroid use include the use of rabbit antithymocyte globulin and anti-CD25 antibody. Regardless, steroid-free arms have higher rejection rates compared to steroid maintenance therapy. In hepatitis C recipients, there was a reduction in viral replication and improved outcome compared to steroid maintenance therapy. CNI avoidance in maintenance therapy is another goal, and recent studies using rabbit ATG as well as everolimus have appeared to be successful with low rejection rates.

The development of spontaneous long-term acceptance of a liver allograft after stopping immunosuppression, referred to "operational tolerance" has been identified in approximately 20% of liver transplant recipients. This state is associated with longer times post transplantation, low dose maintenance immunosuppression, presence of post PTLD, and transplantation for autoimmune diseases. Based on these early observations, there are multiple ongoing trials in adults as well as in children. Recent studies of immunosuppressive withdrawal in pediatric recipients were associated with higher levels of success from 34 to

45% of subjects, demonstrating that pediatric recipients have a propensity to operational tolerance. This may be related to the fact that the immune system is less mature at the time of transplant compared to that in adults, the frequent use of monotherapy for maintenance immunosuppression, and the progressive weaning that occurs due to patient growth in the absence of drug monitoring. Potential biomarkers reported in these recipients include increased numbers of plasmacytoid rather than myeloid dendritic cells. Increased expression of $\gamma\delta$-T cells has also been described with tolerance and gene expression studies in PBMC's of these recipients further demonstrating enhanced expression of genes related to NK- and $\gamma\delta$-T cells. Collectively, these support the notion of organ-specific mechanism of tolerance within the liver. Further insights into the mechanism(s) in liver transplant are needed and could provide important insights for other solid organ recipients.

Hepatitis C (HCV) infection remains a considerable problem in liver transplantation. Between 35 and 41% of recipients are transplanted annually due to HCV (Thuluvath et al., 2010) and the rate is alarmingly increasing. The negative impact of HCV infection on patient survival becomes apparent around 2 years post transplantation, with 5 year recipient survival falling from approximately 85% in those that are not infected to approximately 73% in those infected. A number of recipient factors have a negative impact on graft and patient survival including older age (>65 years), such as African-American race, female gender, diabetes, previous nonliver transplant, prior malignancy, and diagnosis of hepatocellular cancer. Donor factors include older age, with the highest rate of death from donors >64 years, and the use of DCD donor livers.

Recurrent disease is a common complication in recipients. Viremia is nearly uniform and progressive hepatitis C is seen in more than 70% of recipients. While clinical features of recurrent disease are similar to native disease, some important distinctions exist. First and foremost, progression of fibrosis is more rapid in the allograft. This is likely related to rapid viral replication, in part facilitated by the immunosuppression as well as the high degree of HLA mismatches between donor and recipient, which leads to attenuated immunologic control of the virus and alloimmune responses. Fibrosis appears to be related to hepatic stellate cell activation with myofibroblast formation. An additional immunologic contributor may be autoimmune-mediated liver injury similar to that seen in native liver infection. Establishing a diagnosis of recurrent disease versus acute rejection may be difficult. High viral loads >30 million IU/ml are more consistent with recurrence. Clearly, treatment outcome depends on accurate diagnosis as the former suggests immunosuppressive withdrawal and the latter means enhanced treatment.

Challenges in liver transplantation

With graft survival strongly influenced by HCV and recurrent disease, a significant focus of investigation has been related to the immunologic mechanisms of HCV clearance, allograft fibrosis mediated by HCV, and finding effective treatments in this population. As viral replication is associated with intense immunosuppression, immunosuppressive withdrawal has been used in the post-transplant setting with some success. However, too rapid a withdrawal may actually result in rebound disease with more advanced viral replication and further immune activation. Alternatively, with the introduction of new direct antiviral protease inhibitors, the stage is set for the elimination of this virus as well as for reducing its impact on initiating disease in native and transplant tissue (Rice & Saeed, 2014). The major limitation at this time is the high cost.

Similar to other solid organ transplants, long-term graft survival is negatively impacted by the development of other morbidities that are to a large extent related to the toxicities of immunosuppression. The incidence of malignancy increases with time after transplant, ranging at 5 years from 5–15% to 16–42% at 20 years post transplantation, and rates of tumor development are two to four times that of age-matched controls that are not transplanted. There is a 3-fold risk for cardiovascular events and a 2.6-fold risk for cardiovascular death in this population, in part due to the coincident risk factors of diabetes, hypertension, and dyslipidemia that are further associated with immunosuppression and the underlying disease. Finally, chronic kidney disease is quite common in this recipient population. The etiologies include injury prior to transplant, glomerular disease and IgA deposition, hepatitis C, older recipient age, diabetes, and nephrotoxicity due to CNI therapy. In a large registry study, nearly 30% of nonrenal solid organ recipients developed end stage renal disease requiring dialysis or kidney transplantation (Ojo et al., 2003). In liver recipients, nearly 18% will require renal replacement therapy by 5 years after liver transplantation (Table 11.2). Thus, identifying those at risk for renal failure would change their listing strategy and/or post-transplant management, including CNI-free immunosuppression.

Table 11.2 Cumulative incidence of chronic renal failure in other nonrenal solid organ transplant recipients.

Type of organ	Cumulative incidence of chronic failure after transplantation			Relative risk of chronic renal failure (95% CI)
	12 months	36 months	60 months	
Heart	1.9±0.1	6.8±0.2	10.9±0.2	0.63 (0.61–0.66)
Heart-Lung	1.7±0.1	4.2±0.9	6.9±1.1	0.48 (0.36–0.65)
Intestine	9.6±0.2	14.2±2.4	21.3±3.4	1.36 (1.00–1.86)
Liver	8.0±0.1	13.9±0.2	18.1±0.2	1.00 (reference)
Lung	2.9±0.2	10.0±0.4	15.8±0.5	0.99 (0.93–1.06)

Data from Ojo et al. 2003.

Simultaneous liver kidney (SLK) transplantation is a strategy provided for liver failure recipients with irreversible renal disease. While liver transplants increased by 35% from 1999 to 2008, SLK transplants increased by over 279% during the same time, with 379 performed from a total of over 6000 liver transplants. However, defining the extent of irreversible renal disease remains a challenge, even with invasive testing to assess renal reserve and structural abnormalities. This along with the inadequate supply of deceased donor kidneys and that kidney transplant provides a survival benefit to nonliver patients on dialysis, makes organ allocation decisions very difficult. Thus, there is a critical need to identify factors that can predict chronic kidney disease that will continue to progress, not only to determine who to list for a kidney, but also to improve management strategies for those at high risk of renal failure and to identify mechanisms for progression.

Lung

Current status of lung transplantation

Over 1000 individuals with lung disease are currently on the active waiting list for lung transplantation, with another 900 on the inactive (Yusen et al., 2010). As in other countries, in the United States, allocation is based on the lung allocation system (LAS), which incorporates medical urgency and outcome post-transplant to prioritize transplants. This system takes into account not only survival without a transplant for the year after listing but also the outcome expected post-transplant for 1 year. Clinical parameters are also included to determine disease severity in order to most efficiently use a very scarce resource. The impact of this allocation system is that waiting times were dramatically reduced, and in 2008, nearly one-quarter of waiting list patients received a lung graft in 35 days (Yusen et al., 2010). Furthermore, waiting list mortality was reduced, with 128 deaths per 1000 patient years. With effective utilization of organs, about 1400 transplants were performed in 2008, the majority being double-lung transplants. Nearly all the donor grafts were after neurologic determination of death and not DCDD.

Graft survival is shown in Table 11.1, with a 1 year survival of 81.6%, and 5 year of 51.5%. These survivals have not improved significantly over the past decade and are substantially lower than for other solid organs. This is in part affected by recipient age as well as the underlying diagnosis. Immunosuppression in this population uses agents in a similar fashion to other solid organs. About 63% of recipients receive induction therapy, more commonly anti-CD25 (43%), and less commonly depletional induction (Yusen et al., 2010). Maintenance immunosuppression typically includes tacrolimus and mycophenolatemofetil with corticosteroids. This has resulted in 1-year graft rejection rates of only 26%. The majority of these episodes respond to steroid while about 14% required lymphocyte depletion therapy.

Challenges in lung transplantation

As with other solid organs, a major limitation is the lack of donor organs. This is even more complex in the context of lung transplantation, as only 15% of multiorgan donors are acceptable for lung transplantation. This is in part due to injuries associated with brain or cardiac death, barotrauma during ventilation, or other issues including suboptimal gas exchange function or infiltrates on chest x-ray. The use of such organs results in suboptimal graft survival with a high rate of chronic injury. Recent studies using normothermic *ex vivo* perfusion demonstrate that this may be a promising strategy to optimize lung function and facilitate the identification of organs that will provide reasonable clinical results. Other manipulations to limit primary graft dysfunction and related ischemic injury include transfection with IL-10, nitric oxide or carbon monoxide inhalation, soluble complement receptor 1, and platelet-activating factor antagonists. Studies are underway to better understand the mechanisms of injury to expand the donor pool, and provide potential treatment strategies.

Despite early graft success, and the evolution of diagnostics and therapeutics, long-term survival of lung allografts remains quite poor, with less than 30% survival at 10 years. The leading cause of this late graft loss is bronchiolitis obliterans syndrome (BOS). This is characterized clinically by a progressive decline in airway flow that does not appear to be due to acute rejection, infection, or other primary issue. The histology is characterized by patchy submucosal fibrosis involving the bronchioles resulting in occlusion of the airway lumen. Nearly half of the recipients will develop this syndrome by 5 years post-transplant, and while the lesion represents a final common pathway, the presentation, progression, and causes are heterogeneous. Clinical risk factors for BOS include ischemia/reperfusion injury, CMV, and respiratory virus infections; aspergillosis colonization and GI reflux may all stimulate innate activation. A key immune risk factor for disease is acute cellular rejection. Another key contributing factor appears to be antibody-mediated injury. This can include both HLA-donor specific antibodies as well as non-HLA antibodies directed against bronchial epithelium and bronchial wall microvasculature. Limitations here include the ability to detect non-HLA antibodies as well as a lack of effective treatments that suppress antibody production. Autoantibodies may also develop directed against collagen V that resides beneath the basement membrane in the perivascular and peribronchiolar tissues of the lung. As in other organs, the role of Th17 cells in auto and alloimmuneresponses is under investigation. As the lungs represent an interface with the environment, the contribution of innate immune cells is being explored as toll-like receptors (TLRs) are present on pulmonary antigen-presenting cells, as well as the airway epithelium. These may contribute to aggressive immune responses after infections or toxins. Thus, BOS appears to represent an interplay of innate and adaptive immune responses, with undefined genetic susceptibilities and diverse environmental factors.

Heart

Current status of heart transplantation

Despite the rapid advances being made in mechanical support systems, heart transplantation remains the primary therapy for end stage heart disease. About 3100 patients are currently on the active waiting list. Over the past decade, deaths on the waiting list have fallen to 170 per 1000 patient years, in part due to the use of left ventricular assist devices (LVADs). While numbers of older recipients are declining, the prevalence of younger recipients is on the rise due to congenital heart disease and cardiomyopathy, which are leading primary causes of heart failure. A limiting factor again is the availability of suitable organs, as only about 2000 transplants are performed each year. This is in part affected by donor utilization which varies widely among donor service areas. More than 2/3 of candidates on the waiting list require some intensive medical support be it ventilation, intra-aortic balloon pump, ionotropic drugs, or LVAD. In 2008, about 30% of the recipients were bridged from an LVAD, nearly doubling over the past decade (Johnson et al., 2010). As it is not clear if LVAD use affects transplant outcomes, their use is not included in the current allocation policy. However, LVAD appears to provide a survival opportunity for patients on the waiting list (Miller et al., 2007). Patient survival has improved over the past decade at 89%, 75%, and 56% at 1, 5, and 10 years, respectively, post transplantation (Table 11.1). Results are modestly better for those with primary cardiomyopathy compared to those with congenital heart disease. Long-term survival, however, continues to be a major issue.

Induction immunosuppression is used in about half of the recipients with either rabbit ATG or anti-CD25 antibody. Maintenance immunosuppression in the vast majority includes tacrolimus, mycophenolatemofetil, and corticosteroids. Due to the effectiveness of immunosuppression, acute rejection rates in the first year have fallen to 19%, typically treated with corticosteroids and less commonly, with lymphocyte depletion in 17% (Johnson et al., 2010). However, there is a growing interest in and implementation of steroid withdrawal or avoidance with nearly 30% of transplanted recipients in 2007. Moreover, about 10% of the recipients are on mTOR inhibitors by the end of 1 year post-transplant in the attempt to limit the development of transplant vasculopathy.

A unique feature of cardiac transplantation has been the use of ABO incompatible (ABO-I) transplantation in pediatric recipients. Due to the success reported by West and colleagues, infants eligible for ABO-I rose from 0% in 2002 to 50% in 2007. As isohemagglutinins develop later in infancy, transplantation performed prior to the development of these natural antibodies results in B cell tolerance and in the lack of anti-A or anti-B antibodies being formed. The result is similar post-transplant survival compared to infants receiving blood type compatible transplants. This has not resulted in changes in waiting list times, as US allocation places an organ ABO-compatible as the priority, and there has not appeared to be any impact on infant wait list times.

Challenges in heart transplantation

Much like other organs, the lack of available donor organs and the invariable damage from IRI remain the largest hurdles. Thus, strategies aimed at maintaining cardiac function and limiting ischemic damage are of significant interest. Late allograft failure, referred to as cardiac allograft vasculopathy (CAV), is histologically characterized by concentric intimal hyperplasia involving all allograft vessels, resulting in graft ischemia and ultimately failure. Both immune and nonimmune mechanisms may mediate this injury. In particular, innate immune activation appears to be a critical factor, as injury is not altered by current T cell-specific immunosuppression. Much like in kidney and lung transplantation, donor specific alloantibody with attendant complement-mediated endothelial injury is now recognized as a key contributor to vasculopathy. Indeed, histologic criteria for antibody-mediated rejection suffice for diagnosis, even in the absence of cardiac dysfunction or detectable donor specific antibody, and this lesion may further progress to transplant vasculopathy (Kobashigawa et al., 2011). Treatment strategies include those similar to kidney transplants, including plasmapheresis, IVIg, rituximab, as well as the use of mTOR inhibitors. However, effective strategies are a key focus in this field and there are active clinical trials to assess the impact of complement disruption and plasma cell inhibition.

While graft biopsies are used for diagnostic purposes, this may not be the most effective strategy to monitor for disease progression. Intravascular ultrasound (IVUS) is an invasive, but highly sensitive technique to monitor and diagnose disease, providing information on vessel lumen size, intimal thickening, and vessel wall morphology. IVUS can be coupled with noninvasive testing like dobutamine stress echocardiography to further increase diagnostic accuracy. Other biomarkers are under study to assess injury prior to ensuing functional damage.

Small bowel

Current status of small bowel transplantation

About 200 individuals are awaiting small bowel transplantation and the waitlist has doubled over the past 10 years. Not infrequently, a liver transplant or other solid organ may accompany the small bowel. Because of its specialized nature, small bowel transplant is only performed at a limited number of experienced transplant centers. Of those currently wait-listed, the most common etiology of disease is short bowel syndrome (73%), followed by functional abnormalities in 15%. Patient outcomes are similar to other solid organs with a 1 year survival of nearly 90%, followed by a decline to 58% at 5 years, and 46% at 10 years (Table 11.1). Graft survival at 10 years is a dismal 29%. Considerable issues exist in organ allocation and these criteria continue to be refined to be sure there is fairness and equity in providing a very limited resource. A key problem lies in the fact that the relatively small size of the transplant population limits the statistical capabilities of calculating the survival benefits between transplantation and those on the waiting list.

Since 1995, immunosuppression has evolved to include depletional induction followed by triple immunosuppression. Other strategies have included donor bone marrow, infliximab (anti-TNFα therapy), and cyclophosphamide infusion. The inflammatory state of patients and high immunogenicity of the gut, have led to difficulties, as noted later, in suppressing the rejection responses and inflammation adequately.

Challenges in small bowel transplantation

Organ utilization continues to be a considerable issue with about only 3% of organ donors being suitable for small bowel donation. This has translated into significant death rates on the waiting list. The primary reasons for not procuring the small bowel include poor organ function in 25% of the donors, underlying medical history, and refusal by national programs. The last reason is becoming increasingly more common, accounting for 16% in 2008. Strategies currently used include the consideration of living donors, DCD donors, improved donor utilization, expansion of acceptable criteria, and new allocation policies.

The small bowel is a highly immunogenic organ due to a number of factors. These include the presence of intestinal epithelium that can act as antigen-presenting cells, allorecognition that occurs in secondary lymphoid tissue of the graft, the relatively huge numbers of immune cells within the Gut Associated Lymphoid Tissue (GALT), and the state of constant inflammation of the allograft due to exposure to bacterial flora that results in the activation of innate and adaptive immune cells. Thus, T cell-based immunosuppression may be insufficient to control rejection and other mechanisms that lead to chronic rejection and injury. Further insights into this antigenic stimulus could provide new insights into more specific therapies to ensure better graft and patient survival.

Long-term complications in this recipient population include a high rate of renal failure of 21% at 5 years post-transplant. Risk factors for renal failure include low pre-transplant GFR, high-dose CNI therapy, and higher level of disease severity prior to transplantation. PTLD is also more frequently seen in recipients of small bowel allografts with an incidence reported as high as 20% and about half of cases resulting in graft failure and death. Risk factors include the use of OKT3 depletional induction therapy. Further understanding of the etiology of this tumor and its development should lead to improved strategies for prevention and treatment.

Conclusion

While there are similarities in the diagnostics and therapeutics used in each of the organ groups, there is little doubt that they behave differently due to endogenous mechanisms that alter immunogenicity as well as responses to

Table 11.3 Strategies to address key questions in transplantation.

Clinical problem	Scientific problem	Possible subject areas of study
Late allograft failure	Identifying mechanisms of immune injury and potential therapeutic strategies	Immune Regulation
		Tolerance
		Immune reconstitution (homeostatic proliferation)
		Antibody, B cells, endothelial injury
Insufficient donor organs	Identify mechanisms to ameliorate organ injury	Regenerative Medicine
	Synthesis of solid organs	IRI studies
Toxicities including metabolic, infectious, and malignant	Balancing immune system suppression vs toxicities	Immune monitoring assays
		Proteomics, metabolomics, genomics

inflammation and injury. There are considerable insights to be gained by studying the differences. As well, the transplant community must collectively address three critical issues: (i) the inadequate supply of donor organs resulting in long waiting times and death on the waiting list; (ii) long-term graft failure with associated fibrosis, vascular disease, and chronic inflammation; and (iii) recipient morbidity and mortality, which is in large part mediated by toxicities of the chronic immunosuppression. While we are seemingly poised for significant opportunities to investigate these areas (Table 11.3), application of emerging technologies to these problems as well as the identification of new targets and therapeutics is required. Unfortunately, there has been a decline in the investment required for the latter in transplant, due to difficulties in obtaining drug approval, the medical complexity of recipients, and the greater likelihood of adverse events in recipients. More strategic studies, the careful application of existing research tools to well-defined cohorts and push to new therapeutics may provide the much needed long-term benefit to patients.

Acknowledgment

Roslyn B. Mannon was supported in part by grants from the NIH (U01AI084150, U19AI070119, and RO1DK75532). The author has no other relevant affiliations or financial involvement with any organization or entity with a financial interest or conflict with the subject matter discussed in this manuscript. We appreciate the excellent administrative support of Ms. Wendy Bailey.

References

El-Zoghby ZM, Stegall MD, Lager DJ, Kremers WK, Amer H, Gloor JM, et al. Identifying specific causes of kidney allograft loss. *Am J Transplant.* 2009;9(3):527–35.

Fishman JA. Infection in solid-organ transplant recipients. *N Engl J Med.* 2007;357(25):2601–14.

Gentry SE, Montgomery RA, Segev DL. Kidney paired donation: fundamentals, limitations, and expansions. *Am J Kidney Dis.* 2011;57(1):144–51.

Johnson MR, Meyer KH, Haft J, Kinder D, Webber SA, Dyke DB. Heart transplantation in the United States, 1999–2008. *Am J Transplant.* 2010;10(4 Pt 2):1035–46.

Kobashigawa J, Crespo-Leiro MG, Ensminger SM, Reichenspurner H, Angelini A, Berry G, et al. Report from a consensus conference on antibody-mediated rejection in heart transplantation. *J Heart Lung Transplant.* 2011;30(3):252–69.

Mannon RB. Therapeutic targets in the treatment of allograft fibrosis. *Am J Transplant.* 2006;6(5 Pt 1):867–75.

Mannon RB, Kirk AD. Beyond histology: novel tools to diagnose allograft dysfunction. *Clin J Am Soc Nephrol.* 2006;1(3):358–66.

Marfo K, Lu A, Ling M, Akalin E. Desensitization protocols and their outcome 1. *Clin J Am Soc Nephrol.* 2011;6(4):922–36.

Miller LW, Pagani FD, Russell SD, John R, Boyle AJ, Aaronson KD, et al. Use of a continuous-flow device in patients awaiting heart transplantation. *N Engl J Med.* 2007;357(9):885–96.

Ojo AO, Held PJ, Port FK, Wolfe RA, Leichtman AB, Young EW, et al. Chronic renal failure after transplantation of a nonrenal organ. *N Engl J Med.* 2003;349:931.

OPTN/SRTR 2013 annual data report. *Am J Transplant.* 2015;15(S2):4–13.

Organ Procurement and Transplantation Network (OPTN) and Scientific Registry of Transplant Recipients (SRTR).

OPTN/SRTR 2011 Annual Data Report. Department of Health and Human Services, Health Resources and Services Administration, Healthcare Systems Bureau, Division of Transplantation; 2012.

Racusen LC, Colvin RB, Solez K, Mihatsch MJ, Halloran PF, Campbell PM, et al. Antibody-mediated rejection criteria—an addition to the Banff 97 classification of renal allograft rejection. *Am J Transplant.* 2003;3(6):708–14.

Rice CM, Saeed M. Hepatitis C: treatment triumphs. *Nature.* 2014;510(7503):43–4.

Thuluvath PJ, Guidinger MK, Fung JJ, Johnson LB, Rayhill SC, Pelletier SJ. Liver transplantation in the United States, 1999–2008. *Am J Transplant.* 2010;10(4 Pt 2):1003–19.

Yusen RD, Shearon TH, Qian Y, Kotloff R, Barr ML, Sweet S, et al. Lung transplantation in the United States, 1999–2008. *Am J Transplant.* 2010;10(4 Pt 2):1047–68.

CHAPTER 12

Transplant-related complications

Leonardo V. Riella and Anil Chandraker

Transplant Research Center, Renal Division, Brigham and Women's Hospital, Harvard Medical School, Boston, USA

CHAPTER OVERVIEW

- Cardiovascular diseases are the leading cause of death after transplantation, which are caused by compromised graft function and metabolic complications.

- Hyperglycemia is observed in >60% of transplant recipients and is associated with adverse patient and graft outcomes. Post-transplant bone mineral disorder increases the risk of fractures and cardiovascular calcification.

- Infections are related to time after transplant, epidemiologic exposures, and the state of immune suppression.

- Malignancy is the third most common cause of death after transplantation. The most common cancers are skin cancer, renal cell cancer, and post-transplantation lymphoproliferative disorders.

- Impaired immune surveillance and oncogenic viral infections play a major role in the development of cancer in this population.

Introduction

With newer immunosuppressive regimens and better patient management, short-term graft survival has been greatly improved over the years in transplant patients. However, this advancement has not been translated into better long-term outcomes. In kidney transplantation, for example, the half-life of kidneys from deceased donors has only marginally improved from 8 years in 1995 to 8.8 years in 2005. These data indicate that more than 50% of kidney allografts are lost within 10 years of transplantation. With the increasing number of potential recipients on the waiting list, this translates into an ever-growing waiting time for organs, which presents an enormous challenge for the field of organ transplantation.

Transplant Immunology, First Edition. Edited by Xian Chang Li and Anthony M. Jevnikar.
© 2016 John Wiley & Sons, Ltd. Published 2016 by John Wiley & Sons, Ltd.
Copyright ® American Society of Transplantation 2016.
Companion website: www.wiley.com/go/li/transplantimmunology

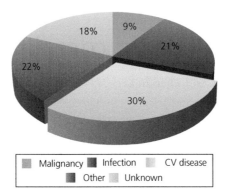

Figure 12.1 Causes of death with a functioning allograft. Source: Adapted from USRDS data (2004–2008).

In a recent study involving a cohort of 1317 kidney transplant patients with a mean follow-up of 50 months (±32), two major causes of allograft loss have been identified, which are death with a functioning allograft (41.8%) and late allograft loss (46.3%) due to recurrent glomerular disease, and rejection or progressive fibrosis. Among the causes of death with a functioning allograft, cardiovascular disease was the leading one, followed by infection and malignancy. These findings are also in accordance with recent USRDS data as depicted in Figure 12.1; similar observations have also been reported with other solid organ transplants. Thus, the control of immunologic responses should not be the sole goal for the long-term improvement of graft survival and special attention should also be given to possible metabolic, infectious, and cancer-related complications in transplant patients. In this chapter, we highlight the most common post-transplant complications, their pathogenesis, and potential management strategies.

Infections

Transplant recipients are at increased risk of infections primarily related to broad immunosuppression that limits responses against viral, bacterial, and fungal pathogens. These infections affect allograft function and cause significant morbidity and mortality. In general, the clinical presentation of infection in transplanted recipients is not always typical, as immunosuppressive medications increase the risk of opportunistic infections, but dampen the signs and symptoms of their presence. There are certain clues that might help in the differential diagnosis of post-transplant infection, including the timing after transplantation, degree of immunosuppression, history of exposure, pre-transplant serologies, and the infectious history of the recipient. Furthermore, the possibility of donor-originated infections should also be considered. Early and specific microbiologic diagnosis is essential, often requiring invasive procedures for accurate and timely diagnosis. There is no objective clinically useful test to quantify the risk of infection in an immunosuppressed patient. As a result, drug dosages or levels are used as poor surrogates of immunotherapy intensity.

Common infections in transplant patients

Urinary tract infection is the most common infection following kidney transplantation with the classic presentation of dysuria sometimes being absent. Renal ultrasound examination is usually performed to rule out any obstruction of the urinary tract. Treatment consists of either trimethoprim-sulfamethoxazole or a fluoroquinolone for 7 days. Based on current available data, guidelines do not recommend either screening for, or treatment of, asymptomatic bacteriuria in renal transplant or other solid organ transplant recipients. However, some retrospective studies suggest that treatment of asymptomatic bacteriuria results in a potential reduction in pyelonephritis; and in most transplant centers, it is common practice to treat a first episode of bacteriuria even in the absence of symptoms.

In general, infections occur in a predictable pattern following solid organ transplantation (Figure 12.2). A caveat is that the timeline for a given patient is reset with each episode of rejection or intensification of immunosuppression and a high degree of suspicion should always be present, especially with the high frequency of atypical presentations.

Cytomegalovirus

Cytomegalovirus (CMV) is the single most important viral infection following transplantation and was traditionally predominant in the first 6 months post transplantation. However, with the use of prophylactic antivirals, its presentation

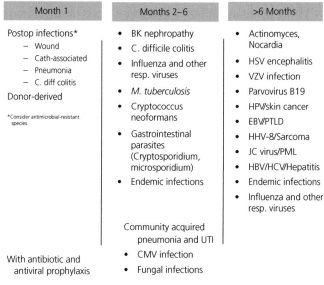

Figure 12.2 Timeline of post-transplant infections.

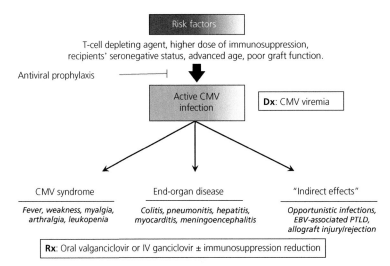

Risk factors

T-cell depleting agent, higher dose of immunosuppression,
recipients' seronegative status, advanced age, poor graft function.

Antiviral prophylaxis

Active CMV infection

Dx: CMV viremia

CMV syndrome

Fever, weakness, myalgia, arthralgia, leukopenia

End-organ disease

Colitis, pneumonitis, hepatitis, myocarditis, meningoencephalitis

"Indirect effects"

Opportunistic infections, EBV-associated PTLD, allograft injury/rejection

Rx: Oral valganciclovir or IV ganciclovir ± immunosuppression reduction

Figure 12.3 CMV infection in solid organ transplant recipients. Dx denotes diagnosis, Rx treatment.

has been occurring later in the transplant course. More than 50% of the world's population has a history of prior CMV infection and the virus tends to remain latent in myeloid cells. Risk factors for infection include induction therapy with T cell depleting agent, higher dose of immunosuppression, recipient's sero-negative status, advanced age, acute rejection, and poor allograft function. CMV disease may present as the classic CMV syndrome with fever, weakness, myalgia, arthralgia, and leukopenia or an end-organ disease, including colitis, pneumonitis, hepatitis, myocarditis, or meningoencephalitis (Figure 12.3). In addition, CMV infection can lead to "indirect effects" on the immune system, raising the overall risk for additional infections (Epstein–Barr virus (EBV), fungal, and bacterial), potentiating the post-transplant lymphoproliferative disorder (PTLD) effect of EBV mismatches and increasing the risk of allograft rejection. These "indirect effects" are mediated by several mechanisms that help the virus evade detection by the host immune system, including decreased HLA expression by antigen-presenting cells, a reduction in antigen presentation and T cell proliferation, and an increase in Fc receptor expression, among others. Renal disease directly caused by CMV infection remains a controversial issue; nevertheless, there have been case reports linking CMV infection with transplant glomerulopathy and thrombotic microangiopathy.

Diagnosis of CMV infection is based on CMV viremia, which can be detected by an antigenemia assay (CMV phosphoprotein 65) or quantitative nucleic acid testing (QNAT). In patients with neurologic manifestations (including chorioretinitis) and gastrointestinal disease (colitis and gastritis), blood-based CMV assays may be negative. Thus, invasive procedures such as colonoscopy and lumbar puncture may be necessary.

Oral valganciclovir has become the treatment of choice for prophylaxis and for mild-to-moderate CMV disease, while intravenous ganciclovir is preferred in patients with severe or life-threatening CMV disease. The length of treatment is best determined by monitoring viremia on a weekly basis and treating the patient until one or two consecutive negative samples are obtained.

Relapse of CMV disease following treatment is frequent. The two recommended approaches are close clinical and viral titer monitoring in the first few months following treatment (pre-emptive) or the use of secondary prophylaxis for up to 6 months following transplantation. High-risk factors for relapse include primary CMV infection, deceased donor transplantation, high baseline viral load, multiorgan disease, and treatment of rejection. Because of the poor correlation of CMV viremia with intestinal disease, a more prolonged course of antiviral is usually recommended after clearing the viremia. Concomitant reduction of immunosuppression should be considered in patients with severe CMV disease, a very high viral load or resistant strains, clinically refractory disease, leukopenia or late/recurrent disease. Adjuvant therapies include CMV immunoglobulin, adoptive infusion of CMV-specific Tcells and leflunomide. Leflunomide is an antiproliferative agent that inhibits pyrimidine synthesis and interferes with CMV virion assembly, in addition to a mild immunosuppressive effect. Nevertheless, there are no consistent trials reporting a superiority of these adjuvant therapies compared to standard treatment. Finally, oral ganciclovir, acyclovir, or valacyclovir should not be used as the initial treatment of CMV disease.

CMV resistance to ganciclovir is uncommon, but when present, it is most often due to mutations in the CMV UL97 gene (a viral protein kinase that phosphorylates the drug) or the UL54 gene (CMV DNA polymerase). CMV resistance should be considered if viremia fails to decrease after 2–3 weeks of treatment. Potential risk factors for resistance include the use antivirals at low dose, D+/R- transplants, prolonged antiviral therapy, increased immunosuppression, severe tissue-invasive CMV disease and/or high viral loads.

Currently, there is no effective vaccine available, although trials are currently underway for a new CMV vaccine that has shown promise. The main modalities employed to prevent active CMV disease are universal prophylaxis or pre-emptive therapy. For the latter, laboratory tests are performed at regular intervals to detect early, asymptomatic viral replication in transplant recipients. Based on the available data from a few small trials comparing both strategies, the use of prophylaxis is favored over pre-emptive therapy in the highest risk transplant recipients (D+/R-), due to better graft survival and clinical outcomes. The most widely used antiviral agent for CMV prophylaxis is valganciclovir at 900 mg once daily for at least 6 months, with dose adjustments if administered with a GFR < 60 ml/min. The use of leuko-depleted blood products and CMV-sero-negative blood products is recommended for sero-negative recipients to decrease the risk of transfusion transmitted CMV. Re-initiation of CMV prophylaxis for 1–3 months should also be considered after treatment of acute rejection (consensus recommendation).

BK (polyoma) virus

The incidence of BK-associated nephropathy has increased remarkably in the past 15 years, correlating with the use of more potent immunosuppressive agents. The greatest challenge is that between 30 and 65% of patients that develop BK-associated nephropathy lose their kidney allograft within 1 year of diagnosis.

Primary BK infection in humans typically occurs in childhood and commonly presents as a limited respiratory viral infection. Latency of the virus in tubular epithelial cells of the kidney is frequent. By adulthood, more than 80% of the general population is seropositive for BK. However, reactivation of the virus is only evident in immunosuppressed states with a special predilection in renal allografts compared to other solid organ transplants. Reactivation of the BK virus is commonly characterized by asymptomatic deterioration of kidney allograft function usually 3–6 months after transplant. In contrast to CMV infection, the serologic BK status of the donor/recipient pair does not help in predicting the risk of developing the disease. The only widely accepted risk factor is the degree of overall immunosuppression and thus BKV may be viewed as a biomarker of sorts, of excessive immunosuppression. Diagnosis relies on evidence of viral replication in the blood (quantitative polymerase chain reaction (PCR) of BK DNA) and confirmatory histologic examination. Since BK nephropathy can be focal and difficult to distinguish from acute rejection, at least two cores should be obtained with the inclusion of the medullary tissues for polyomavirus-specific histologic analysis (SV40 nuclear stain). Urinary viral levels and decoy cells are not routinely used anymore due to their poor specificity (low positive predictive value). Identification of BK viremia is the best positive predictor of BK virus-associated nephropathy.

There is no effective antiviral therapy against BK virus and effective treatment is largely limited to reduction of immunosuppression. The most effective approach is screening for the presence of BK viremia and a decrease or elimination of one of the immunosuppressive agents if viremia is detected. Indeed, the detection of BK viremia is regarded by some as a biomarker of excessive immunosuppression. After reduction in immunosuppression, BK viral load is followed every 2–4 weeks until negative. A decrease is usually seen in the following weeks to months; however, kidney function can temporarily deteriorate further. Adjuvant therapies considered include IVIg, leflunomide, and fluoroquinolone antibiotics. The first can be considered in cases where tubulitis or C4d staining is concomitantly seen on biopsy, suggesting concurrent acute rejection. Often, the rejection is treated as a primary goal and then BK, secondarily. However, since BK virus has a glucorticoid-responsive element (GRE), the use of pulse dose steroids for rejection should be balanced with the risk of worsening BK infection.

Based on the stepwise progression of BK infection and the poor allograft recovery rates when BK-associated nephropathy is diagnosed in the setting of decreased renal function, screening for BK in asymptomatic recipients is indicated if estimated prevalence is greater than 2%. The most accepted strategy is serial blood BK viral loads at months 1, 2, 3, 6, 9, and 12. If very high levels of BK virus are detected on screening, kidney biopsy should be considered to determine the presence and degree of BK nephropathy as well as any concurrent process such as rejection. A BK viral load should also be considered in any patient with unexplained deterioration of kidney allograft function.

Patients who lose their allografts due to BK-associated nephropathy may be considered for re-transplantation after the clearing of viremia. Case reports have documented favorable outcomes, especially with the avoidance of intense immunosuppression upon subsequent transplant.

Other infections

Parvovirus infection should be suspected in immunosuppressed patients presenting with unexplained, isolated anemia associated with a low reticulocyte count. In comparison with non-immunosuppressed individuals, rash, arthropathy, and fever are not as common. Diagnosis requires measurement of parvovirus by PCR in the serum. Treatment consists of IVIg since it contains high levels of parvovirus-specific antibodies as well as monitoring of the reticulocyte count to gauge a response as a positive PCR might persist for several months.

Herpes Zoster should be considered in the differential of atypical skin lesions/rashes. A swab of the lesion for viral DFA and culture is the diagnostic test of choice with prompt institution of antiviral therapy. Central nervous system infection in a transplanted recipient is a medical emergency requiring empirical therapy, while the results of imaging studies, lumbar puncture, and blood cultures are pending. The differential diagnosis is broad and includes Listeria, HSV, JC virus, and *Cryptococcus neoformans*.

Chronic intestinal infection with *Strongyloides stercoralis* is usually asymptomatic in patients from endemic areas with eosinophilia sometimes being the only finding. In these patients, initiation of immunosuppression may lead to hyperinfection with devastating dissemination of infection involving both gastrointestinal and pulmonary symptoms, with a high mortality rate (50–85%). Therefore, screening in patients who have lived or traveled to endemic areas is essential.

Post-transplant malignancy

Cancer is more common among solid organ transplant recipients than it is in the general population or in patients on dialysis; one study found that after 20 years of immunosuppressive therapy, 40% of recipients had cancer. In fact, malignancy after kidney transplantation is the third most common cause of death in renal transplant recipients. One interesting aspect about transplant recipients is that they have an increased risk for specific malignancies, but they may not be broadly predisposed to all cancers. Lastly, the incidence and prevalence of cancer in transplant patients have increased in the past 10 years, partly because of the older age of recipients as well as more potent immunosuppressive drugs. Therefore, further understanding of the aspects of cancer in transplantation has become essential for the long-term care of transplant recipients.

Epidemiology

The malignancies with the highest incidence after solid-organ transplantation are non-melanoma skin cancers, renal cell carcinoma, and non-Hodgkin lymphomas. In one study, their incidence was found to be more than 20-fold higher than in the general population. Also, with high incidence post-transplantation are Kaposi's sarcoma (KS), melanoma, leukemia, cancers of the pharynx and oral cavity, cervical/vulvovaginal cancers, and a variety of sarcomas. In contrast, the incidence of most common solid tumors in the general population (lung, prostate, breast, and colorectal) is only modestly increased or similar to the nontransplanted population. Among different solid organ transplants, lung transplants have the highest risk of malignancy, followed by heart, liver, and kidney transplantation. It has been suggested that this effect may be related to higher doses of immunosuppressive drugs used in lung and heart transplantation. Compared with patients on the waiting list, the relative risk of various malignancies can be seen in Table 12.1.

Overall, cancer rates in kidney recipients are similar to the nontransplanted population 20–30 years older as can be viewed in Figure 12.4; however, absolute risks differ based on additional risk factors such as race, viral infections, and environmental exposures.

Clinical characteristics

The time of presentation of malignancies following transplantation seem to vary depending on the nature of the cancer; but on average, malignancy occurs at approximately 3 years after transplantation and its course tends to be more aggressive in transplant recipients than in the general population.

Non-melanoma skin cancer is the most common type of cancer following solid-organ transplantation, occurring at an average of 8 years after renal transplantation in recipients less than 40 years and at 3 years in recipients >60 years. Compared to the general population, the risk of squamous cell carcinoma is 100 times greater in transplant recipients, while it is 10 times higher for basal cell carcinoma. These skin cancers also tend to occur at a younger age and at multiple sites. The most important risk factors are cumulative exposure to ultraviolet radiation, history of prior non-melanoma skin cancer, fair skin, and susceptibility to sunburn and type/degree of immunosuppression.

Kaposi's sarcoma (KS) is caused by human herpesvirus 8 (HHV-8), and its prevalence follows the geographic distribution of this virus (Middle Eastern, Mediterranean, and sub-Saharan Africa populations). Classically, it presents as angioproliferative lesions involving the lower extremity, leading to lymphedema.

Table 12.1 Relative risk of cancer after transplantation compared to waiting list population and adjusted for age, gender, race/ethnicity, primary cause of kidney failure, and prior duration of end-stage kidney disease ($n = 35,765$ kidney recipients and 46,106 patients on waiting list).

Type of malignancy	Relative risk (95% CI)	p-Value
Skin		
Skin	2.55 (2.26–2.88)	<0.0001
Melanoma	2.19 (1.31–3.65)	0.0028
Other any non-skin	1.17 (1.07–1.28)	0.0004
Gastrointestinal		
Colon	0.75 (0.54–1.01)	0.0860
Genitourinary		
Bladder	1.12 (0.73–1.70)	0.6098
Cervix (women)	1.28 (0.48–3.36)	0.6230
Kidney	1.39 (1.10–1.76)	0.0058
Ovary (women)	0.34 (0.12–0.97)	0.0439
Prostate (men)	0.79 (0.62–1.00)	0.0460
Vulvovaginal (women)	2.19 (0.67–7.12)	0.1936
Lymphomas		
Hodgkin's	2.60 (1.01–6.68)	0.0471
Non-Hodgkin's	3.29 (2.40–4.51)	<0.0001
Others		
Bone	0.91 (0.40–2.04)	0.8145
Breast (women)	0.82 (0.57–1.17)	0.2648
Kaposi's sarcoma	9.03 (2.58–31.60)	0.0005
Lung	1.05 (0.79–1.40)	0.7241
Mouth	2.19 (1.33–3.61)	0.0022
Myeloma	0.92 (0.57–1.49)	0.7338

Source: Adapted from Kasiske et al. (2004). Reproduced by permission of John Wiley & Sons, Ltd.

In some recipients, it involves the mucosal surfaces and lymphoid tissue, but rarely shows visceral involvement.

Post-transplantation lymphoproliferative disorders (PTLDs) are a heterogeneous group of diseases characterized by an abnormal lymphoid proliferation following organ transplantation. The most common type is a non-Hodgkin lymphoma

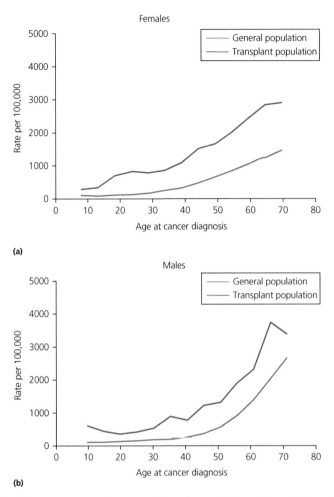

Figure 12.4 Incident cancer rates for women (a) and men (b) in a cohort of kidney transplant recipients ($n = 15,183$), compared to age-matched general population. Source: Data from Webster et al. (2007).

with approximately 50% extranodal involvement. Infection with EBV is strongly associated with PTLD, since it is believed that oncogenes expressed by EBV-infected cells (e.g., LMP1) help the lymphoma cells to evade host immunity through a variety of measures, including by the enhancement of antiapoptotic and growth signals of malignant cells. Risk factors for PTLD include recipient's EBV-negative status, high degree of immunosuppression, and CMV co-infection. Belatacept, a recently FDA-approved drug that blocks T cell costimulation may be associated with increased risk of PTLD in EBV sero-negative recipients. Typically, PTLD presents with fever and mono-like symptoms and other variable characteristics depending on the area of involvement, including abdominal mass, gastrointestinal bleeding, CNS disease, or allograft infiltration. The average time to development of PTLD is 32 months after transplantation; however, the incidence is highest during the first year after transplantation and can be driven by infection with EBV, especially in EBV sero-negative recipients who are more susceptible to EBV infection. Diagnosis is performed through imaging studies and tissue specimen with staining for EBV.

Renal cell carcinoma has also an increased prevalence post transplantation, in particular in kidney transplant recipients. It may present as asymptomatic hematuria, erythrocytosis, abdominal mass, and/or weight loss. Treatment involves surgical resection and prognosis is usually good.

Pathogenesis

There are several factors that seem to be associated with the development of malignancy after transplantation: impaired immune surveillance secondary to immunosuppression; increased invasiveness of cancers by a direct effect of the drugs; carcinogenic factors like sun exposure; and host factors such as genetic predisposition to cancer, presence of oncogenic viral infections, and prolonged dialysis (Figure 12.5). In rare cases, malignancy can be transplanted from the donor.

Immunosuppression: The intensity and duration of immunosuppression can significantly affect the risk of development of post-transplant malignancy. Immunosuppressive drugs can severely disrupt immune function, affecting immune surveillance of cancers cells and importantly dampening antiviral immunity. This latter effect increases the likelihood of infection by oncogenic viruses such as EBV, HCV, HBV, HPV, or HHV-8, predisposing the patient to malignancies. Moreover, certain immunosuppressive drugs also seem to have some direct effects on tumor development. For example, both azathioprine (AZA) and cyclosporine (CSA) have been shown to lower the repair rate of

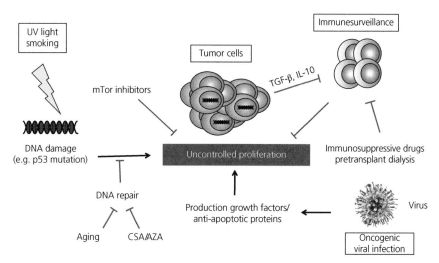

Figure 12.5 General pathogenesis in the development of malignancies in transplant recipients.

DNA damage induced by solar UV radiation (Figure 12.5). In addition, AZA's incorporation of 6-thioguanine pseudobases in the DNA enhances mutagenicity from solar UV exposure and CSA is capable of enhancing angiogenesis and tumor growth. On the contrary, mTOR inhibitors have been shown to inhibit tumor growth, despite their immunosuppressive effect, suggesting that the unique characteristics of the drug are also important in determining cancer risk. Its antiproliferative effect seems to be mediated by both the blockade of the PI3K-Akt-mTOR pathway, which is frequently activated in cancer, and by angiogenesis inhibition. Finally, incidence of tumor can also be influenced by growth factors produced by tumor cells that modulate the tumor microenvironment.

Environmental factors The correlation of sun exposure and skin cancer after transplantation is well documented in the literature, with extreme cases as in Australia, where the high sun exposure rates in susceptible individuals have led to a very high incidence of skin cancers. Smoking is also a known risk factor that is especially relevant for lung cancers.

Host factors: Genetic predisposition, as evident by a prior history of malignancy or strong family history of cancer, plays an important role in the development of post-transplant malignancy. Additional host factors that play an important role after transplantation include a history of prolonged dialysis therapy, which has been shown to significantly increase the risk of kidney and urinary tract malignancies. Finally, certain viral infections have been shown to be associated with the development of different neoplastic disorders after transplantation (Table 12.2). As an example, PTLD can be associated with EBV infection and induction therapies such as anti lymphocyte globulin preparations and the now discontinued OKT3 appears to especially render the host susceptible to EBV infection, leading to an increased risk of PTLD. HHV-8 is another virus also directly related to another malignancy after transplantation, namelyKS. HHV-8 is necessary, but by itself is not sufficient for the development of KS. The presence of viral oncogenes in the HHV-8 genome explains the capacity of the virus to induce tumors, by affecting cell-cycle and apoptosis regulation. Lastly, human papillomavirus (HPV) has also been associated with a greater risk of skin and

Table 12.2 Common viral-associated malignancies.

Infectious agent	Viral-associated cancers
Epstein-Barr virus	Lymphoproliferative disorder
Hepatitis B virus, Hepatitis C virus	Hepatocellular carcinoma
Human Herpes virus 8	Kaposi sarcoma
Human papillomavirus	Cancer of the cervix, vagina, penis, anus, tongue, mouth, oropharynx
Merkel cell polyomavirus	Merkel cell carcinoma

anogenital cancers; however, a causative role for HPV in secondary skin cancers among transplanted patients has not been proven.

Metabolic disorders

With improvement in graft survival, death with a functioning allograft has become a major concern in the transplant field. The main cause of death following transplantation is cardiovascular disease. Transplant recipients are at increased risk due to both traditional as well as nontraditional risk factors (Figure 12.6). Among the nontraditional risk factors, the duration of pre-transplant dialysis, history of delayed graft function, and/or acute rejection are important predictors of cardiovascular events. In the following text, we discuss three major post-transplant disorders: transplant-associated hyperglycemia, dyslipidemia and bone mineral disorder.

Transplant-associated Hyperglycemia (TAH)

Disorders of glycemic control are very common after transplantation and the term "transplant-associated hyperglycemia" (TAH) has been used to encompass both new-onset diabetes after transplantation (NODAT) and pre-diabetic states, since both lead to higher rates of cardiovascular events, infections, death, and allograft loss (Figure 12.7a and b). The prevalence of NODAT is believed to be approximately 15% by 1 year following transplantation, while impaired glucose tolerance (pre-diabetes) is present among 30–45% of recipients at a similar time point. NODAT is defined by a fasting plasma glucose higher than 126 mg/dl (7 mmol/l) or a 2 h plasma glucose level greater than 200 mg/dl (11 mmol/l) during an oral glucose tolerance test (75 g of anhydrous glucose dissolved in water). On the other hand, impaired glucose tolerance is diagnosed by a fasting

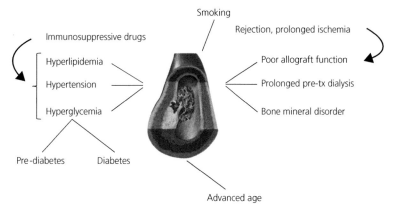

Figure 12.6 Risk factors for cardiovascular disease in kidney transplant recipients.

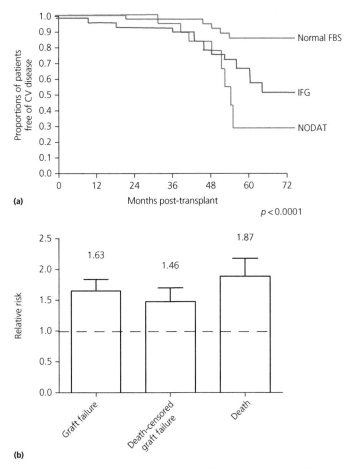

(a)

(b)

Figure 12.7 Transplant-associated hyperglycemia (TAH). (a) *Association of TAH and cardiovascular events in a cohort of 351 patients, stratified by* glycemic status at 1 yr after transplantation: normal fasting blood glucose (Normal FBS), impaired fasting glucose (IFG) and NODAT. Source: Adapted from Cosio et al. (2005). Reproduced by permission of Macmillan Publishers Ltd. (b) Glycemic status after oral glucose tolerance test 1 year after transplantation in a cohort of 114 kidney transplant recipients who were confirmed to be euglycemic before transplantation.

glucose between 110 and 125 mg/dl or a 2 h plasma glucose level between 140 and 200 mg/dl after glucose load.

The pathogenesis of TAH involves both a decreased production of insulin by pancreatic β cells and insulin resistance. Numerous risk factors predispose patients to TAH (Table 12.3). The choice of immunosuppression drugs plays a major role in the development of TAH, as glucocorticoids are known to affect glucose metabolism by increasing hepatic glucose production and by reducing peripheral tissue insulin sensitivity. Using a reduced dose of steroids or withdrawing it from maintenance immunosuppression results in a significant reduction in NODAT. Among the

Table 12.3 Risk factors for transplant-associated hyperglycemia.

General	Transplant-specific
Family history of diabetes	Immunosuppression (glucocorticoids, calcineurin inhibitors, mTor inhibitors)
Nonwhite race	
Advanced age	Weight gain after transplantation
Male gender	Certain viral infection (e.g., HCV and CMV)

calcineurin inhibitors (CNIs), tacrolimus use is associated with a higher risk of NODAT compared to cyclosporine and the mechanism is related to inhibition of glucose-stimulated insulin secretion by β cells and increased peripheral resistance to insulin. This adverse effect seems to be dose-related and the current use of lower-dose tacrolimus has seen a decrease in the rates of glucose intolerance compared to a higher dose. mTOR inhibitors are also diabetogenic through several mechanisms, including direct β cell toxicity and impairment of insulin-mediated suppression of hepatic glucose production. Finally, the weight gain that commonly occurs after transplantation due to steroids and reversal of the uremic state (improved appetite) may also augment both hepatic and peripheral insulin resistance.

When NODAT or glucose intolerance is diagnosed, lifestyle changes should be the primary intervention, including increasing exercise and following an appropriate diet for a goal HbA1c<7%. Adjustment of immunosuppression should be weighed against the risk of allograft rejection, with reducing steroids being a common approach followed by decreasing the tacrolimus dose or possibly switching to cyclosporine. It is important to note that reversal of diabetes is not predictably achieved with any drug alteration. If additional interventions are needed, oral hypoglycemics like sulfonylureas (e.g., glipizide), biguanides (e.g., metformin) or insulin may be considered in a step-up approach if blood sugars are still uncontrolled (insulin is usually required when fasting glucose is above 200 mg/dl or 11 mmol/l). If metformin is chosen, close monitoring should be performed in the setting of renal dysfunction due to the risk of lactic acidosis and it should be avoided if the GFR < 30 ml/min. Dose adjustments should be performed when the GFR is between 30–60 ml/min. Despite the rare possible complications, metformin has a number of potential benefits for solid-organ transplant recipients in addition to its glycemic effect, like lack of weight gain, attenuation of metabolic syndrome, diabetes prevention, and cardiovascular protection. Further studies are needed to clarify the best management strategy for diabetes control after transplantation.

Dyslipidemia

Due to the high incidence of atherosclerotic disease events in transplant recipients, hyperlipidemia should be aggressively managed. Data from the 1990s reported that the prevalence of an elevated total cholesterol (>200 mg/dl or

5 mmol/l) was between 80 and 90% at 1 year post-transplant, with elevated LDL levels (>100 mg/dl or 2.5 mmol/l) in more than 90% of recipients. However, the changes in immunosuppressive agents in the past decade have altered this picture. Immunosuppressive drugs play a major role in the development of dyslipidemia after transplantation, with glucocorticoids indirectly affecting lipid metabolism by stimulation of hepatic VLDL synthesis via hyper-insulinemia and downregulation of LDL receptors, possibly through adrenocorticotropic hormone (ACTH) suppression. With similar deleterious effects, cyclosporine directly leads to an increased total and LDL cholesterol level in a dose-dependent manner, while tacrolimus does not seem to have such a significant effect. Lastly, mTOR inhibitors lead to significant hypertriglyceridemia by blockade of insulin-stimulated lipoprotein lipase. Secondary causes of hyperlipidemia, including nephrotic syndrome, hypothyroidism, diabetes, excessive alcohol intake, chronic liver disease and other medications should also be evaluated.

General screening recommendations are to check lipid profiles within 6 months of transplant, at 1 year post transplant, and annually thereafter. Target lipid levels in recipients have been extrapolated from the general population: LDL-C <100 mg/dl or 2.5 mmol/l, triglycerides <200 mg/dl and non-HDL-C <130 mg/dl or 3.8 mmol/l. Recipients with elevated LDL-C are treated with dietary and exercise changes followed by statin initiation if still not at goal. There has only been one prospective randomized trial (ALERT) with statins (fluvastatin) in kidney transplant recipients, which showed lower cholesterol levels in the treatment arm compared to placebo, with relatively few side effects. However, there was only a nonsignificant trend towards reduction of composite cardiovascular events in the initial trial, but treatment achieved significance in the composite end point of stroke and myocardial infarcts with extended 5 year follow-up. Nonetheless, secondary outcomes of this trial, observational and post hoc analyses in other trials have suggested a beneficial effect.

Statins are metabolized by hepatic cytochrome P450 3A4, similarly to cyclosporine, tacrolimus, and mTOR inhibitors. In the presence of these immunosuppressive agents, statin levels are raised and the risk of myopathy is increased. Therefore, statins should be started at a low dose and increased progressively, and monitored closely for signs of toxicity. The dose should not be higher than half the usual maximum prescribed dose in the setting of CNI use. Furthermore, the FDA has recently issued a warning, recommending against the use of simvastatin with cyclosporine and to cap the dose of simvastatin to 20 mg in patients taking amlodipine. Among the statins, fluvastatin and pravastatin have minimal interaction with CNIs and are generally well tolerated in transplant recipients. Rosuvastatin, a newer drug in the class with greater antilipid action, is also an alternative, since it does not undergo metabolism by P450. Atorvastatin carries a risk of interaction though it is believed to be slightly lower than simvastatin.

Post-transplant bone mineral disorder

Bone mineral disorders after transplantation encompass a number of disturbances that range from bone pain/fractures, and electrolytes disturbances (calcium/phosphate) to avascular necrosis. These disorders differ between renal and non-renal solid organ transplants. In the latter, steroid-induced osteoporosis is the predominant finding, with some additional risk for osteomalacia related to low 25-hydroxylase activity in liver allograft recipients. In contrast, bone disease after kidney transplantation is more complex since it arises from a combination of factors that include pre-existing renal osteodystrophy, immunosuppressive therapy, reduced renal allograft function, and elevated PTH/FGF-23 post-transplantation (Figure 12.8). Additional nontransplant-specific risk factors for bone loss include advanced age, history of previous fracture, post-menopause, low body weight (<58 kg), inactivity, diabetes, smoking, and excessive alcohol intake.

In general, there are two features that determine bone strength: its quality and its density. The latter can be determined by bone mineral density tests (BMDs), while the first is usually unmeasured. This is important since BMD has been shown to be a poor predictor of fractures in the transplant population. After kidney transplantation, BMD falls rapidly in most patients during the first 6 months with subsequent stabilization after that. The overall fracture risk after transplantation is more than 300% higher than in healthy individuals, though minimization of steroids has been shown to reduce this risk significantly. Interestingly, in one survey of 600 patients, the most common site of fracture in transplant recipients was the foot.

The two major classes of immunosuppressive drugs that contribute to bone loss are glucocorticoids and CNIs, which decrease osteoblast proliferative activity and increase bone resorption through ostoclasts. Glucocorticoids, in particular, are strongly associated with the most worrisome bone complication in transplant

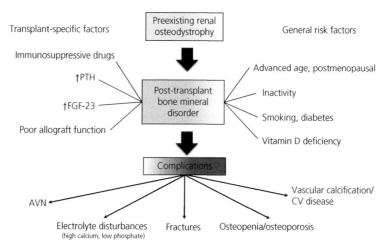

Figure 12.8 Risk factors for post-transplant bone-mineral disorders.

patients: avascular necrosis (AVN). AVN incidence is about 5.5% and usually presents with hip or groin pain exacerbated by weight bearing. Diagnosis requires an MRI and more than 60% of patients that develop AVN of the hip will need a total hip replacement. The role of bisphosphonates or other therapies in early AVN has not been defined yet.

Guidelines recommend measuring BMD in patients with a GFR > 30 ml/min in the first 3 months after kidney transplant if they receive corticosteroids or have risk factors for osteoporosis. A low BMD in the first 12 months after transplant should be managed initially according to the abnormal levels of calcium, phosphorus, PTH, and 25(OH)-vitamin D. Nevertheless, PTH levels have been shown not to correlate with bone histopathologic findings. Therefore, a biopsy is recommended if biphosphonates are being considered or in the setting of recurrent fractures to rule out adynamic bone disease. A trial with pamidronate in kidney recipients showed that it was able to preserve BMD in this population, though it led to 100% adynamic bone disease after treatment. The long-term consequences of bisphosphonates and terparatide in post-transplant bone mineral disorders are still unclear. Similar uncertainty also exists regarding the use of cinacalcet in transplant recipients. In general, most centers stop this agent on the day of transplantation and monitor PTH/Calcium afterwards for the need of reinstitution, since PTH levels are known to progressively decrease during the first year after transplantation. Since BMD is not a good predictor of fractures on transplant recipients, trials with hard end-points like fracture should be used to indicate the benefits of therapy in this population as well as possible inclusion of cardiovascular events as an outcome.

Among the bone mineral electrolyte disorders, hypophosphatemia is a common complication after kidney transplantation (>90% of patients) due to a decrease in tubular reabsorption of PO_4 by the allograft. Its etiology is likely multifactorial related to increased PTH level and activity; increased levels of FGF-23; and side effects from immunosuppressive drugs. In the majority of patients, the hypophosphatemia regresses spontaneously. We recommend a conservative management of hypophosphatemia in transplant recipients, geared toward increasing the phosphate intake through dietary changes. Oral supplementation with potassium phosphate should only be used in symptomatic patients or when persistent severe hypophosphatemia (<1.0 mg/dl; 0.3 mmol/l) is present despite nutritional interventions. This cautious approach differs from the general recommendation for the management of hypophosphatemia, since kidney allografts have a higher risk of calcium phosphate deposition upon phosphate supplementation, which has been linked to worse graft outcomes. Initial dosage should be 1000 mg of oral phosphate/day, distributed in small doses throughout the day in order to avoid an acute rise of serum phosphate.

Hyperparathyroidism is an important component of hypophosphatemia and cinacalcet has been shown to correct phosphate levels in short-term small trials by decreasing PTH levels, in addition to controlling hypercalcemia. However, long-term trials with a larger number of patients and hard outcomes (fracture risk and survival) are warranted to guide this therapy. If cinacalcet is started, a trial starting at low dose and a gradual reduction and eventual discontinuation at a later time point is recommended. Likewise, the role of parathyroidectomy in renal transplant recipients is unclear and should be likely delayed until 1–2 years after transplantation, due to the progressive reduction of PTH with time on most patients.

Hypertension

Post-transplant hypertension develops in about approximately 60–80% of transplant recipients and is associated with higher cardiovascular burden and allograft loss. CNIs play an important role in its pathogenesis and cyclosporine seems to be more hypertensive than tacrolimus. CNI raises significantly both systemic and renal vascular resistance through multiple mechanisms including activation of the sympathetic nervous system, upregulation of endothelin and inhibition of inducible nitric oxide by the endothelium. Glucocorticoids can also contribute to hypertension, especially at higher doses. Resistant hypertension should raise suspicion for possible renal artery stenosis, which tends to develop between 3 months and 2 years post transplant. The gold standard for diagnosis is arteriography, but MRA or CTA have been increasingly utilized lately. Ultrasound has good specificity, however sensitivity is variable and the procedure is highly operator dependent.

Post-transplant hypertension should be aggressively treated to protect against cardiovascular disease and against possible hypertensive injury to the graft. Guidelines recommend blood pressure goals <130/80 mmHg in transplant recipients. First, reduction of the CNI should be considered if possible. If the patient remains hypertensive, therapy with a calcium channel blocker (e.g. amlodipine) or a diuretic should be started. The first appear to improve CNI-induced vasoconstriction, improving renal blood flow. The role of ACEI/ARB is not well established and its use is usually avoided early after transplantation in order to prevent confusion in the interpretation of a rise in serum creatinine. However, if the clinical course is stable at 6 months, these agents should be considered as good alternatives, especially in diabetics and in patients with proteinuria or history of heart failure/myocardial infarction. Careful monitoring of potassium should be performed, especially if in combination with a CNI.

Hematologic disorders

Anemia after transplantation affects approximately 20% of recipients at 1 year after transplantation. Its etiology can be variable including iron or vitamin B12 deficiency, poor allograft function (low EPO production), immunosuppression

(MMF, AZA, or mTOR inhibitors), parvovirus B19 infection or thrombotic microangiopathy (TMA). TMA post-transplantation is commonly associated with CNI, though several factors such as vascular rejection, viral infection, complement abnormalities or other drugs may play a contributory role. It typically presents with anemia in combination with low platelets and schistocytes in the peripheral smear. Its management involves mainly interruption of the CNI. Nonetheless, there is accumulating evidence suggesting that in some cases plasmapheresis might be beneficial and the role of Eculizumab (monoclonal antibody against C5) still needs further exploration in the transplant setting. Finally, a low reticulocyte count and persistent anemia might suggest parvovirus infection, which is usually diagnosed by measuring B19 viral load in the blood.

Post-transplant erythrocytosis is characterized by a hematocrit >51% after transplantation and it affects approximately 5% of kidney recipients. Its etiology is not well defined, but is believed to be a combination of increased responsiveness to erythropoietin (EPO) and/or increased EPO production. The most important condition to exclude in this setting is renal cell carcinoma, which can lead to high secretion of EPO levels. Work-up involves renal ultrasound of both native and transplanted kidneys and urine cytology. The presentation of this condition is variable involving malaise, headache, plethora, or the more worrisome complication of thromboembolism (10–30% of patients). Treatment consists of administration of ACEI or ARB for a goal hemoglobin below 17.5 g/dl. These agents are capable of reducing EPO production and inhibiting erythroid progenitor cells. In resistant patients, phlebotomy is a potential alternative.

Leukopenia is also a common hematologic complication after transplantation and may affect 20–50% of recipients in the first year post-transplant. Its etiology is multifactorial, but the leading culprits are the use of the antiproliferative agent MMF, which has strong myelosuppressive effects, and the use of valganciclovir for CMV prophylaxis. The increased use of induction therapy with thymoglobulin also significantly contributes to leukopenia in transplant recipients. Among other immunosuppressive agents, mTOR inhibitors have demonstrated some mild myelotoxicity, while prednisone and calcineurin inhibitors are not considered important contributors, though tacrolimus' inhibition of MPA glucuronidation might increase the availability of the active form of MMF, exacerbating leukopenia. Bactrim, frequently used as antibiotic prophylaxis in the first 6 months after transplantation, can also exacerbate leukopenia. One of the important conditions to exclude in the setting of leukopenia is CMV infection, which can present with isolated leukopenia in patients at risk (e.g., CMV-negative recipients), and measuring CMV viral load is warranted. The major consequence of leukopenia is the increased risk of bacterial infections, especially if significant neutropenia is present (<500). There are no specific guidelines in transplantation for the management of leukopenia, but the most effective way to improve it is to cut down the MMF dose. Some centers also consider stopping the infectious prophylaxis (valganciclovir/bactrim) until white blood counts have recovered. In cases where leukopenia is refractory to those approaches, G-CSF could be considered, though data from the oncology literature suggests that despite shortening the duration of neutropenia, it does not affect the number of culture-positive infections or the rate of hospitalizations and it might be associated with an increased risk of rejection in transplantation.

Summary

Post-transplant complications play a major role in allograft loss in the long-term and prevention of these conditions should be an area of major focus in transplant care. The three leading causes of death after transplantation (cardiovascular disease, malignancy, and infections) remain unchanged. In all these conditions, immunosuppressive regimens used to prevent rejection play a major role in such complications, suggesting that individualization of the therapy of transplant recipients should be considered, based on a pre-emptive risk stratification. As additional immunosuppressive drugs become available, physicians should favor drugs that have a lower side effect profile, in addition to good graft function outcomes. Finally, most of the complications after transplantation are managed using data extrapolated from the general population, and clinical trials specific to the transplant population are warranted to provide evidence-based medicine in the field.

References

Kasiske BL, Snyder JJ, Gilbertson DT, Wang C. Cancer after kidney transplantation in the United States. *Am J Transplant.* 2004;4(6):905–13.

Webster AC, Craig CJ, Simpson JM, Jones MP, Chapman JR. Identifying high risk groups and quantifying absolute risk of cancer after kidney transplantation: a cohort study of 15183 recipients. *Am J Transplant.* 2007;7: 2140–51.

Further reading

Asberg A, Humar A, Rollag H, Jardine AG, Mouas H, Pescovitz MD, et al. Oral valganciclovir is noninferior to intravenous ganciclovir for the treatment of CMV disease in solid organ transplant recipients. *Am J Transplant.* 2007;7(9):2106–13.

Ayus JC, Achinger SG, Lee S, Sayegh MH, Go AS. Transplant nephrectomy improves survival following a failed renal allograft. *J Am Soc Nephrol.* 2010;21(2):374–80.

Coco M, Glicklich D, Faugere MC, Burris L, Bognar I, Durkin P, et al. Prevention of bone loss in renal transplant recipients: a prospective, randomized trial of intravenous pamidronate. *J Am Soc Nephrol.* 2003;14(10):2669–76.

Conley E, Muth B, Samaniego M, Lotfi M, Voss B, Armbrust M, et al. Bisphosphonates and bone fractures in long-term kidney transplant recipients. *Transplantation.* 2008;86(2):231–7.

Cosio FG, Kudva Y, van der Velde M, Larson TS, Textor SC, Griffin MD, et al. New onset hyperglycemia and diabetes are associated with increased cardiovascular risk after kidney transplantation. *Kidney Int.* 2005;67(6):2415–21.

Crutchlow MF, Bloom RD. Transplant-associated hyperglycemia: a new look at an old problem. *Clin J Am Soc Nephrol.* 2007;2(2):343–55.

Fishman JA. Infection in solid-organ transplant recipients. *N Engl J Med.* 2007;357 (25):2601–14.

Humar A, Limaye AP, Blumberg EA, Hauser IA, Vincenti F, Jardine AG, et al. Extended valganciclovir prophylaxis in D+/R-kidney transplant recipients is associated with long-term reduction in cytomegalovirus disease: two-year results of the IMPACT study. *Transplantation.* 2010;90(12):1427–31.

Johnston O, Rose C, Landsberg D, Gourlay WA, Gill JS. Nephrectomy after transplant failure: current practice and outcomes. *Am J Transplant.* 2007;7(8):1961–7.

Kaplan B, Meier-Kriesche HU. Death after graft loss: an important late study endpoint in kidney transplantation. *Am J Transplant.* 2002;2(10):970–4.

Kasiske BL, Snyder JJ, Gilbertson D, Matas AJ. Diabetes mellitus after kidney transplantation in the United States. *Am J Transplant.* 2003;3(2):178–85.

Kasiske BL, Zeier MG, Chapman JR, Craig JC, Ekberg H, Garvey CA, et al. KDIGO clinical practice guideline for the care of kidney transplant recipients: a summary. *Kidney Int.* 2010;77(4):299–311.

Kiberd BA, Rose C, Gill JS. Cancer mortality in kidney transplantation. *Am J Transplant.* 2009;9(8):1868–75.

Kotton CN. Management of cytomegalovirus infection in solid organ transplantation. *Nat Rev Nephrol.* 2010;6(12):711–21.

Kotton CN, Kumar D, Caliendo AM, Asberg A, Chou S, Snydman DR, et al. International consensus guidelines on the management of cytomegalovirus in solid organ transplantation. *Transplantation.* 2010;89(7):779–95.

Malluche HH, Monier-Faugere MC, Herberth J. Bone disease after renal transplantation. *Nat Rev Nephrol.* 2010;6(1):32–40.

Mangray M, Vella JP. Hypertension after kidney transplant. *Am J Kidney Dis.* 2011;57(2): 331–41.

Monier-Faugere MC, Mawad H, Qi Q, Friedler RM, Malluche HH. High prevalence of low bone turnover and occurrence of osteomalacia after kidney transplantation. *J Am Soc Nephrol.* 2000;11(6):1093–9.

Martinez OM, de Gruijl FR. Molecular and immunologic mechanisms of cancer pathogenesis in solid organ transplant recipients. *Am J Transplant.* 2008;8(11):2205–11.

Opelz G, Dohler B. Improved long-term outcomes after renal transplantation associated with blood pressure control. *Am J Transplant.* 2005;5(11):2725–31.

Randhawa P, Brennan DC. BK virus infection in transplant recipients: an overview and update. *Am J Transplant.* 2006;6(9):2000–5.

Webster AC, Wong G, Craig JC, Chapman JR. Managing cancer risk and decision making after kidney transplantation. *Am J Transplant.* 2008;8(11):2185–91.

CHAPTER 13

Biomarkers of allograft rejection and tolerance

Choli Hartono, Thangamani Muthukumar, and Manikkam Suthanthiran

Department of Medicine, Weill Cornell Medical College, New York, USA

CHAPTER OVERVIEW

- The development of noninvasive diagnostic and prognostic biomarkers for allograft rejection and for allograft tolerance is critical to the advancement of transplant medicine.

- Biomarkers related to the functional attributes of T cells, B cells, and innate cells have shown great promise in predicting transplant outcomes in selected cohorts of patients.

- Whether biomarkers in the clinical settings are stable and enduring remain unknown.

- Biomarker validation is strengthened by data from large-scale clinical trials.

- Further technologies to interrogate the genomes, transcriptomes, proteomes, and metabolites should facilitate new biomarker discovery, validation, and qualification.

Introduction

Transplant outcomes, especially in the short term, have dramatically improved in the past five decades, and graft loss due to acute rejection is considerably rare now in the clinic. Despite this remarkable progress, for reasons that have not been fully resolved, long-term allograft survival has not improved *pari passu*. The potential contributors to poor long-term outcomes include inadequately treated acute rejection, undetected acute rejection (subclinical rejection), chronic rejection (CR), and calcineurin inhibitor (CNI)-related nephrotoxicity. Cardiovascular morbidity and mortality, infections, and malignancies undermine long-term outcome as well. It is intuitive that an approach that avoids allograft rejection while minimizing the side effects of immunosuppressive drugs would go "a long way" to improve long-term outcomes. Consequently, immunologic tolerance

---

Transplant Immunology, First Edition. Edited by Xian Chang Li and Anthony M. Jevnikar.
© 2016 John Wiley & Sons, Ltd. Published 2016 by John Wiley & Sons, Ltd.
Copyright ® American Society of Transplantation 2016.
Companion website: www.wiley.com/go/li/transplantimmunology

remains the "holy grail" in transplantation. Achieving this elusive goal will be a significant step towards realizing the promise of transplantation.

New insights into the molecular pathways of organ rejection and of tolerance and invention of innovative technologies such as polymerase chase reaction (PCR) to detect biologic signals during an episode of rejection have heralded the burgeoning field of biomarkers in transplantation. Success in this new endeavor is clearly essential if we aim to achieve the state of detectable and predictable tolerance in solid organ transplantation. In this chapter, we will review the evolving knowledge regarding biomarkers of kidney allograft rejection and of tolerance.

Biomarkers

The need for diagnostic and prognostic biomarkers

The clinical application of the Banff classification of transplant rejection enables transplant clinicians to standardize and tailor treatment based on the severity and type of rejection. Determination of rejection however requires the examination of the allograft by needle core biopsy, which may be imprecise since biopsy specimens represent only a small portion of the entire allograft; moreover, diagnostic inaccuracies may be augmented by the patchy nature of the rejection process and by the suboptimal concordance rate in the histologic interpretation. Since biopsy procedures are invasive, a surrogate blood or urine test might serve as a noninvasive or minimally invasive alternative, allowing for multiple sampling. Profiling messenger ribonucleic acid (mRNA) in transplant recipients fulfills various important objectives as summarized in Table 13.1, and conceptually can be applied to solid organ transplants as well as cellular transplants.

The advantages and disadvantages of sampling blood, kidney allograft (or other solid organs), and urine for mRNA expression patterns are summarized in Table 13.2. In kidney transplants, a rise in serum creatinine is often an indication of allograft dysfunction, but is neither sensitive nor specific to diagnosing clinical acute rejection, and is uninformative of subclinical acute rejection. The serum creatinine test does allow for ease of sampling to identify abnormally functioning allografts and to follow the outcome of therapy for rejection. Thus, it is routinely used in practice and as an endpoint in clinical trials. In contrast to measurement of serum creatinine, noninvasive molecular biomarkers such as urinary cell levels of mRNA for *perforin* and *granzyme B* have improved sensitivity and specificity for detecting acute rejection compared to creatinine alone, and also allow for frequent testing as well as providing mechanistic insights. A signal detected by molecular biomarkers is expectantly "earlier" in the course of immunologic activation and thus, prior to changes in histology or any signs of elevation in serum creatinine (Figure 13.1). In this way, biomarkers might also serve to predict a rejection in the allograft prior to permanent injury.

Table 13.1 Objective of mRNA profiling in organ graft recipients.

1. Diagnose rejection by noninvasive means and obviate the need for the invasive procedure of allograft biopsy

2. Anticipate the subsequent development of rejection before the development of tissue injury

3. Prognosticate the outcome of an episode of rejection, and responsiveness to antirejection therapy

4. Predict subsequent allograft function

5. Help develop mechanism-based therapy

6. Facilitate individualization or optimization of immunosuppressive drug therapy including weaning or reintroduction of therapy

Reprinted with permission from Anglicheau and Suthanthiran (2008).

Table 13.2 The advantages and disadvantages of blood, kidney tissue or urine as a source of RNA for biomarker discovery.

Source of RNA	Advantages	Disadvantages
Peripheral blood	1. Ease of frequent sampling 2. May detect blood-borne immune events	1. May not detect intragraft immune events 2. May not detect immune events in Secondary lymph nodes 3. Semi-invasive
Kidney tissue	1. Highly specific to detect intragraft-immune events 2. Gold standard for rendering a Diagnosis	1. May not detect immune events in secondary lymph nodes 2. Sampling error 3. Frequent sampling is invasive and risky
Urine	1. Noninvasive 2. Ease of frequent sampling 3. Detect intragraft immune Events	1. May not detect blood-borne immune events 2. May not detect immune events in secondary lymph nodes 3. Dependent on urine output

The practice of "one size fits all" when prescribing antirejection medications inevitably leads to serious unwanted side effects in transplants recipients. We suggest that different individuals have distinctive immune repertoires and can mount varying degrees of immunologic response against their allografts. With the aid of biomarkers, the ability to profile and phenotype an individual's immune response will bring us closer to the goal of personalized medicine for the transplant patient.

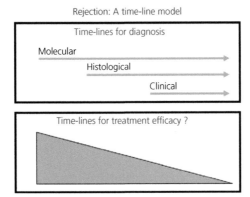

Figure 13.1 Rejection: A time-line model. Reprinted with permission from Anglicheau and Suthanthiran (2008).

Biomarkers associated with allograft rejection
Messenger RNA-based biomarkers

For more than a decade, investigators have shown that levels of mRNAs in the urine or blood of allograft recipients may serve as biomarkers of allograft rejection (Table 13.3). In these studies, PCR assays, microarrays or a combination of both have been used to detect mRNAs of interest. Quantitative PCR assays are commonly used to quantify a panel of mechanistically informative mRNAs in urine collected from kidney transplant recipients and acute rejection can be noninvasively diagnosed with a high degree of accuracy by measuring urinary cell levels of mRNA for perforin, granzyme B, IP-10, CXCR3, and PI-9. The urinary cell level of Foxp3 mRNA was also diagnostic of acute rejection and very importantly the levels predicted the reversal of an episode of acute rejection and of allograft failure.

In the Clinical Trials in Organ Transplantation 04 (CTOT-04) study, 4300 urine specimens were collected from 485 kidney transplant recipients prospectively at scheduled times for mRNA profiling. In this observational study, urinary cell levels of mRNAs were measured using real-time quantitative PCR assays. CTOT-04 study validated the diagnostic utility of urinary cell mRNA levels for the noninvasive diagnosis of acute cellular rejection. Moreover, a combination of CD3ε mRNA, IP-10 mRNA, and 18S rRNA was predictive of the future development of acute cellular rejection.

Urinary cell mRNA profile can also be used to noninvasively diagnose the presence of fibrosis in human renal allografts. We studied 48 kidney transplant recipients with allograft fibrosis, and 66 with normal biopsies. A discovery set of 76 recipients (32 Fibrosis and 44 Normal) were used to develop a diagnostic signature, and an independent set of 38 recipients (16 Fibrosis and 22 Normal) were used to validate the diagnostic signature. In the discovery set, a 4-gene model of vimentin, e-cadherin, NKCC2, and 18S rRNA was diagnostic of intragraft fibrosis. Using a composite score based on the 4-gene model, allograft fibrosis was diagnosed with

Table 13.3 mRNA profiles diagnostic of acute rejection of kidney allograft.

R*n**	Urinary cell mRNA levels during acute rejection as compared with no acute rejection
151/85	Perforin and granzyme B higher
95/87	PI-9, granzyme B, and perforin mRNAs higher
99/99	Granzyme B higher; UTI did not increase granzyme B levels
89/79	CD 103 higher
221/26	Granulysin higher
63/58	IP-10 and CXCR3 mRNAs higher
83/83	FOXP3 mRNA higher
–/76	IP-10 mRNA higher
162/37	Perforin, granzyme B, and FasL mRNAs high during AR, UTI, CMV and DGF
–/117	NKG2D mRNA higher
72/72	Tim-3 and IFNγ mRNAs higher
165/115	Tim-3 higher
48/35	Perforin, granzyme B, FasL, PI-9, and FOXP3 higher
64/64	Perforin, granzyme B, granulysin higher; granzyme B, granulysin but not perforin higher in AR as compared with bacteriuria; perforin but not granzyme B and granulysin higher in AR as compared with CMV
	Peripheral blood cell mRNA levels during acute rejection as compared with no acute rejection
31/25	Granzyme B, perforin, and FasL mRNAs increased
–/21	IL-4, IL-5, IL-6, IFNγ, granzyme B, and perforin mRNAs increased
–/57	CD40L mRNA increased in AR, CAN, or both
27/27	Granzyme B, perforin, and HLA-DRA mRNAs increased
206/29	Granzyme B, perforin, and FasL mRNAs increased
364/67	Granzyme B and perforin mRNAs increased
88/15	Perforin mRNA increased
268/46	Granzyme B and perforin mRNAs increased
64/–	Granzyme B, perforin, and FasL mRNAs increased
165/115	Tim-3 higher
48/35	Perforin, granzyme B, FasL, PI-9, and FOXP3 higher

Source: Reprinted with permission from Hartono et al. (2010).
AR, acute rejection; CAN, chronic allograft nephropathy; CMV, cytomegalovirus; CXCR3, chemokine (CXC motif) receptor 3; DGF, delayed graft function; FasL, Fas ligand; FOXP3, forkhead box P3; IFN, interferon; HLA, human leukocyte antigen; IL, interleukin; IP-10, inducible protein 10; PI-9, proteinase inhibitor-9; Tim-3, T-cell immunoglobulin domain; UTI, urinary tract infection.
* Number of samples/number of patients.

a sensitivity of 93.8% and a specificity of 84.1% ($p<0.0001$). In the validation set of 38 renal allograft recipients, the 4-gene signature was diagnostic of allograft fibrosis with a sensitivity of 77.3% and a specificity of 87.5% ($p<0.0001$).

AlloMap® was the first US Food and Drug Administration (FDA)-approved *in vitro* diagnostic assay for use in heart transplant recipients. It is intended to aid, in conjunction with standard clinical assessment, the identification of heart transplant recipients having stable allograft function with a low probability of acute cellular rejection at the time of testing. AlloMap tests a panel of 20 genes from the peripheral blood of heart transplant recipients by PCR assays and calculates a score that has a high negative predictive value for rejection in the cardiac allograft.

Microarrays use a high throughput approach to search for biomarkers of allograft status. Microarray investigation typically requires a test set and a validation set with subsequent verification of gene expression data using real-time (RT)-PCR assays. The study from Stanford University reported on the global gene expression of 67 kidney allograft biopsy samples obtained for acute or chronic allograft dysfunction (n=52), at the time of engraftment from donors (n=8), and stable graft function (n=7). The 52 samples obtained from patients with graft dysfunction displayed gene expression patterns that could be divided into three clusters: cluster A—acute rejection, cluster B—toxicity and infection, and cluster C—chronic allograft nephropathy. Of the 26 samples collected from patients with acute rejection, 12 fell into cluster A (AR-I), 9 into cluster B (AR-II), and 5 into cluster C (AR-III). The authors found a 385 gene-set that was differentially expressed in AR-I versus AR-II and AR-III. The gene-set mostly reflected cellular functions such as apoptosis, infiltration by immune cells, and lymphocyte activation by NF-κB and IFN-γ. Other lymphocyte-related genes such as interleukin-2 (IL-2)–receptor chains and T-cell–receptor chains, natural-killer–cell transcript 4, matrix metalloproteinase-7, and macrophage receptors were also represented. Heightened expression of genes reflecting effector functions of T cells such as granzyme A and RANTES (regulated upon activation normal T-cell expressed and secreted), adhesion molecules, cytokines, cytokine receptors, and growth factors were also observed. Interestingly, the study identified mRNA for prominent B cell proteins such as CD20, CD74, immunoglobulin heavy and light chains, and other molecules associated with B-cell receptors in the group AR-I as compared to the groups AR-II and AR-III. The validation of B-cell involvement was made by CD20 immunohistochemical staining of infiltrating lymphocytes in the biopsy samples with rejection. In the study, the finding of CD20 cellular infiltration correlated with steroid-resistant acute rejection that mostly clustered in AR-I.

An up-to-date assessment of microarrays in kidney transplant rejection was recently completed. We have summarized the advantages and disadvantages of using microarray as a biomarker discovery platform when compared to RT-PCR and other-omics in Table 13.4.

Table 13.4 Comparison of Major Platforms for Biomarker Discovery and Validation.

Platforms	Features
Real-time PCR	1. Hypothesis testing (vs. hypothesis generating) 2. Simple to perform and analyze data 3. Cost effective 4. Rapid turnaround 5. Highly sensitive and specific 6. High-throughput
Microarray	1. Hypothesis generating 2. Requires expertise for performance and data analyses 3. Expensive 4. Lacks sensitivity and specificity 5. High-throughput 6. Allows study of tens of thousands of genes rapidly 7. Prior knowledge of DNA sequence required
Sequencing	1. Hypothesis generating 2. Prior knowledge of DNA sequence not required 3. High-throughput 4. Technically challenging to perform and analyze data 5. Requires expertise for performance and data analysis 6. Expensive at this time but costs rapidly falling
Metabolomics	1. Hypothesis generating 2. High-throughput 3. Study of wide variety of chemically diverse compounds and wide dynamic range of concentrations is analytically challenging
Proteomics	1. Hypothesis generating 2. Highly sensitive 3. Lacks specificity 4. Technically challenging 5. High-throughput

MicroRNA-based biomarkers

MicroRNAs (miRNAs) are a newly discovered class of RNAs that are not translated to proteins. They are evolutionarily conserved and are produced from noncoding regions or from the introns of the protein-coding regions of DNA. They regulate gene expression by destabilizing mRNAs or by inhibiting translation. miRNAs are 20–25 nucleotides long and a single miRNA can regulate hundreds of functional targets within a single cell type while each mRNA can be targeted by multiple miRNAs. To date, more than 1000 miRNAs have been described.

We studied intragraft miRNA expression pattern in 33 kidney allograft biopsies. Global expression profiling was done on 7 of the 33 biopsies using TaqMan® low density array human miRNA panel containing primers and probes for 365 mature human miRNAs (discovery/training set), and the remaining 26 biopsies (validation set) were profiled using PCR assays for the subset of miRNAs identified in the training set to be diagnostic of allograft status. Unsupervised hierarchical clustering and principal component analysis of intragraft miRNA expression patterns correctly differentiated AR from normal biopsies, without any *a priori* sample classification (Figure 13.2). Supervised analysis identified 17 miRNAs ($p < 0.01$) that discriminated acute rejection biopsies from normal allograft biopsies expressed. We chose 6 of the 17 miRNA for validation based on their expression patterns and potential relevance, and differential expression of 5 the 6 miRNAs was validated using PCR assay while the remaining one miRNA was marginally significant ($P = 0.08$) between AR and normal biopsies. To ascertain the basis for the altered expression of miRNAs in acutely rejecting kidney allografts, we measured the miRNA expression in activated and inactivated human peripheral blood mononuclear cells (PBMCs) as well as in cultured human renal tubular epithelial cells treated with concentrated cell-free supernatants of activated and inactivated human PBMCs. Our studies revealed that (i) miRNAs expressed in high abundance in human PBMCs are present at high levels in acutely rejecting allografts; (ii) a strong positive association exists between intragraft levels of overexpressed miRNAs and mRNA for T cell CD3 mRNA and B cell CD20 mRNA; and (iii) a strong positive relationship between renal tubule-specific NKCC-2mRNA and miR-30a-3p and miR-10b expressed in high abundance in human renal tubular epithelial cells. Our observations were consistent with the interpretation that the altered expression of miRNAs during AR is most likely because of the relative proportions of graft-infiltrating immune cells and resident renal parenchymal cells. Our *in vitro* studies showing that some, but not all, of the differentially expressed miRNAs are also regulated by stimulation raises the possibility that there may be altered regulation of miRNAs within the cells themselves during an episode of acute rejection.

We used a novel barcoded deep sequencing of cDNA libraries of small RNAs to characterize miRNA transcriptome of human kidney allograft biopsies. Our analyses revealed that the total miRNA content is 50% lower in the RNA isolated from biopsies showing fibrosis compared with normal biopsies. Several miRNAs including miR-21, miR-30b, and miR-30c were differentially expressed between biopsies with fibrosis and normal biopsies. This distinction between the two groups, that is, fibrosis versus normal was also noted in the pattern of nucleotide sequence variations. We used RT-PCR to confirm the differential expression of miRNAs in an independent set of 18 allograft biopsies.

Proteomic biomarkers of allograft status

Proteomic technology examines proteins in a defined biologic compartment such as blood or urine. This approach is complementary to the genomic approach as there is no linear relation between the genome and the proteome, and indeed proteins can change without a change in gene expression and gene expression can change without an associated increase in detected protein. Mass spectrometry

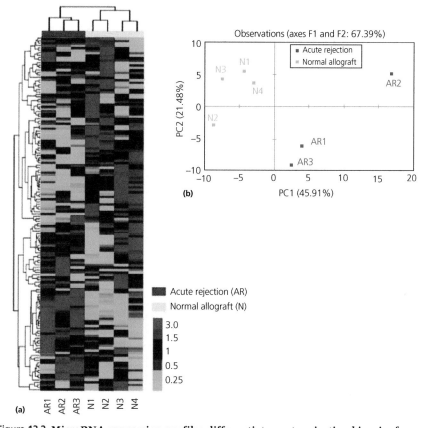

(a)

(b)

Observations (axes F1 and F2: 67.39%)

PC2 (21.48%)

PC1 (45.91%)

Acute rejection (AR)
Normal allograft (N)

3.0
1.5
1
0.5
0.25

Figure 13.2 MicroRNA expression profiles differentiate acute rejection biopsies from normal allograft biopsies of human renal allografts. (a) miRNA expression patterns of 7 human kidney allograft biopsies (3 showing histologic features of acute rejection [AR] and 4 with normal allograft biopsy results [N]) were examined using microfluidic cards containing TaqMan probes and primer pairs for 365 human mature miRNAs. A total of 174 ± 7 miRNAs were expressed at a significant level (i.e., CT<35) in all samples. The biopsies were grouped by unsupervised hierarchical clustering on the basis of similarity in expression patterns. The degree of relatedness of the expression patterns in biopsy samples is represented by the dendrogram at the *top*. Branch lengths represent the degree of similarity between individual samples (*top*) or miRNA (*left*). Two major clusters (*top*) accurately divided AR biopsies from normal allograft biopsies. Each column corresponds to the expression profile of a renal allograft biopsy, and each row corresponds to an miRNA. The *color* in each cell reflects the level of expression of the corresponding miRNA in the corresponding sample, relative to its mean level of expression in the entire set of biopsy samples. The increasing intensities of *red* mean that a specific miRNA has a higher expression in the given sample, and the increasing intensities of *green* mean that this miRNA has a lower expression. The scale (shown at *bottom right*) reflects miRNA abundance ratio in a given sample relative to the mean level for all samples. (b) Principal component analysis of 7 kidney allograft biopsies based on the expression of 174 small RNAs significantly expressed (i.e., CT<35) in all the samples. Principal component analysis (PCA) is a bilinear decomposition method designed to reduce the dimensionality of multivariable systems and used for overviewing clusters within multivariate data. It transforms a number of correlated variables into a smaller number of uncorrelated variables called PCs. The first PC accounts for as much of the variability in the data as possible, and each succeeding component accounts for as much of the remaining variability as possible. PCA showed evidence of clustering and confirmed the separation of AR samples from normal allograft biopsies. Samples were accurately grouped by PC1, which explained 45.91% of the overall miRNA expression variability, whereas PC2 explained 21.48% of variability and did not classify the samples according to their diagnosis. Source: Reprinted with permission from Anglicheau et al. (2009).

(MS) is the commonly used method to analyze the samples with regards to protein and peptide characterization, identification, and quantification. The classic proteomic study in transplantation identified urinary β2-microglobulin as a marker for acute rejection. Subsequent validation studies showed that it was not a specific marker, but rather a signature for tubular injury. Several laboratories have reported the use of urine and blood proteomic based approach for the diagnosis of kidney transplant rejection, cardiac allograft rejection, drug-free tolerance in liver transplants, graft-versus-host disease, and BK virus nephropathy. One study used aqueous humor proteins to diagnose acute corneal rejection while another found peptides isolated from bronchoalveolar lavage to be diagnostic of chronic lung allograft rejection. Studies on the utility of proteomics in transplantation merits further evaluation.

Biomarkers associated with allograft tolerance

Tolerance is defined as a lack of a graft-destructive immune response despite the absence of immunosuppressive medications. Allograft tolerance is donor specific and, thus, capable of rejecting a third-party allograft. In the clinic, it is extremely difficult to show donor-specific tolerance. Instead, the term "operational tolerance" is used to describe the clinical state where, in kidney transplantation, a recipient is not on immunosuppressive therapy and has stable graft function. The potential pathways contributing to tolerance are listed in Table 13.5. It is likely that multiple pathways operate to maintain immune tolerance. Furthermore, tolerance to an allograft may be complete or partial, and permanent or transient.

Table 13.5 Classification of tolerance.

A. Based on the major mechanism involved
1. Clonal deletion
2. Clonal anergy
3. Suppression
B. Based on the period of induction
1. Fetal
2. Neonatal
3. Adult
C. Based on the cell tolerized
1. T cell
2. B cell
D. Based on the extent of tolerance
1. Complete
2. Partial, including split
E. Based on the main site of induction
1. Central
2. Peripheral

Source: Suthanthiran et al. (2007). Reproduced by permission from Wolters Kluwer Health.

B cell signatures associated with operational tolerance

A multicenter study at four US transplant centers (Emory University, NIH, Swedish Medical Center, and University of Wisconsin) sponsored by the Immune Tolerance Network (ITN) examined whether blood- or urine-based signatures are associated with kidney transplant tolerance. In this study, 25 kidney transplant recipients (17 living-related donors; 5 deceased donors; 1 living-unrelated; and 2 donors, type unknown) with operational tolerance (TOL) were enrolled between 2004 and 2007. TOL patients had stopped taking immunosuppressive medications for at least 1 year with 20 of the 25 patients not on immunosuppressive therapy due to nonadherence, and the remaining 5 due to medication-related complications. The comparison groups included 33 clinically stable kidney transplant recipients on triple CNI-based immunosuppression regimen (SI) and 42 normal healthy individuals (HCs). This study found five unique tolerance-associated genes (*TUBB2A, TCL1A, BRDG1, HTPAP*, and *PPPAPDC1B*) after a false discovery rate correction was applied to the analysis to be statistically significant. Hierarchical clustering of 30 genes expressed greater than twofold in the TOL versus the SI group, which showed 22 genes to be B cell-specific. Urinary cell profiling of TOL patients showed that out of 18 genes tested only the urinary cell levels of *CD20* were significantly higher in TOL versus SI patients. The urinary cell levels of mRNA for *CD20, CD3, perforin*, and *FOXP3* were all significantly lower in HC individuals when compared to TOL patients. Multiplex RT-PCR testing of whole blood revealed 31 genes that were differentially expressed at a higher level ($p<0.05$) when comparing TOL and SI patients, but none between TOL patients and HC individuals. Again, most genes expressed were B cell-specific, encoding κ and λ immunoglobulin light chains.

Using the linear discriminate analysis (LDA) predictive model, a 3-gene signature of *IGKV4-1, IGLL1*, and *IGKV1D-13* distinguished the TOL group from the SI group with a positive predictive value (PPV) of 83% and a negative predictive value (NPV) of 84%. This 3 gene-set encode for κ and λ immunoglobulin light chains, which are upregulated when pre-B cells transition to mature B cell and during classswitching and receptor editing following antigenic activation of mature B cells. Consistent with this, flow cytometry analysis of whole blood from the TOL subjects showed greater number of total B cells (CD19+) and naïve B cells (CD19+CD27-IgM+IgD+) compared to SI subjects. Notably, transitional B cells (CD19+ CD38+CD24+IgD+) were also increased in the TOL group when compared to the SI group. Altogether, these studies implicated B cells in clinical tolerance, but many unanswered mechanistic questions remain.

The indices of tolerance (IOT) consortium in Europe, in conjunction with ITN, examined whether across-platform approach resolves signatures associated with kidney transplant tolerance. In this study, the 35 kidney transplant recipients classified as operationally tolerant were immunosuppressive drug-free for at least 1 year (TOL-DF), and included a training set comprising 11 subjects enrolled by IOT and a test set comprising 23 subjects enrolled in the ITN study.

The pertinent findings from this investigation were: (i) flow cytometric analysis of whole blood from the TOL-DF group showed greater number of B cells (CD19$^+$) in the TOL-DF groups than the nontolerant groups; (ii) both the training and test sets showed TOL-DF patients to be associated with a higher ratio of peripheral blood *FOXP3 mRNA* to α-1, 2-mannosidasemRNA when analyzed using RT-PCR assay; and (iii) microarray analysis of whole blood RNA identified gene probes that were differentially expressed between all the groups of the training and test sets at a significant level. Genes within B cell–related pathways were significantly associated with tolerance and of the top 11 ranked probes, 6 were known to be expressed by B cells or have related B cell function. The cross-platform biomarker study developed a multiparameter model of: (i) ratio of B to T lymphocytesubsets, percentage of CD4$^+$CD25^{int} T cells, (ii) ratio of antidonor to antithird party ELISPOT frequencies, (iii) ratio of *FOXP3mRNA* to α-1, 2-mannosidase mRNA, and (iv) a multigene signature of the top 10 ranked genes; this model predicted tolerance with an area under the curve of 1.0 for the training set (threshold of 0.01, PPV, and NPV of 100%) and for the test set, with a specificity of 0.923 and a sensitivity of 0.903 (threshold of 0.27, PPV of 80%, and NPV of 96%). That the thresholds for the training set and test were different raises challenges for the clinical applicability of the multiparameter prediction model.

A European study investigated the specific role of B cells and B cell signatures in patients with TOL. This study enrolled 12 patients with TOL), and 9 out of 12 TOL discontinued immunosuppressive therapy on their own, that is, to nonadherence, 2 due to post-transplant lymphoproliferative disease (PTLD), and the remaining one due to CNI toxicity. These 12 TOL patients were compared to 34 clinically stable kidney transplant recipients (STAs) on standard immunosuppression regimen, 31 patients with deteriorating allograft function while on standard immunosuppression regimen (CR), and 29 age-matched healthy volunteers (HVs). The study used the Bm1–Bm5 classification system to identify B cell developmental stages in the blood of study participants. Bm3 and Bm4 were absent in the blood and were not included in data analysis.

Flow cytometric analysis found that TOL patients displayed a significantly higher number of peripheral B cells due to a significant increase in IgD$^+$CD38$^+$ (activated Bm2 cells) and IgD$^-$CD38$^{+/-}$ subsets (EBm5/Bm5 memory B cells that express CD27). B cells of TOL patients displayed a higher level of CD80 ($p < 0.05$), CD86 ($p < 0.01$), CD40 ($p < 0.05$), and CD62L ($p < 0.05$) than STA and CR participants. The mean fluorescence intensity (MFI) of CD40 was higher in the IgD$^-$CD38$^{+/-}$memory populations from TOL patients compared to STA and HV participants suggesting that TOL patients exhibit a high number of circulating B cells expressing an activated-memory phenotype with a heightened expression of costimulatory molecules.

Gene enrichment analysis of microarray data to showed that seven major sets of genes related to B cell pathways were significantly enriched (false discovery rate < 25%, $p < 5\%$) in the TOL group compared to the STA groups. Biologic functions analysis indicated that regulation of several B cell functions with upregulation of genes related to cell cycle (*CCNA2, CCND2, BIRC5, CDC2, CDKN3, CKS2, PCNA*), proliferation (*CCNA2, CDC20, BUB1*), development, and maturation. B-cell scaffold protein with ankyrin repeats 1 (BANK1) in the blood of TOL patients were higher than in STA patients ($p < 0.01$). TOL patients had a significantly reduced CD32a/CD32b ratio compared to CR patients ($p < 0.05$) and a trend for a reduced CD32a/CD32b ratio was also observed at the level of CD19$^+$ B cells. The significant increase in CD32b mRNA transcript expression in PBMC is consistent with a higher expression at the protein level by flow cytometry both in absolute value and in the MFI of CD32b in TOL patients. Flow cytometry analyses of CD1d and CD5 expression among CD19+ cells were performed and 11 TOL patients were found to have a significantly higher number of B cells expressing CD5 and CD1d compared to STA patients ($p < 0.05$). The reduced CD32a/CD32b ratio and heightened BANK1 expression suggest that the B cells of TOL patients display an inhibitory profile. Also, TOL patients displayed an increased BAFF-R/BAFF ratio compared with STA patients ($p < 0.01$), HV participants ($p < 0.05$), and CR patients ($p < 0.05$), suggesting that TOL patients are characterized by a transcriptional profile favoring B-cell survival, thus contributing to their elevated peripheral B-cell count.

T cell signatures associated with operational tolerance

A study by investigators at the Stanford University and the Nantes Hospital examined whether peripheral blood cells analyzed using microarrays and RT-PCR assays resolves signatures associated with kidney transplant tolerance. In this study, 17 patients with TOL were enrolled between 2000 and 2006 and among the 17 TOL patients, 15 had stopped taking immunosuppressive medications for at least 2 years on their own (nonadherence), 1 due to PTLD and 1 due to CNI-induced nephrotoxicity. Prediction analysis of microarrays (PAM) applied to the training set of TOL (n = 5), CR (n = 11), and N (n = 8) identified a tolerance signature of 49 genes that accurately distinguished TOL patients from the other groups. RT-PCR assays were performed testing transcripts of *FOXP3, GITR*, and *Neuropilin-1* in the RNA extracted from the PBMC of 6 TOL-Test patients and 6 CR-Test patients, none of whom were included in the microarray analysis, and seven patients randomly chosen among the 12 STA patients. Profiling confirmed heightened expression of *FOXP3* ($p = 0.009$) in TOL-Test relative to CR-Test. Expression of *neuropilin-1* and *GITR* transcripts was also approximately twofold and eightfold greater, respectively, in TOL-test versus CR-Test, ($p = $ NS). When comparing TOL-Test with CR-Test, several transcripts from the 49 gene-set were statistically significant by RT-PCR assays ($p < 0.001$ for *CCL20, TLE4, CDH2, PARVG*, and *SPON1*; $p < 0.006$ for *RAB30, BTLA*, and *SMILE*; $p < 0.03$ for *SOX3, CHEK1, HBB*, and *DEPDC1*; $p = 0.045$ for *CDC2*).

A model of 33 of 49 tolerant gene signatures used in a blind cross-validated PAM, correctly classified TOL-Test 7-11 as tolerant and CR-Test 6-11 as CR, with a single misclassification (TOL-Test 12 as CR). The unique composite 33 gene transcripts was used to classify 7 STA post-transplant patients as either TOL or CR and a single stable patient was predicted to share the TOL phenotype with a classification score of greater than 99%. Thus, in the study, RT-PCR-based gene expression evidence of TOL remains strong across a modest number of genes. The study found that TGF-β regulates the function of 27% of the genes that differentiate tolerance from CR. These TGF-β-regulated genes include latent TGF-β-binding protein 4($LTBP4$) (2.6-fold increase), which functions to convert latent TGF-β protein into the active form; N-cadherin ($CDH2$) (5-fold increase), which enhances the ability of TGF-β to induce cell-cycle arrest in the G1 phase and $CD9$, a surface antigen that initiates the TGF-β signaling pathway and is expressed at a 40% higher level in TOL patients. Another significant finding was that T cell costimulatory genes were underexpressed in TOL patients when compared with CR. The study also confirmed that in TOL patients there was an absence of upregulation of genes associated with T cell activation ($CD69$, $TACTILE$, $LAG3$, or $SLAM$) and reduced levels of cytotoxicity-associated genes ($granzyme$, $perforin$, fas, and $granulysin$), and genes associated with pro-inflammatory responses (e.g., TNF-α).

Innate immunity and operational tolerance

Innate immunity has been increasingly recognized recently for augmenting adaptive immune responses leading to rejection, as well as for inducing allograft injury directly. A European study investigated the role of peripheral blood toll-like receptor 4 (TLR4) in TOL. The study groups included eight patients considered operationally tolerant and drug-free, eight patients with stable kidney graft function (N) treated with standard immunosuppressive therapy, 26 patients with CR, 10 patients with nonimmune causes of renal failure (NIRF), and 22 healthy volunteers (HV). Twenty-two of the 26 CR biopsies were C4d-positive, and 24 of the 26 patients had anti-HLA antibodies as well. Thirty-six biopsies from a separate cohort of 36 kidney transplant patients showed transplant glomerulopathy (TG, n = 10), CR (CR-Bx, $n = 18$), or were normal (N-Bx, $n = 8$). Myeloid differentiation factor 88 (MyD88) mRNA, and TLR4 mRNA in PBMC collected from the patients were measured. MyD88 mRNA was overexpressed in the PBMC from the CR patients compared to TOL or N patients. CR patients had heightened MyD88 mRNA expression compared to HV and NIRF participants. Heightened expression of TLR4 mRNA was observed in the CR group when compared to the TOL, N, and HV groups. The investigators showed also that TLR4 blood levels were not affected by concomitant infections. Intragraft expression of TLR4 mRNA was also higher in the biopsies from the CR-Bx group compared to the TG and N-Bx groups. Since the TOL patients did not undergo biopsy, intragraft levels of mRNA for MyD88 or TLR4 were not characterized.

Identification of tolerance signatures in clinical transplant tolerance trials

Kidney transplant tolerance accomplished via donor and recipient mixed hematopoietic stem cell (HSCT) chimerism has been advanced to the clinic. Analysis of total RNA from kidney allograft biopsy specimens of tolerant, HLA-mismatched patients with transient chimerism and 5-year follow-up using RT-PCR assays revealed high intragraft levels of *FOXP3* mRNA and the absence of the acute cellular rejection biomarker, *granzyme B* mRNA. Four of the original five tolerant patients continued to have functioning grafts up to 11 years following transplantation.

mRNA analysis of urinary cells of tolerant patients enrolled in the HLA-identical renal transplant tolerance study achieved by HSCT at Northwestern University revealed significantly lower levels of CD25, CD3ε, granzyme B, perforin, IP-10, CXCR3, and CD103 compared to patients on immunosuppressive drugs. In kidney transplant tolerance trials achieved by HSCT, other markers identified as potential signature for tolerance include sustained T-cell chimerism and increased production of regulatory natural killer T cells.

We have summarized clinically informative biomarkers of tolerance in Table 13.6. With the advent of microarray and RT-PCR technologies, previously unidentified molecular mechanisms underpinning clinical tolerance have begun to be resolved. Most of the biomarker signatures point to upregulation of B cell-related function and pathways in patients with TOL. This finding may merely be a consequence of being off immunosuppression; hence, the choice of comparative groups is important when investigating biomarkers in tolerance. For example, in expression of a key modulator gene for hyperactive B cell responses, BANK1 transcript was significantly higher in tolerant patients when compared to healthy volunteers who were also not receiving any immuno-modulating drugs suggesting an active immune component to the maintenance of spontaneous tolerance after withdrawal of immunosuppression. In the future, there is a significant opportunity for biomarker-driven investigation in tolerant patients to contribute to mechanistic-based tolerance-induction trials.

The description of biomarker results to date in patients with TOL not only reflects some commonalities in T cell signatures, but also highlights an unexpected presence of many B cell signatures. Obviously, this will need to be addressed not only in our concepts of tolerance induction, but also in our use of anti-B cell therapies.

New and emerging technologies
Next-generation sequencing

Sequencing is a way of determining the primary structure of the genome. For more than 30 years the chain-termination method developed by Frederick Sanger at the University of Cambridge has been the gold standard for determining the order of nucleotide bases in a chain of DNA. In the past few years, we have witnessed the emergence of a second-generation of high throughput

Table 13.6 Biomarkers of kidney allograft tolerance.

Authors	Sites	Tolerant sample size	Platforms	Samples	Main biomarker findings in tolerant patients
Newell et al. (2010)	4	25	Microarray	Blood	↑*IGKV4-1*, *IGLL1*, and *IGKV1D-13* (encode κ/λ light chain)
			RT-PCR		↑Transitional B cells (CD19⁺CD38⁺CD24⁺IgD⁺)
			Flow	Urine	↑ Urinary CD20 transcript
Sagoo et al. (2010)	Consortium	35	Microarray	Blood	↑ Blood CD19⁺ cells
			RT-PCR		↑ Blood *FOXP3* to α-1,2-mannosidase ratio
			Flow		↑ 6 Genes enriched in B cell function and related pathways
			ELISpot		4 biomarkers and 10 genes (see text)
Pallier et al. (2010)	European	12	Microarray	Blood	↑ IgD⁺CD38⁺ activated Bm2 and CD27+ Memory B cells
			RT-PCR		↑ 7 Sets of genes enriched in B cell related pathways
			Flow		↑ Blood BANK1 in B cells
					↓ CD32a/CD32b ratio at the level of CD19⁺ cells
					↑ BAFF-R/BAFF ratio for B cell survival (see text)
Brouard et al. (2007)	2	17	Microarray	Blood	↑ Blood *FOXP3*
			RT-PCR		↑ *TGF-β* regulated genes (*LTBP4*, *CDH2*, *CD9*)
					↓ Cytotoxic genes (*granzyme*, *perforin*, *fas*, and *granulysin*)
					↓ Pro-inflammatory genes (*TNF-α*, *IL-4*, and *IL-10*)
Braudeau et al. (2008)	1	8	RT-PCR	Blood	↓ Blood *TLR4* and *MyD88*
Kawai et al. (2008)	1	5	RT-PCR	Intragraft	↑ Intragraft *FOXP3*

parallel sequencing technologies. Overcoming the inherent limitations of the Sanger sequencing, "next-generation" sequencing methods allow sequencing of the complete genome, transcriptomes (expressed genes) and known exomes in a short period of time and at substantially reduced cost—characteristics that are essential for clinical utility. The major platforms currently used for sequencing are (1) HiSeq2500 (Illumina), (2) GS FLX+ System (Roche/454 Life Sciences), (3) SOLiD 5550XL System (Applied Biosystems), and (4) HeliScope Single Molecule Sequencer (Helicos Biosciences).

The Illumina sequencer is the most commonly used platform worldwide. Illumina sequencing consists of fragmentation of DNA and addition of 5′ and 3′ universal adapters to the fragmented DNA. The DNA molecules are then immobilized on a glass slide (flow cells). The "flow cell" surface is coated with single-stranded oligonucleotides that correspond to the sequences of the adapters. DNA is amplified by solid-phase bridge PCR on the flow cell surface, resulting in an array of clonal clusters. These clusters are then sequenced by successively incorporating fluorescent-labeled reversible terminators picked one at a time from a mixture of four nucleotides. The sequence is read in real-time by four-channel fluorescent scanning with each signal corresponding to a single nucleotide at a single position. The forward strand of each cluster is usually read, but reading both the forward and reverse templates of each cluster, also known as paired-end reading, is also possible. Translating the reads into meaningful information is done in multiple stages. Analyzing the images from the sequencers and converting them into sequence reads, alignment reads can be done either by *de novo* assembly or by mapping to a reference database, and finally using the mapped and unmapped reads in experiments for specific downstream applications.

Depth of coverage is the average number of times a given DNA nucleotide is represented in sequence reads. The Lander–Waterman equation is used to determine the coverage: $C = LN/G$, where $C = $ coverage, $L = $ read length, $N = $ number of reads and $G = $ haploid genome length. The level of coverage to detect mutations, single nucleotide polymorphisms or rearrangements in human genome requires about 10×–30× depth of coverage. For RNA sequencing however, the fact that different transcripts are expressed at different levels complicates the calculation. Instead, determining the total number of mapped reads is a more useful metric. In general, about 25–30 million mapped reads are recommended for differential expression studies in humans.

DNA sequencing can identify structural alterations in the human genome such as single nucleotide polymorphisms (SNPs) and copy number variations. Sequencing is advantageous compared to other techniques like microarray in the sense that the latter requires hybridization probes and hence are limited by the design of probes, which requires prior knowledge of the DNA sequence (see Table 13.4). In a recent report, Snyder and colleagues showed that cell-free DNA could be used to detect an organ-specific signature that correlates with rejection. Among heart transplant recipients, they monitored donor DNA levels over time to detect the onset of rejection. DNA sequencing was used to identify reads with donor and recipient SNPs to calculate the percentage of donor DNA in the recipient plasma.

Studies in mice have shown that epigenetic modifications via DNA methylation might provide a molecular basis for perpetuated fibroblast activation and fibrogenesis in the kidney.

RNA sequencing is an alternative approach for high-throughout transcriptome analyses. It is advantageous to microarray technology as its higher resolution improves discovery of novel transcripts, differential allele expression, alternate splice variants, post-transcriptional mutations and isoforms. Moreover, no prior knowledge of transcript sequences is required. RNA sequencing can also compare the differential expression between test samples. An RNA sequencing-based approach has been used for biomarker discovery. For example, in cancer, RNA sequencing was used to quantify papillary serous ovarian cancer transcriptomes. Insulin-like growth factor binding protein (IGFBP-4) was consistently present in the top 7.5% of all expressed genes in all tumor samples. In a larger independent validation set, IGFBP-4, as measured by enzyme-linked immunosorbent assay (ELISA), was significantly increased.

Metabolomics

The *metabolome* is the complete pool of all endogenous and exogenous small molecular metabolites in a biologic compartment. The goal of metabolomics is to identify and quantify the metabolome in a high-throughput manner. The metabolome contains a wide variety of chemically diverse compounds that includes lipids, organic acids, carbohydrates, amino acids, and nucleotides. Identification of the metabolome can either be targeted or untargeted. In an untargeted approach, the goal is to identify as many metabolites as possible in a sample and classify phenotypes based on a metabolic pattern. In a targeted approach, a predetermined set of metabolites is measured. The workflow of metabolomics consists of sample preparation, separation and detection of metabolites either by nuclear magnetic resonance (NMR) or by mass spectrometry, data mining, extraction, and analysis. Studies in kidney transplants have mainly used untargeted approach with NMR-based platforms. Kim and colleagues applied NMR-based metabolomics to study the serum metabolic profiles of transplant recipients with cyclosporine- or tacrolimus-based immunosuppression and were able to identify unique changes in serum metabolic profiles.

Over the past two decades, a new field of science called systems biology has emerged. The goal of systems biology is to characterize an organism at multiple levels that include genomic, transcriptomic, proteomic, and metabolomics information. Such integration of -omics will provide a powerful platform not only for the discovery of biomarkers, but also to understand the response of a biologic system to disease, abnormal genetic make-up, pharmacologic therapy, and environmental insults.

Current status and outlook

Despite the recent gains from biomarker discovery and validation related to acute T cell—mediated rejection, biomarkers diagnostic of humoral/antibody-mediated rejection remain to be fully defined. The discovery process for new biomarkers has been facilitated by new high-throughput technologies and platforms (Table 13.7). Biomarker signature discovery by cross-platform composite efforts from RT-PCR to microarray and flow cytometry may improve the accuracy and predictive values for diagnosing allograft rejection and tolerance. The molecular basis and science behind biomarkers is still ahead of available tools to swiftly implement the discovery process even though this is much improved in recent years. For the clinician, the benchmark of obtaining a serum creatinine measurement is both intuitively and in practice faster than ordering a biomarker test to diagnose allograft dysfunction. The gold standard of obtaining histologic confirmation, albeit invasive, remains important for clinical management. Despite the progress made on diagnosing rejection, a robust assay to diagnose and predict tolerance in a transplant recipient is not available, thus making the impact of finding a biomarker signature for tolerance far more reaching and critical.

Table 13.7 Platforms for biomarker discovery and validation.

Test		Platform	Examples of potential biomarkers
Gene transcripts	Single gene	RT-PCR	mRNA: granzyme B, perforin, FoxP3; miRNA; miR155, miR223
	Multiple genes	DNA microarray	
Proteins	Single protein	ELISA	Fractalkine, amyloid A, β2 microglobulin
	Multiple proteins	Protein microarray	
Lymphocyte function	Cytokine-producing cells	ELISPOT	IFNγ
	ATP levels in activated T cells	Immuknow	ATP
Alloantibodies	Single or multiple antibodies	Luminex xMAP	Anti-HLA antibody, anti-MICA antibody

Source: Reprinted with permission from Hartono et al. (2010).
FoxP3, forkhead box P3; HLA, human leukocyte antigen; IFNγ, interferon gamma; MICA, major histocompatibility complex (MHC) class I-related chain A; miRNA, microRNA; RT-PCR, real-time PCR; enzyme-linked immunosorbent assay, ELISA; enzyme-linked immunosorbent spot assay, ELISPOT.

Translating new knowledge from bench to the bedside remains an arduous process. Several issues such as funding and regulatory challenges beyond the customary barrier to implementation still exist in the field. The tolerance trials described in this chapter required almost a decade from design to execution and for obtaining meaningful results. For tolerance research, achieving an adequate sample size and recruiting enough subjects to meet the inclusion criteria is time consuming and poses logistic hurdles. Also, the biomarkers identified in a subject with TOL may not yield mechanistic insights. It is also not clear if the tolerance signature is stable and enduring. Hence, carefully designed long-term validation studies are needed.

Summary

Much has been accomplished in the development and validation of biomarkers of allograft rejection and of tolerance. Research in the biomarker arena is sure to benefit from systematic interrogation of the graft recipient with high-throughput assays and multiple platforms capable of fully characterizing the genome, transcriptome, proteome, and metabolome. An emphasis on noninvasive approaches has high merit. The clinical utility of discovered biomarkers needs to be validated in appropriately designed clinical trials.

References

Anglicheau, D and Suthanthiran M. Noninvasive prediction of organ graft rejection and outcome using gene expression patterns. Transplantation 2008;86:192–199.

Anglicheau D, Sharma VK, Ding R, et al. MicroRNA expression profiles predictive of human renal allograft status. Proc Natl Acad Sci U S A 2009;106:5330–5335.

Braudeau C, Ashton-Chess J, Giral, M, et al. Contrasted blood and intragraft toll-like receptor 4 mRNA profiles in TOL versus CR in kidney transplant recipients. Transplantation 2008;86:130–136.

Brouard S, Mansfield E, Braud C, et al. Identification of a peripheral blood transcriptional biomarker panel associated with operational renal allograft tolerance. Proc Natl Acad Sci U S A 2007;104:15448–15453.

Hartono C, Muthukumar T, and Suthanthiran M. Noninvasive diagnosis of acute rejection of renal allografts. Curr Opin Organ Transplant 2010;15:35–41.

Kawai T, Cosimi AB, Spitzer TR, et al. HLA-mismatched renal transplantation without maintenance immunosuppression. N Engl J Med 2008;358:353–361.

Newell KA, Asare A, Kirk AD, et al. Identification of a B cell signature associated with renal transplant tolerance in humans. J Clin Invest 2010;120:1836–1847.

Pallier A, Hillion S, Danger R, et al. Patients with drug-free long-term graft function display increased numbers of peripheral B cells with a memory and inhibitory phenotype. Kidney Int 2010;78:503–513.

Sagoo P, Perucha E, Sawitzki B, et al. Development of a cross-platform biomarker signature to detect renal transplant tolerance in humans. J Clin Invest 2010;120:1848–1861.

Suthanthiran M, Hartono C, and Strom TB. Immunobiology and Immunopharmacology of Renal Allograft Rejection" Chapter 96 in: *Diseases of the Kidney and Urinary Tract*, 8th Edition Robert W. Schrier, Editor. Lippincott Williams & Wilkins, Philadelphia, 2007.

Further reading

Bechtel W, McGoohan S, Zeisberg EM, et al. Methylation determines fibroblast activation and fibrogenesis in the kidney. Nat Med 2010;16:544–550.

Kim CD, Kim EY, Yoo H, et al. Metabonomic analysis of serum metabolites in kidney transplant recipients with cyclosporine A- or tacrolimus-based immunosuppression. Transplantation 2010;90:748–756.

Leventhal JR, Matthew JM, Salomon DR, et al. Genomic biomarkers correlate with HLA-identical renal transplant tolerance. J Am Soc Nephrol 2013;24:1376–1385.

Li B, Hartono C, Ding R, et al. Noninvasive diagnosis of renal-allograft rejection by measurement of messenger RNA for perforin and granzyme B in urine. N Engl J Med 2001;344:947–954.

Lorenzen JM, Volkmann I, Fiedler J, et al. Urinary miR-210 as mediator of acute T-cell mediated rejection in renal allograft recipients. Am J Transplant 2011;10:2221–2227.

Metzker ML. Sequencing technologies—the next generation. Nat Rev Genet 2010;11:31–46.

Mosig RA, Lobl M, Senturk E, et al. IGFBP-4 tumor and serum levels are increased across all stages of epithelial ovarian cancer. J Ovarian Res 2012;5:3–11.

Muthukumar T, Dadhania D, Ding R, et al. Messenger RNA for FOXP3 in the urine of renal-allograft recipients. N Engl J Med 2005;353:2342–2351.

Nankivell BJ and Alexander SI. Rejection of the kidney allograft. N Engl J Med 2010;363:1451–1462.

Nankivell BJ, Borrows RJ, Fung CL, et al. The natural history of chronic allograft nephropathy. N Engl J Med 2003;349:2326–2333.

Sarwal M, Chua MS, Kambham N, et al. Molecular heterogeneity in acute renal allograft rejection identified by DNA microarray profiling. N Engl J Med 2003;349:125–138.

Snyder TM, Khush KK, Valantine HA, et al. Universal noninvasive detection of solid organ transplant rejection. Proc Natl Acad Sci U S A 2011;108:6229–6234.

Solez K, Colvin RB, Racusen LC, et al. Banff 07 classification of renal allograft pathology: updates and future directions. Am J Transplant 2008;8:753–760.

Suthanthiran M, Schwartz JE, Ding R, et al. Urinary-cell mRNA profile and acute cellular rejection in kidney allografts. N Engl J Med 2013;369:20–31.

Weiss RH, Kim K. Metabolomics in the study of kidney diseases. Nat Rev Nephrol 2011;8:22–33.

CHAPTER 14

Emerging issues in transplantation

Rupert Oberhuber, Guangxiang Liu, Timm Heinbokel, and Stefan G. Tullius

Division of Transplant Surgery and Transplant Surgery Research Laboratory, Brigham and Women's Hospital, Harvard Medical School, Boston, USA

CHAPTER OVERVIEW

- Elderly patients represent the fastest growing population among waitlisted transplant candidates, and age-related issues have become a significant concern in transplantation.

- The demand for donor organs has lead to increased use of marginal donors, raising issues related to organ age, organ injury and repair, and overall organ quality.

- The impact of immunosenescence in the elderly on alloimmune responses, immunosuppressive therapy, incidence of drug-related complications, and overall transplant outcomes remains poorly understood.

- There remains a considerable interest in the area of xenotransplantation as an alternative approach to resolving the issue of organ shortage.

- Other areas of significant interest include artificial organs, devices for transplantation, stem cells, and organ regeneration.

Introduction

Over the past 50 years, organ transplantation has experienced an unparalleled advancement from an experimental procedure to an established treatment for patients with end-stage organ failure. With greatly improved quality of life and reduced morbidity rates after transplants, indications for transplantation have been substantially broadened and age limits have been essentially eliminated. Thus, more patients than ever before are currently awaiting organ transplants. In renal transplantation, for example, about 100,000 patients were on waiting lists in the United States in 2011, representing a 90% increase over the past decade. Consequently, median waiting times have increased dramatically for transplant patients.

Transplant Immunology, First Edition. Edited by Xian Chang Li and Anthony M. Jevnikar.
© 2016 John Wiley & Sons, Ltd. Published 2016 by John Wiley & Sons, Ltd.
Companion website: www.wiley.com/go/li/transplantimmunology

At the same time, availability of donor organs has been stagnant at best, or even slightly declining despite intensive efforts to increase organ donations. Similar trends are observed in living donations. While rates were increasing in the early nineties with the advent of minimal invasive procedures for donor nephrectomies, a slight decline has been observed recently for living donations. Thus, a significant discrepancy between demand and supply for organ transplants has emerged. To meet these demands, marginal and older organs or organs procured from donors with circulatory arrest prior to organ retrieval (so-called donation after cardiac or circulatory death or DCD donors) have been increasingly used in the clinic in an attempt to expand the donor pool. Indeed, marginal donor organs and those retrieved from DCD donors have shown the highest proportional increase in the recent past. Both aggressive neurosurgical approaches for craniotomies and demographic developments toward an aging population may lead to further increases in the use of DCD and marginal donor organs in the future. Thus, with concerns of reduced organ availability and quality, it will be critical to further explore the clinical implications of using marginal donor organs.

Aspects of organ senescence and compromised repair capacities may be involved in mediating inferior outcome of marginal donor organs. To improve outcomes of marginal donor organs, it will be important to understand the mechanisms of senescence and to explore proper treatment options during organ perfusion, organ preservation, and in the early post-transplant period. With relevance to aging patients on waitlists, we have learned from nontransplant disease models that the immune response is subject to profound changes in the process of aging. Indeed, age seems to affect almost all compartments of the immune system. As older individuals undergo transplantation more frequently, it will be important to understand the complexity of age-related changes of the immune system and their impact on immunosuppression and organ survival.

With an ever-increasing demand for organ transplants, alternative approaches to address organ shortage are once again experiencing strong interest. Xenotransplantation has gained momentum along with the development of bio-artificial organs, which have made great strides in the recent past. These two fields merging as xenogeneic organs are being explored as a means to provide scaffolds for bioengineered organs, reconstituted with human stem cells. The current demand for donor organs is representing an impetus to explore and review recent development in this area (Figure 14.1).

Age and immune responses

Age-related changes in immune responses are multifactorial and not all compartments seem to be affected in a uniform fashion. Thymic involution as a hallmark of the aging immune system exerts a profound influence on phenotypes and functions of all T cell compartments. Functional aspects of the innate

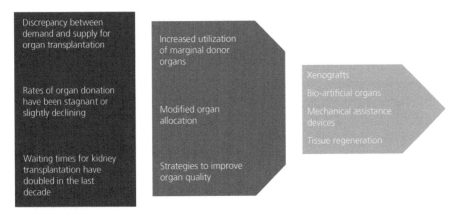

Figure 14.1 Pressing issues in organ transplantation: current and future approaches.

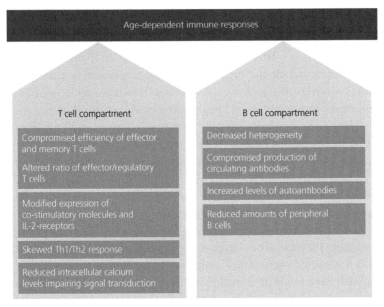

Figure 14.2 Age-dependent aspects of the alloimmune response.

immune system including complement activity, chemotaxis, and phagocytotic properties seem to be well preserved with aging. In addition to the decline in numbers of certain T cell subsets, there are significant changes in the expression of certain cell surface markers (Figure 14.2). For example, the expression of costimulatory molecules on T cells from older adults is altered, potentially interfering with the clinical use of agents to block costimulatory pathways. The emerging concept of T cell "exhaustion" through altered expression of PD-1 is particularly intriguing, particularly as there is great interest in this area by cancer researchers to enhance anti tumor immunity.

Aging causes a shift from a Th1 to a Th2 cytokine profile: production of INF-γ is reduced, while Th2-related cytokines such as IL-4 and IL-10 gain prominence in elderly patients. Older individuals show higher frequencies of T cells with an effector/memory phenotype; however, these cells seem to be less efficient in mounting immune responses *in vivo*. "Older" T cells also show reduced intracellular calcium levels, possibly impacting the signal transduction and activation of downstream proteins such as protein kinase C, MAPK, and MEK. Several studies have reported a decreasing density of IL-2 receptors on T cells and a compromised synthesis of IL-2 upon stimulation. Interestingly, higher numbers of regulatory cells are observed in the elderly.

Likewise, the B cell compartment undergoes extensive modifications with increasing age and demonstrates decreased heterogeneity and lower levels of antibodies, along with increasing levels of autoantibodies. Metabolic and gender-related differences may also play a role when dissecting the consequences of the aging immune response. As shown recently, age-related hormonal changes seem to influence the immune response and are, at least in part, responsible for immune senescence, as sex hormones are, among others, involved in thymic involution. It is important to note that most of our knowledge on the aspects and mechanisms of the aging immune response to date is based on disease processes outside of transplantation. However, it appears that the preservation of regulatory capacities and compromised effector functions might explain the less frequent acute rejection rates in elderly recipients. This may serve as a guide in the management of immunosuppression in elderly patients.

Marginal donor organs

In the wake of the growing shortage of organ donors, marginal organs are increasingly being used for transplantation. While previous allocation systems in the United States differentiated expanded from standard criteria organs, the current allocation system that has been introduced since the end of 2014 assesses the quality of organs based on the so-called KDPI (Kidney Donor Profile Index). This measure provides a continuous scale estimating the likelihood of graft failure based on 10 donor factors represented on a 0–100 graduation. In general, outcomes of organs with a higher KDPI are inferior, illustrated by higher rates of delayed or primary nonfunction and compromised long-term graft survival. Delayed graft function (DGF), as a consequence of ischemia/reperfusion injury, is more frequent following transplantation of older organs and may be a result of greater age-related injury and attenuated repair processes. In many recent studies, DGF has been linked to increased rates of acute rejection and graft failure. However, the precise impact of DGF on long-term survival continues to be debated using registry data, reflecting the complex biology with many variables that are not tracked, and perhaps problems inherent to registry analyses. Marginal donor organs are less well defined for other organ allocation systems, but age in addition to organ injuries subsequent to brain death, prolonged ischemia or the consequences of previous diseases that affect the quality of transplants.

Transplantation of organs from marginal donors has led to an overall increased utilization of available organs. However, it is worth noting that most clinical studies have shown significant lower 1- and 5-year patient and graft survival rates for extended criteria donors (ECDs) or higher (>85) KDPI kidneys. It is important to recognize that the transplantation of marginal kidneys provides a significant survival benefit for *selected* patients compared to staying on the waiting list, but that this benefit may not be universal. Indeed, some patients may do better on optimized dialysis than those with a marginal kidney transplant in the short term. This, of course, remains in the realm of clinical judgment rather than established optimal protocols. Of note, in renal and in liver transplantation, excellent patient and graft survival rates have been reported with organs from donors over the age of 80.

With respect to marginal donor organs, some organ-specific aspects seem to be of particular relevance. Aging is linked to loss of functional capacity and, therefore, donor age is an important risk factor for poor long-term graft function. Donor age has also been linked to increased rates of both acute and chronic rejection, suggesting an increased immunogenicity as a consequence of aging *per se*. Additionally, an age-related decline in repair mechanisms may also contribute to inferior graft outcomes. However, it may be difficult to discriminate between changes related to chronic rejection such as interstitial fibrosis and tubular atrophy (IFTA) or glomerulosclerosis, and changes caused by physiological aging.

In contrast to the kidney, the liver seems to be less susceptible to senescence *per se*, especially in healthy individuals. This may be related to a large functional reserve and significant regenerative capacity of the liver. However, older livers have been found to have a decreased capacity to synthesize adenosinetriphosphate (as a surrogate marker of synthetic capacity) and liver grafts procured from old donors showed increased endothelial cell injury post transplantation. Recipients of marginal liver grafts are at a higher risk for primary nonfunction, especially with prolonged cold ischemia times. Older livers also have an increased incidence of pre-existing steatosis, thereby accelerating the detrimental effects of ischemia/reperfusion injury. As a consequence, careful selection should be applied to organs from older donors, and organ allocation should consider risk factors related to both donor and recipient age (Figure 14.3).

Organs from donors after cardiac or circulatory death (DCD)

Organ-specific susceptibility to prolonged ischemia plays a critical role in the use of DCD donor organs. In renal transplantation, warm ischemia times of up to 1 h (defined as the time period between cardiac arrest and commencement of cold

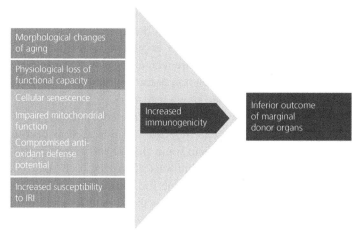

Figure 14.3 Organ quality impacts transplant outcomes.

perfusion) are currently accepted. While kidneys from DCD donors demonstrate increased rates of DGF, their outcome after 1 year seems comparable to the outcome of kidneys procured from neurologically determined death (NDD) donors. Interestingly, age seems to aggravate deteriorating effects of prolonged warm ischemia, as kidneys from older DCD donors seem to fare less well than those from older NDD donors.

As livers appear to be more susceptible to damage subsequent to warm ischemia, the maximally tolerated warm ischemia time in general does not exceed 30 min. Moreover, livers from older DCD donors are rarely used. Pancreata are commonly used only from young donors with brief warm ischemia times and the use of hearts and lungs from DCD donors has so far been a rare exception. Successful cases of lung transplantations have recently been reported following normothermic *ex-vivo* perfusion, allowing for a detailed assessment and improvement of organ quality prior to transplantation. Overall, it should be stressed that DCD donation represents a valuable "end-of-life option" for patients in the intensive care unit and an appropriate and necessary approach to increase the availability of donor organs. Of note, while DCD donation has contributed to an overall increase of donors, organ transplantation on the whole has not necessarily increased, as organs other than kidneys are less frequently used.

Organ age and its roles in immunogenicity, injury/repair, and immune responses

In general, organ age is linked to compromised repair processes following unspecific injury. Unspecific injuries subsequent to ischemia/reperfusion injury (IRI) or brain death are inherent components of the transplantation procedure. There is a growing body of evidence suggesting that organs from elderly donors are particularly susceptible to these injuries. Antioxidant defense potentials and regenerative capacities are limited in older organs and contribute to the more detrimental consequences observed. Moreover, older grafts show impaired mitochondrial function, resulting in a depletion of intracellular energy contents, thus attenuating repair capacities further.

Recent clinical studies have shown that increased donor age is associated with more frequent episodes of acute rejection. Donor age has been linked to more potent host immune responses in some clinical and experimental reports. Moreover, compromised repair mechanisms following ischemia/reperfusion injury or brain death may aggravate nonspecific graft injuries when transplanting older organs. These nonspecific injuries activate pattern recognition receptors (PRRs) on antigen-presenting cells (APCs) through pathogen associated molecular patterns (PAMPs) such as peptidoglycans or lipopolysaccharides. Toll-like receptors (TLRs) representa major subgroup of PRRs and are expressed on macrophages/monocytes, dendritic cells (DCs), and natural killer (NK) cells. Engagement of TLRs by their ligands trigger the release of pro-inflammatory cytokines, in turn, recruiting and activating critical components of the innate immune system such as neutrophils and macrophages; these cells then activate and modulate adaptive immune responses. Moreover, TLRs also recognize products of damaged and injured cells. Graft injury subsequent to prolonged ischemia, reperfusion injury, or brain death may therefore not only activate innate, but also adaptive immune responses. Most recently, regulated forms of cell necrosis, termed "necroptosis," have been implicated in promoting allorejection in kidney and cardiac transplant models. As new therapeutics targeting the endogenous pathways of cell death are emerging, these findings may open up exciting new perspectives for the pharmacological influence of organ injury and repair.

Donor alloantigens are processed and presented by donor and host APCs. When T cells are cocultured with old APCs, an increased proliferation of responder calls has been observed, suggesting that senescent APCs may have an enhanced antigen presenting capacity with the potential to increase graft immunogenicity. Thus, aspects of age-dependent antigen presentation in concert with age-specific injuries and compromised repair mechanisms may be responsible for the enhanced immune responses observed when transplanting older organs (Figure 14.4).

Recipient age and transplant outcome

Older individuals show the highest proportional increase among patients awaiting organ transplantation. In renal transplantation, for example, the majority of transplant recipients is now in individuals older than 50 years. Moreover, current demographic changes show a rising proportion of the elderly in our society,

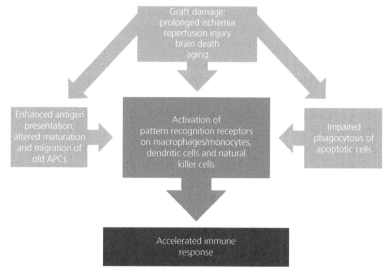

Figure 14.4 Graft injury will determine immune responses.

which will likely translate into a further increase in older donors and older recipients in the future. Indeed, those older than 65 years awaiting renal transplantation have tripled during the past decade.

When analyzing graft survival, it is important to distinguish between death-censored and uncensored graft survival rates, as death is obviously more frequent in the elderly. More recent clinical data suggest that renal transplantation in patients older than 65 years led to doubled life expectancy compared to patients remaining on dialysis. These data emphasize the clinical benefit of transplanting older individuals. For liver transplantation, even though still controversial, most authors agree that patient survival rates start to decline when transplanting recipients older than 60 years. However, patients older than 70 years have undergone transplantation with promising survival rates. Critical to improving outcomes when transplanting older organs is the careful analysis of donor and recipient risk factors, as they are linked in an additive or even synergistic fashion.

Infections after transplantation are more common in elderly recipients. Aging itself is one of the leading risk factors for infections, responsible for almost 50% of all deaths within the first year after transplantation in patients over 50 years. Moreover, rates of malignancies are higher in the elderly, potentially related to a compromised immune surveillance. *De novo* malignancies and particularly nonskin malignancies are more frequent and are an important cause for poorer outcome after transplantation in the elderly. With immunosuppression being a major risk factor for future malignancies and infections, it is critical to gain a more in-depth understanding of the consequences of immunosenescence and how immunosuppression can be adjusted to better suit the elderly.

Immunosenescence is defined as a dysfunction of the immune system, which is caused by aging. It is believed that cellular senescence of nonimmune cells has evolved as a physiologic strategy to prevent uncontrolled cell divisions. The senescence of immune competent cells, at the same time, limits tumor surveillance and subsequently allows malignant cells to escape elimination. The shortening of telomeres, a specific region of repetitive DNA sequences at the end of chromosomes, is a hallmark of aging. Once the telomere length reaches a critical limit, cells lose the ability to replicate and become senescent. Senescent cells show greater morphologic heterogeneity, accumulation of lipofuscin granules, and, per definition, a reduced capacity to respond to mitogenic stimuli and expression level changes of genes involved in cell cycle such as p16INK4a. Besides replicative senescence, stress-induced premature senescence (SIPS) may also contribute to the detrimental effect of injuries observed in older organs.

Immunosuppression in the elderly

Current immunosuppressive drugs increase the risk for post-transplant malignancies and infections, and these effects appear to be more pronounced in the elderly.

Drug metabolism, compromised kidney function, reduced hepatic and splanchnic blood flow, and a redistribution of body fat toward a prominence of abdominal fat may impact not only absorption but also drug distribution and elimination in the elderly. Additional factors that impact absorption and metabolization of immunosuppressants in the elderly include a shift towards a more alkalotic gastric milieu, compromised gastric motility, and a less-efficient cytochrome IIIa system. Of note, many clinical trials have mostly excluded older transplant recipients.

The benefits of using induction agents have been well established in renal transplantation. However, with an increased risk for infections and malignancies linked particularly to antilymphocytic agents, their use needs to be carefully assessed in the elderly. Although prospective clinical trials remain lacking, IL-2 receptor antibodies have been used successfully in older kidney transplant recipients, resulting in reduced frequencies of post-transplant lymphoproliferative disease (PTLD) and infections compared to more aggressive induction therapy (Figure 14.5).

Mycophenolate-mofetil (MMF) and prednisone, along with calcineurin inhibitors (CNIs) are the most common immunosuppressive drugs currently used in elderly transplant recipients. To this point, dose adjustments or specific preferences among available drugs for elderly transplant recipients, based on altered aging immune response, have not been explored sufficiently. In theory, side effect profiles and the antiproliferative properties of mammalian target of rapamycin (mTOR) inhibitors seem, at least in theory, well suited for their use in

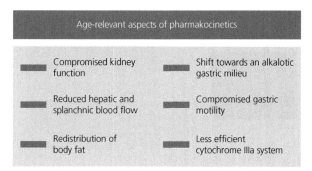

Figure 14.5 Factors leading to altered absorption and metabolism of immunosuppressants in the elderly.

the elderly. Sirolimus has the potential to reduce the risk for malignancies while preserving renal function. However, impaired wound healing, interstitial pneumonitis, thrombocytopenia, and lipid abnormalities may limit the use of this drug in the elderly.

Belatacept, an inhibitor of CD28 costimulation, has been approved for clinical use. Promising 1- and 2-year allograft survival rates with reduced nephrotoxicity and cardiovascular risk profiles make the application of belatacept attractive. However, the efficacy of the drug in the elderly will require detailed studies in this population.

Xenotransplantation

Xenotransplants, that is, organs, tissues, or cells originating from other species, have been considered to be an ideal way to overcome organ shortage in clinical transplantation. Nonhuman primates and pigs may be suited for xenotransplantation. However, besides immunological obstacles, infectious risks as well as differences in physiology need to be addressed prior to clinical application. There also remain legal and ethical issues that will require further clarification.

There are key biologic barriers hindering xenotransplantation, with the most significant being hyper-acute rejection (HAR) mediated by pre-existing antibodies that occur within 24 h after engraftment. Xenoantibodies are directed against Galα1-3Galβ1-4GlcNAc (αGal) carbohydrate residues. α-Gal is present on vascular endothelial cells of nonhuman primates, but absent in humans. These anti-αGal antibodies, mostly of the IgMiso type, comprise approximately 1% of the total immunoglobulins in the circulation. When these antibodies bind to the vascular endothelial cells in xenografts, the complement system is activated through the classical pathway leading to graft rejection within minutes to hours. Histologic features of HAR are interstitial hemorrhages and

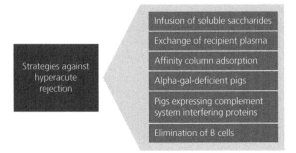

Figure 14.6 Strategies preventing hyperacute rejection after xenotransplantation.

edema, accompanied by thrombosis of blood vessels. These changes occur as soon as blood supply to the graft is restored. Toward preventing HAR, inhibition of antibody binding to porcineαGal by "soluble saccharide" has been tested. Unfortunately, the large amounts of sugar needed led to toxic side effects and were able to block only 30% of injurious antibodies. In order to reduce the titers of xenoantibodies, exchange of recipient plasma with albumin, fresh frozen plasma, or other volume replacement fluids has been attempted. Although a prolongation of graft survival has been achieved with this approach, many biologically important immunoglobulins were also eliminated, thus limiting its clinical application. Selective elimination of xenoantibodies through affinity column adsorption has also been tested, but did not sufficiently reduce antibody titers (Figure 14.6).

As an alternative strategy, deletion of αGal in donor grafts substantially prolonged xenograft survival. For example, pig hearts deficient ofα-1,3-galactosyltransferase(αGalT) survived for up to 6 months when transplanted into baboons. Pigs lacking the 1,3 galactosyltransferase gene thus may represent a source for xenografts. Transgenic pigs expressing proteins interfering with the human complement system have also been tested. As the complement cascade is responsible for cell lysis and activation of the coagulation cascade during HAR, genetic manipulations of CD55 (human decay accelerating factor [hDAF]), CD59 (protectin; blocking the membrane attack complex), and CD46 (membrane cofactor 1) have been tested and more recently triple transgenic pigs have become available. Indeed, these approaches were able to prevent hyperacute rejections in a pig to baboon transplant model. Eliminating B cells responsible for the production of xenoantibodies has also been explored in conjunction with gene manipulation and immunosuppression. In some models, heart xenografts survived up to 50 days in which a graft from α-1,3-galactosyltransferase knockout pigs transgenic for hDAF were transplanted into baboons treated with Rituximab (anti-CD20), tacrolimus, sirolimus, MMF, and prednisone.

Besides HAR, acute xenoantibody-mediated rejection (AXR) occurs within days or weeks after transplantation based on very low levels of αGal-specific antibodies in addition to antibodies against other porcine antigens. AXR has even been observed in αGalT deficient transgenic pigs, indicating that non-αGal antigens are, at least in part, responsible for AXR. Strategies to prevent AXR still remain limited. However, the concept of "accommodation" has shown promising results, at least in minor disparate combinations. Accommodation, defined as graft survival in the presence of antibodies, was first observed clinically in ABO-incompatible transplantation. Survival of grafts in the presence of antidonor antibodies include a process of downregulating antigenic determinants on endothelial cells, a change in the antibody repertoire, and the induction of protective genes.

Cellular xenograft rejection, in contrast to HAR and AXR, is mediated mainly by NK cells and T cells. NK cells play a prominent role in rejection of xenografts and human T cells are able to recognize porcine major histocompatibility complex (MHC) II antigens through the direct pathway. Moreover, recipient APCs can activate recipient T cells through the indirect pathway of xenorecognition. Cellular rejections of xenografts are even more potent than those observed in allografts with a dense and diverse presence of antigens. Different strategies to overcome T cell-mediated xenograft rejection have been investigated, including the use of different immunosuppressive and tolerance regimens. The concept of physical isolation by encapsulation has been tested for islets with limited success.

Strategies of tolerance induction using hematopoietic chimerism have shown promising results. In this approach, donor stem cells reconstituting the host immune system are transplanted into the recipients following intense preconditioning. During this process, T cells responsive to donor xenoantigens are deleted in the thymus, leaving behind only cells that are tolerant to the graft. Using hDAF pigs as donors of hematopoietic stem cells allowed induction of xenomicro chimerism in irradiated baboons. However, the achieved low-level chimerism was only transient. More recently, progenitor cell engraftment has been achieved following nonmyeloablative conditioning and subsequent transplantation of large doses of bone marrow (1–2×10^9 cells/kg) from GalT-KO pigs. However, even less toxic recipient conditioning regimens allowing the engraftment of porcine progenitors are in need.

Besides a broad spectrum of immunologic issues, xenotransplantation also faces a potential risk for infection. Particularly, Xenozoonosis, the transmission of infectious agents through xenografts, represents a risk in heavily immunosuppressed recipients. Moreover, it has been shown that human complement regulators such as CD46, CD55, and CD59 expressed by transgenic pigs can serve as virus receptors, allowing the infection of host cells. Porcine endogenous retroviruses (PERVs), an entity of at least three different subgroups, have, at least in theory, the potential to integrate into the human genome. Although no transmission has been documented thus far, PERV transmission remains a major concern.

Artificial or biologic organ replacement

Artificial kidneys

The attempts to construct an artificial kidney were initiated by Rowntree and Turner in 1913 using celloidin tubes contained in a glass jacket as a blood cleansing device. Anticoagulation was achieved using hirudin obtained from leeches. This device served as a model for subsequent attempts, and the first clinical applications were reported in 1924 (Figure 14.7). Kolff, Berk, and Watschinger developed a hemodialysis device in 1943, which consisted of a rotating drum with 30–40 m of cellophane tubing in a stationary tank. This device came into clinical application following further refinements in 1945. Despite these early successes, devices were not clinically usable for long-term treatment as adequate blood flow could only be obtained via large catheters, which damaged veins and arteries in patients.

The next key step in hemodialysis was the development of arterio-venous shunts, and in 1952 the first program for the dialysis treatment of patients with chronic renal failure was initiated in Seattle. As a result of the evolved technologies in dialysis, millions of patients suffering from end-stage kidney disease are currently undergoing routine periodic dialysis at local dialysis centers throughout the world. Although dialysis represents one of the most successful organ replacement therapies, it remains inferior to renal transplantation, thus demonstrating the enormous challenge of replacing organs entirely by artificial systems.

Artificial organs for the replacement of nonrenal organs, although attempted with some success, have so far been less effective.

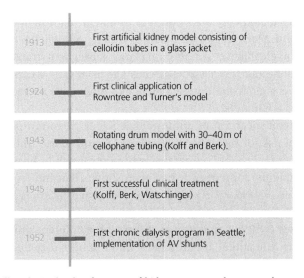

Figure 14.7 Hallmarks in the development of kidney organ replacement therapy.

Liver support systems

Artificial liver-supporting systems have the potential to temporarily assume metabolic and excretory functions while removing hepatotoxic substances, and in some cases they can stabilize patients with liver failure. If sufficient numbers of hepatocytes remain following liver injury, regeneration and subsequent recovery of liver function has been reported. Two main strategies have been pursued for the replacement of failing livers: comparable to the principle of hemodialysis, membrane and adsorbents have been designed to achieve detoxification. Charcoal filters may serve as an example to absorb many of the circulating toxins present in liver failure. Protein-bound toxins, however, could not be removed until the molecular adsorbent recycling system (MARS) was developed. MARS has been shown to remove water-soluble and albumin-bound low- and middle-molecular-weight toxins with high selectivity and currently represents the most widely used extracorporeal liver support technique. Three artificial liver supporting systems have undergone randomized controlled trials, including the MARS device (Gambro, Stockholm, Sweden), Prometheus (Fresenius Medical Care, Bad Homburg, Germany), and the BioLogic-DT/Liver Dialysis Unit. Most clinical trials have shown that the devices are safe and some reports suggest rapid improvements in patient's conditions when compared to a standard medical care (Figure 14.8).

Biologic devices using live hepatocytes represent an alternative approach. Bioartificial systems incorporate either human hepatoblastoma cells or porcine hepatocytes into bioreactors to perform both detoxification and synthetic liver functions. A permeable barrier between the patient's blood isolates cells from immunoglobulins and leucocytes, thus avoiding immune responses, while smaller sized particles such as toxins, metabolites, and synthesized proteins can be filtered. Randomized controlled trials have been performed for two bioartificial liver systems, the HepatAssist which uses porcine hepatocytes and the Extracorporeal Liver Assist Device based on human hepatoblastoma cells. Clinical reports indicate an improvement in liver function parameters and in some cases clinical symptoms. The impact on patient outcome, however, will need to be confirmed.

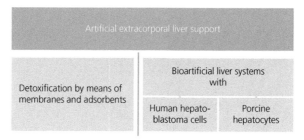

Figure 14.8 Principles of artificial liver support systems.

Ventricular assist devices and cardiac regeneration

Mechanical devices for the temporary support for heart failure have been developed. These devices are mainly designed as a short-term support and are placed either intra- or extra-corporeal. Right ventricular (RVAD), left ventricular (LVAD) or biventricular assist devices (BiVADs) are currently used. An ideal VAD system should cover a wide range of needs including durability, sufficient systemic flow, low risks for thrombosis, bleeding, or hemolysis. More recently, so-called third-generation VADs based on continuous-flow pumps have been developed. Despite recent advancements, almost all devices are composed of nonbiologic materials and therefore predispose to clotting, thus requiring anticoagulation. A more recent device, the HeartMateXVE, addresses this issue by using a biologic surface derived from fibrin, which does not require anticoagulation.

In most cases, VADs are implanted as bridge-to-transplantation devices. In some cases, however, a marked improvement in heart function was observed, even allowing the devices to be removed. This concept, coined "bridge to recovery," is most successful in patients with postsurgical cardiac failure, acute myocarditis, and acute myocardial infarction.

Tissue engineering, organ scaffolds, and stem cells

There is tremendous excitement about the possibility that organs can be rebuilt on engineered extracellular matrices called scaffolds. The extracellular matrix (ECM) guides organ development, cellular repair and regeneration, and is therefore of special interest in the field of tissue engineering. ECM scaffolds with intact 3D anatomical architecture and vasculature have been assembled using a nanofiber and decellularization technique (Figure 14.9).

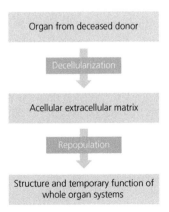

Figure 14.9 Organ scaffolds to build whole organ systems.

Decellularization of human or xenogeneic organs generates an acellular ECM scaffold with intact anatomic structures and vasculature conduits, which can then be used for recellularization. Recently, whole organ scaffolds have been generated from deceased hearts, lungs, livers, pancreata, and kidneys in small as well as in large animal models. Importantly, these scaffolds are free of DNA and nuclei while preserving ECM components such as collagen I, III, laminin, fibronectin, and glycosaminoglycans. Studies have shown that decellularized scaffolds can be repopulated by stem cells or progenitor cells to form structures of whole organ systems, which can restore at least partial organ function (e.g., of liver, kidney) or structure (i.e., bladder, trachea). With an almost inexhaustible number of possible applications for stem cells, the crucial challenge to harness their potential still remains. Recently, functional liver elements generated from induced pluripotent stem cells successfully repopulated organ scaffolds that then showed partially restored liver functions. Regenerative medicine holds great promises for the future, but requires new insights into basic stem cell biology as well as continued immunologic studies, as immune responses to artificial or xenogeneic scaffolds and the human cells they support will no doubt emerge.

Summary

Organ transplantation has evolved over a rather short time period to an evidence-based therapeutic approach, providing enormous benefits for patients with end-stage organ failure. As a result of this success, more patients than ever before are being wait-listed for organ transplantation, which is in turn imposing great challenges to deal with the shortage of donor organs. While exploring alternative sources for organs, optimization of the quality of organs, and better appreciation of variance in immune responses with donor/recipient age as well as new ways of modulating organ repair, programs will be critical for further improvements in transplant outcomes.

Further reading

Aspinall R, Andrew D. Thymic involution in aging. *J Clin Immunol* 2000;20: 250–256.

Bernardo JF, McCauley J. Drug therapy in transplant recipients: special considerations in the elderly with comorbid conditions. *Drugs Aging* 2004;21: 323–348.

Danovitch GM, Gill J, Bunnapradist S. Immunosuppression of the elderly kidney transplant recipient. *Transplantation* 2007;84: 285–291.

de Fijter JW. The impact of age on rejection in kidney transplantation. *Drugs Aging* 2005;22: 433–449.

Gourishankar S, Halloran PF. Late deterioration of organ transplants: a problem in injury and homeostasis. *Curr Opin Immunol* 2002;14: 576–583.

Kim IK, Bedi DS, Denecke C, Ge X, Tullius SG. Impact of innate and adaptive immunity on rejection and tolerance. *Transplantation* 2008;86: 889–894.

Martins PN, Pratschke J, Pascher A et al. Age and immune response in organ transplantation. *Transplantation* 2005;79: 127–132.

Merion RM, Ashby VB, Wolfe RA et al. Deceased-donor characteristics and the survival benefit of kidney transplantation. *JAMA* 2005;294: 2726–2733.

Orlando G, Baptista P, Birchall M et al. Regenerative medicine as applied to solid organ transplantation: current status and future challenges. *Transpl Int* 2011;24: 223–232.

Pierson RN, III, Dorling A, Ayares D et al. Current status of xenotransplantation and prospects for clinical application. *Xenotransplantation* 2009;16: 263–280.

Pomfret EA, Sung RS, Allan J, Kinkhabwala M, Melancon JK, Roberts JP. Solving the organ shortage crisis: the 7th annual American Society of Transplant Surgeons' State-of-the-Art Winter Symposium. *Am J Transplant* 2008;8: 745–752.

Port FK, Bragg-Gresham JL, Metzger RA et al. Donor characteristics associated with reduced graft survival: an approach to expanding the pool of kidney donors. *Transplantation* 2002;74: 1281–1286.

Rao PS, Schaubel DE, Guidinger MK et al. A comprehensive risk quantification score for deceased donor kidneys: the kidney donor risk index. *Transplantation* 2009;88: 231–236.

Soto-Gutierrez A, Yagi H, Uygun BE et al. Cell delivery: from cell transplantation to organ engineering. *Cell Transplant* 2010;19: 655–665.

Stutchfield BM, Simpson K, Wigmore SJ. Systematic review and meta-analysis of survival following extracorporeal liver support. *Br J Surg* 2011;98: 623–631.

The 2009 OPTN/SRTR Annual Report: Transplant Data 1999–2008. Available from: www.srtr.org/annual_Reports/archives/2009/2009_Annual_Report. Accessed July 21, 2014.

Timsit MO, Tullius SG. Hypothermic kidney preservation: a remembrance of the past in the future? *Curr Opin Organ Transplant* 2011;16: 162–168.

Tullius SG, Garcia-Cardena G. Organ procurement and perfusion before transplantation. *N Engl J Med* 2009;360: 78–80.

Tullius SG, Tran H, Guleria I, Malek SK, Tilney NL, Milford E. The combination of donor and recipient age is critical in determining host immunoresponsiveness and renal transplant outcome. *Ann Surg* 2010;252: 662–674.

Yang YG, Sykes M. Xenotransplantation: current status and a perspective on the future. *Nat Rev Immunol* 2007;7: 519–531.

CHAPTER 15

New frontiers and new technologies

Haval Shirwan[1], Yiming Huang[1], Kadiyala Ravindra[1], and Suzanne T. Ildstad[2]

[1] Institute for Cellular Therapeutics, University of Louisville, Louisville, and Duke University, Raleigh, USA

[2] Department of Surgery, Physiology, Immunology, University of Louisville, Louisville and Duke University, Raleigh, USA

CHAPTER OVERVIEW

- Stem cells have great potential in tissue repair/regeneration. This will have significant impact on transplantation in the future.

- Vascularized composite allotransplantation is rapidly moving to the clinical arena, which will require new protocols that can support transplant tolerance.

- Nanotechnology is a rapidly evolving area that will provide new drug delivery systems as well as new diagnostic tools, with great relevance to transplantation.

- The rapid evolution of new generation real-time imaging technology will dramatically advance transplantation research.

- The current strategies, limitations and future directions of gene therapy in organ transplantation will have significant impact on clinical transplantation.

Regenerative medicine: past, present, and future possibilities

Regeneration is defined as a process of renewal, restoration, and/or replacement of a lost part of the body due to injury. The history of regeneration can be traced to the early seventeenth century when Rene-Antoine Ferchault de Reaumur observed that crayfish could regenerate damaged limbs and claws. This triggered a century-old debate as to the application of regeneration to patients. Stem cells are pluripotent and by definition exhibit "self-renewal" capability, giving rise to progenitor and eventually differentiated cells of tissue or organ derivation from all three primary germ layers. Endogenous stem cells and exogenous stem cells can both contribute to tissue repair and regeneration. Remarkably, they can replace specific tissue in organs such as brain, heart, liver, kidney, pancreas,

---

Transplant Immunology, First Edition. Edited by Xian Chang Li and Anthony M. Jevnikar.
© 2016 John Wiley & Sons, Ltd. Published 2016 by John Wiley & Sons, Ltd.
Companion website: www.wiley.com/go/li/transplantimmunology

retina, and skeletal muscle and have the capacity to rebuild complex structures such as limbs (Figure 15.1). The general strategy for tissue engineering is to combine stem cells with a three-dimensional (3D) scaffold, which provides the support and structure for stem cells, which enable the reorganization of cells to form a functional tissue or organ (Figure 15.2). This of course has enormous implications in transplantation in the future, where insufficient organ donation, rejection, recurrence of disease, and premature failure of organs remain the greatest challenges. This section will highlight the recent advancements in stem cell-based therapeutic applications in tissue repair/regeneration in experimental studies and, more recently, in the clinic.

Definition of stem cell concepts

Stem cells: classified by their developmental potential as totipotent, pluripotent, multipotent, oligopotent, and unipotent
Totipotent: able to give rise to all embryonic and extraembryonic cell types
Pluripotent: able to give rise to all cell types of the embryo proper
Multipotent: able to give rise to a subset of cell lineages
Oligopotent: able to give rise to a more restricted subset of cell lineages than multipotent stem cells
Unipotent: able to contribute to only one mature cell type
Ectoderm: able to give rise to skin and neural lineages
Mesoderm: generates blood, bone, muscle, cartilage and fat
Endoderm: contributes to tissue of respiratory and digestive tracts
Dedifferentiation: conversion of a fully differentiated cell to a progenitor-like phenotype before potential redifferentiation to a different cell type
Transdifferentiation: conversion of one mature cell phenotype to another
Reprogramming: induces differentiated cells into reverting to pluripotency

Sources of stem cells

Embryonic stem cells (ESCs) are derived from the inner cell mass of blastocyst-stage embryos. These cells have self-renewal capabilities as well as the ability to differentiate into all adult cell types derived from the three embryonic germ layers: endoderm, mesoderm, and ectoderm. A pluripotent mouse ESC line was first established in 1981 by Evans and Kaufman (1981). ESCs hold great therapeutic promise in the generation of functional cell types relevant for neurons, cardiomyocytes, hematocytes, lung epithelium, pancreatic beta cells, and retinal pigment epithelium. It is of concern that ESCs have been associated with teratoma formation and have also been reported to produce benign or malignant tumors if transplanted in an undifferentiated type. In addition, many political,

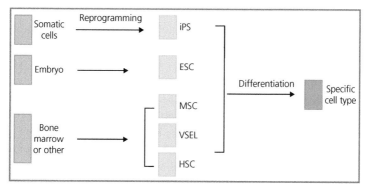

Figure 15.1 The source of stem cells. The figure outlines the origin of different types of stem cells. The mechanisms of stem cells involved in cell or tissue regeneration includes reprogramming, dedifferentiation, and transdifferentiation.

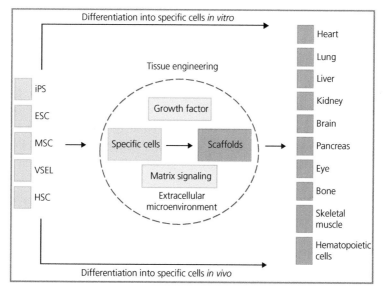

Figure 15.2 Stem cell-based therapy in regenerative medicine. Stem cells can be differentiated into specific cell types *in vitro* or *in vivo*, which offer a potential therapy for cell regeneration and tissue repair. Specific cell types can be seeded onto natural or artificial scaffolds, relying on matrix signaling and growth factor stimulation to support specific organ cells' differentiation and maturation.

ethical, and religious issues have limited the use of human ESCs in clinical applications.

Mesenchymal stem cells (MSCs) were discovered in the bone marrow by Friedenstein et al. (1968). Other sources of MSCs have been reported including adipose tissue, muscles, placenta, cord blood, and liver. *Ex vivo* expanded MSC express CD105, CD90 and CD73and lack CD45, CD34, CD14, and major histocompatibility complex (MHC) class II expression. MSC have the ability to self-renew as well as differentiate into mesoderm-type cells and nonmesoderm cells. In addition, MSCs appear to provide a powerful immunomodulatory effect *in vitro* and *in vivo* by inhibiting T cell activation, dendritic cell differentiation, B cell proliferation, and natural killer cytolytic function.

Induced pluripotent stem cells (iPS) derived from adult tissue were first described by Takahashi and Yamanaka (2006). The technology offers an approach to resolve the current limitations of ESC pools and provide specific stem cells derived from specific patient tissue. iPS cells have been generated from patients with a variety of genetic diseases. iPS are pluripotent ESC-like cells reprogrammed *in vitro* from terminally differentiated somatic cells by retroviral transduction of four transcription factors: Oct3/4, Sox2, K1f4, and c-Myc. iPS can be cultured *in vitro* and differentiated into cardiomyocytes, hematopoietic cells, hepatocyte-like cells, retinal cells, neurons, adipocytes, and osteoblasts. iPS may also provide an option that is less constrained by ethical, political, and practical considerations. However, these cells have similar developmental potential as ESCs with respect to morphology, proliferation, and the limitation of teratoma formation.

Bone marrow-derived very small embryonic-like stem cells (VSELs) are a rare homogenous small cell population in the bone marrow that exhibit morphologic characteristics similar to that of ESC and express several markers also expressed by ESC. VSEL cells are capable of differentiating into cells from all three germ layers *in vitro*. The phenotypic markers of VSEL cells are CD45$^-$/Sca-1$^+$/CXCR4$^+$/lineage$^-$. They also express early embryonic transcription factors. VSEL cells are a mobile pool of stem cells that are mobilized into peripheral blood following acute myocardial infarction (AMI) in mouse and human; stroke in mouse and human; liver injury, skeletal muscle injury, streptozotocin-(STZ) induced diabetes, and NaIO$_3$ damaged retinal pigment epithelium. However, the potential involvement of VSEL cells in tumor formation needs further evaluation.

Hematopoietic stem cells (HSCs) were best characterized as multipotent stem cells derived from mouse bone marrow in 1988 by Spangrude et al. (1988). HSCs can self-renew and give rise to all blood cell types including blood myeloid and lymphoid lineages. The phenotype markers of HSC are Sca-1$^+$, c-Kit$^+$, Thy-1.1^{lo} and lineage$^-$ (B220, CD3, CD4, CD8, Mac-1, Gr-1, Ter 119) in mice, or CD34$^+$, Thy-1$^+$, and lineage$^-$ (CD10, CD14, CD15, CD16, CD19, CD20) in humans. Recently, a series of studies suggested that bone marrow cells enriched by various methods to induce increased hematopoietic stem cell activity can contribute to the development of multiple nonhematopoietic tissues including myocardium, lung epithelium, kidney epithelium, liver parenchyma, pancreas, skeletal muscle, and CNS neurons.

Experimental studies and clinical applications

Translation of stem cell therapies to the clinic has occurred in growing abundance in recent years, beginning with neurologic applications.

Brain

Stem cells have great potential in the treatment of stroke, Parkinson's disease, and spinal cord injury. Many different types of stem cells, including ESC, various types of neural stem cells (NSCs), MSC, VSEL, and HSC, the olfactory ensheathing cells, and olfactory nerve fibroblasts have been investigated to determine if they can repair and rescue cells from injury. Early studies showed that undifferentiated ESC, NSC, MSC, and VSEL could proliferate and differentiate into different neurons and glial cell types, which helped the recovery of brain function in a rat stroke model. Additional animal studies have shown that undifferentiated ESC differentiated into dopaminergic neurons and improved functional recovery in unilateral rotation in a rat model for Parkinson's disease. iPS cells can differentiate into neural precursor cells and give rise to neuronal and glial cell types *in vitro* and *in vivo*. iPS-derived neural precursor cells were shown to engraft and integrate in the striatum of rat and were able to improve behavior in a rat model of Parkinson's disease after local injection. Clinical trials of human neuron cells, fetal porcine neural progenitors, and bone marrow-derived MSC have been performed in patients with stroke. Recently, human ESC-derived oligodendrocyte precursor cells and adult neural stem cells derived from fetal tissue were used in a phase 1 clinical trial for the treatment of ischemic stroke and spinal cord injury (Mack, 2011).

Heart

Regeneration of cardiomyocytes and establishment of new blood vessels from stem cells to repair damaged hearts have attracted considerable attention now. Currently, most clinical trials are focused on stem cell-based regenerative therapy for the treatment of acute AMI and congestive heart failure. Several studies have shown that mouse and human iPS can differentiate into cardiomyocytes as well as ESC. Transplantation of cardiomyocytes or cardiac progenitor cells derived from ESC or iPS into infracted rodent hearts has been reported to improve cardiac function. Several clinical trials have shown that bone marrow-derived cells improve myocardial perfusion and contractile performance in AMI, heart failure, and chronic myocardial ischemia. Recent research has reported that a novel method can generate a whole heart scaffold with intact 3D geometry and vasculature (Ott et al., 2008). Rat hearts were decellularized and the decellularized heart scaffold was then repopulated with neonatal cardiac cells or rat aortic endothelial cells, and then cultured under simulated physiologic conditions for organ maturation. Currently, the constructs are able to generate pumping function equivalent to only 2% of adult heart function.

Lung

Stem/progenitor cells can be used to repair lung injury. Bone marrow-derived cells including MSC, HSC, endothelial progenitor cells, circulating fibrocytes, and other cell types have been demonstrated to contribute to the regeneration of mature differentiated airway structures, alveolar epithelial cells, and vascular, endothelial and interstitial lung cells. The ability of MSC in tissue repair and modulating innate and adaptive immunity has promoted interest in MSC as a potential cell-based therapy for diverse lung diseases. Furthermore, the successful *clinical* implantation of tissue-engineered airways used acellular matrix scaffold in 2008 (Macchiarini et al., 2008). A tracheal segment was retrieved from a deceased human donor, the cells were removed, and the scaffold was repopulated by the recipient's own epithelial cells and MSC-derived chondrocytes. The graft was then used to replace the recipient's left main bronchus. The graft resulted in improved function of the airway and quality of life 4 months after transplantation. In another study, decellularized rat lungs repopulated with epithelial and endothelial cells regenerated gas exchange tissue *in vitro* and provided gas exchange *in vivo* for up to 6 h after extubation in a rat model (Ott et al., 2010).

Kidney

The interest in stem cell-based therapy for renal repair has increased in recent years. Evidence suggests that endogenous stem cells such as renal progenitor cells, label-retaining cells, and exogenous stem cells such as HSC, MSC, and ESC may contribute to the replacement of damaged cells. However, the mechanism of action of these stem cells remains unclear. Transplantation of HSC and MSC has been shown to reduce renal injury in an animal model of ischemia reperfusion. Bone marrow-derived cells have been shown to differentiate into mesangial cells, podocytes, and the endothelial cells of glomerular capillaries. Several studies indicated that MSC, which possess potential anti-inflammatory effects, modulate ischemia or reperfusion and lead to an earlier regeneration of damaged renal tissue.

Decellularized rat kidney was recently seeded with murine pluripotent ESC through the renal artery and ureter, and incubated in growth media without prodifferentiation agents. Immunohistochemical results demonstrated that ESC proliferated and differentiated into mature renal cells in this decellularized rat kidney (Uygun et al., 2010).

Liver

Hepatocyte transplantation offers an alternative to orthotopic liver transplants for the treatment of liver failure and/or end-stage liver diseases. A major limitation of cell-based therapies for liver diseases, however, is the production of primary human hepatocytes. Research has focused on how to induce the generation of hepatocyte-like cells from different types of extra hepatic stem or precursor cells from animal and human sources. Several studies have reported that ESC, MSC, bone marrow-derived cells, and liver stem/progenitor cells can be prompted to differentiate into hepatocytes both *in vitro* and *in vivo*.

A recent study demonstrated a novel approach to generate transplantable liver grafts using a decellularized liver matrix in a rat model (Uygun et al., 2010). The recellularized rat liver matrix using rat primary hepatocytes showed liver-specific function, including albumin secretion, urea synthesis and cytochrome

P450 expression at comparable levels to normal liver *in vitro*. The recellularized liver grafts, which can be implanted into rats, support hepatocyte survival and also function with minimal ischemic damage.

Pancreatic beta cell regeneration

Type 1 diabetes mellitus is characterized by the autoimmune destruction of pancreatic beta cells. Strategies to generate pancreatic beta cells from stem/progenitor cells have focused on ESC, iPS, bone marrow-derived cells (MSC and VSEL), organ-specific stem or progenitor cells, pancreatic duct epithelial cells, acinar cells, and liver cells. Transplantation of MSC or VSEL increased levels of serum insulin and reduced blood glucose levels in hyperglycemia in STZ-induced diabetic mice. Human ESC have been shown to secrete insulin in response to glucose after transplantation into STZ-treated immunodeficient mice. Human ESC-like iPS derived from skin cells by retroviral expression of OCT4, SOX2, c-MYC and KLF4 have the potential to differentiate into insulin-producing islet-like clusters. The efficiency of differentiation to functional beta cells from ESC/iPS was low. An approach to promote the formation of functional beta cells may result in alternative regeneration-based approaches to treat diabetes.

Hematopoietic system

Transplantation of HSC for reconstitution of hematopoietic cells and treatment of neoplastic disease has become a clinical reality over the past 40 years. In 1968, the first successful case reports involved hematopoietic cell transplantation for the treatment of severe combined immunodeficiency disease and Wiskott-Aldrich syndrome. More evidence has shown that transplantation of bone marrow cells or HSC can lead to prolonged survival and cure of leukemia, severe combined immunodeficiency, and severe aplastic anemia (Copelan, 2006). Currently, bone marrow cells or HSC transplantation requires the use of nonspecific immunosuppressive agents and irradiation to prevent graft rejection and graft-versus-host disease. Toxicities associated with treatment are substantial and include opportunistic infections and an increased rate of malignancy. Studies have focused on safe procedures for the induction of donor-specific transplantation tolerance. Patient-specific iPS cell-derived HSCs have recently been evaluated in a humanized mouse model of sickle cell anemia where it was shown that autologous genetically corrected iPS-derived hematopoietic progenitor cells phenotypically and functionally corrected the sickle cell defect.

Future challenges

Translation of stem cell-based technology into clinical applications still faces the following formidable challenges: (i) the risk of tumor formation, (ii) gene correction of iPS from patients with genetic disease, and (iii) successful differentiation of iPS cells into target cell types. The cellular source for specific tissue regeneration, for achieving efficient homing to an injured area and maintaining durable engraftment of functional cells to promote the formation of tissues remain unsolved. Fully understanding the biologic mechanism of regeneration, including dedifferentiation, transdifferentiation, and reprogramming, will improve stem cell research outcomes, resulting in the achievement of the full potential of tissue regeneration *in vivo*.

Recently, research has focused on the exploration of 3D nanotechnology culture systems and bioengineering approaches to generate functional tissue. Researchers are currently developing engineered scaffolds that mimic the dimensional scale of the extracellular matrix (ECM), for effective organization of cells and for creating tissue with morphologic and physiologic features similar to natural tissue development *in vivo*. Successful engineering of heart, lung, liver, kidney, skin, and bone has been reported in animals and humans. Several issues associated with tissue engineering, such as the specific extracellular microenvironment, how much maturation *in vitro* is required prior to implantation, and the biocompatibility and biodegradation of engineered scaffolds, still need to be addressed before they can be safely applied in the clinic (Dvir et al., 2011).

Vascularized composite allotransplantation

"Composite tissue allotransplantation" (CTA) has been renamed "vascularized composite allotransplantation" (VCA) to emphasize the distinction from nonvascularized composite tissue transplantation. Despite the first hand transplant that was performed over 15 years ago, progress in the field has been slow. The absence of long-term data on VCA recipients and the need for life-long immunosuppression have slowed clinical application. Only about 100 VCA grafts have been recorded thus far (Brandacher et al., 2010). These include hand/upper extremity, partial face, abdominal wall, larynx/trachea, uterus, penis, knee joints and so on. (Table 15.1). Conventional reconstructive surgery has limitations in subjects with severe defects (such as amputees) and severe facial deformities. The only way to restore form and function in such situations is to "replace like with like."

The lack of widespread application of the VCA procedures is evident from Table 15.2. This analysis, based on the data from the International Registry of Hand and Composite Tissue Transplantation, of the different procedures over the past 13 years underscores the fact that much work still needs to be done before the field gains momentum. Current strategies to prevent rejection of VCA grafts include conventional triple-drug immunosuppression along with antibody induction. The overall degree of immunosuppression is similar to that in pancreas transplantation.

Table 15.1 List of VCA procedures that have been compiled.

Hand/upper extremity	49 in 33 recipients
Face	9
Abdominal wall	15 in 14 patients
Larynx/trachea	14 in 14 patients
Knee	8 recipients
Penis	1
Uterus	1
Tongue	1

Table 15.2 Number of VCA procedures by type and publication over the past 13 years.

Year	1998/1999	2000/2001	2002/2003	2004/2005	2006/2007	2008/2009	2010
Hand transplant	1/3	10/3	5/2	0/1	4/2	4/3	10
Face transplant	—	—	—	—/1	1/1	1/3	4
Other CTA*	—/11	0/0	10/0	0/1	15/0	0/0	2
Publications	7/16	18/12	9/18	24/21	14/28	24/43	20/41

Based on International Registry on Hand and Composite Tissue Transplantation.
* The numbers reflect the year of reporting of single-center series.

Unique challenges

VCA will be subject to higher scrutiny as it is not lifesaving. There is continuing debate on the risk: benefit balance when performing these procedures. There is an urgent need for scientific studies to determine the advantages that VCA provides in terms of quality of life and function.

Visual inspection of VCA grafts enables continuous immunologic monitoring. This may account for the higher rates of acute rejection reported with face and hand allografts. Nearly 85% of hand and nearly all face transplant recipients were reported to have experienced at least one episode of acute rejection in the first year after transplantation. This is higher than that seen in solid organ transplants. Surprisingly, the higher acute rejection in VCA does not seem to adversely impact long-term results.

Solid organ transplants undergo chronic damage of the graft due to many factors including drug toxicity and chronic rejection. The entity of chronic rejection is poorly defined in VCA. There is continuous debate about whether VCA is "privileged" and immune to chronic injury. Experimental data, however, suggest that vasculopathy may develop following multiple episodes of acute cellular rejection. The hand allografts that were lost following cessation or noncompliance with immunosuppression showed features suggestive of chronic rejection. Chronic rejection of VCA grafts is not defined in the current Banff classification schema (Cendales et al., 2008).

Complications

As of 2011, three hand grafts were lost (excluding combination with face) in the western world: one lost due to noncompliance at 29 months, one lost in the immediate post-operative period and another from vascular rejection at 9 months (Kanitakis et al., 2003). More have been lost since then. However, there have been no mortalities among the hand allograft recipients. In contrast, face transplants have been complicated by serious complications resulting in a high mortality rate of 20%. Immunosuppression-related complications in VCA are similar to those seen in solid organs transplantation. Infections, metabolic complications, renal impairment, and neoplasia have been reported in hand transplant recipients. Cytomegalovirus infections have posed serious problems in some of the hand and face transplant recipients.

Current research

The challenges faced in the field of solid organ transplantation are under sharper focus in VCA due to the perception that its primary role is improvement in quality of life. Because of the unique accessibility of the graft, VCA is ideal to test innovative immunosuppression therapies. Many questions in VCA remain unanswered, including those pertaining to (i) optimal preservation methods and limits of cold and warm ischemia, (ii) the role of the bone marrow component of VCA grafts in immune modulation, (iii) the role of topical immunosuppression, (iv) the occurrence of chronic rejection, and (v) the induction of donor specific tolerance. In conclusion, VCA is still evolving and future research will enhance and improve graft outcomes.

Nanotechnology

The goal of tissue engineering is to develop functional substitutes that will replace damaged tissues and organs. Engineering functional tissue requires the organization of cells containing morphologic and physiologic features into tissue. One major challenge has been to identify supporting structures to direct stem cell-mediated regeneration to differentiate into functional structures such as organs. Recently, nanotechnology-based strategies for tissue engineering have proven beneficial (Figure 15.3). To put things in perspective, the terminology surrounding nanotechnology must be defined. *Nanoparticles* are typically 50–500 nm per particle in diameter (i.e., smaller than DNA). *Nanostructures* are of similar diameter and size. A typical cell is 25 μm or 25,000 nm.

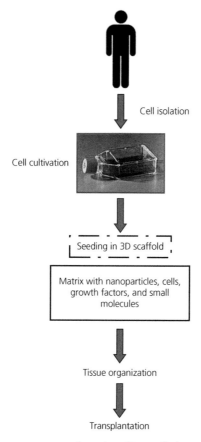

Cell isolation

Cell cultivation

Seeding in 3D scaffold

Matrix with nanoparticles, cells, growth factors, and small molecules

Tissue organization

Transplantation

Figure 15.3 Specific tissue or organ engineering. Stem cells from various sources are isolated and cultivated in growth factor-enriched medium. After expansion/activation, they are seeded on a 3D scaffolding impregnated with nanoparticles, growth factors, and small molecules to allow tissue and organ organization. The long-term goal is to generate an organ replacement structure for implantation.

Conceptually, the ECM is a dynamic and hierarchically organized nanocomposite that regulates critical cellular functions, including differentiation and cell proliferation. The signaling involved in this 3D structure is not yet fully understood. It is believed that the ECM plays an essential role in guiding morphogenesis. Indeed, the loss of ECM signaling to cells can result in deprivation-induced cell death termed anoikis.

Understanding the role of the porous nanoscale topography of the ECM has prompted tissue engineers to take advantage of nanotechnology over previously used, much larger macroporous scaffolds. *Electrospinning* and *molecular self-assembly* are common nanofabrication approaches used to prepare 3D scaffolds composed of interwoven fibers. Electrospinning uses an electric field to deposit polymer fibers on a target substrate. The scaffold can be simultaneously impregnated with growth factors, peptides, enzymes, drugs, PNA, and RNA to promote tissue regeneration by stem cells. One limitation is that this approach only promotes the assembly of thin tissues, which do not allow infiltration of the cells to the core of the matrix. To address this limitation, electrospinning has been combined with 3D microprinting to prepare a macroporous structure with interconnected pores that more closely resemble the ECM. However, these technologies seldom reach a range lower than 500 μm.

To better replicate the ECM, *molecular self-assembly* has been used to prepare much smaller pore sizes. With this approach, the 3D scaffolds have a fiber diameter as low as 10 nm and pore sizes between 5 and 200 nm. This structure has been shown to promote the rapid differentiation of cells into neurons. Further research is needed to optimize success in this area.

Nanotechnologies have had a significant impact on tissue engineering and initiatives in regenerative medicine, providing the first biomimetic chimerism to developing tissue. It has moved the file one major step closer to clinical transplantation.

Imaging of allografts: nanotechnology and beyond

Until recently, the diagnosis of rejection was made with biopsy procedures, which are invasive and error-prone. At the early stages of rejection, the infiltrates are patchy and inconsistent, and sampling error is a major limitation due to the small sample size that can safely be taken from most vascularized organ grafts. Over the past two decades, a number of imaging modalities have been developed to allow noninvasive detection of rejection at the cellular level, including echocardiography, positron emission tomography, computed tomography, optical and magnetic resonance imaging (MRI). These modalities can also serve as powerful research tools to follow the fate of individual cells *in vivo*.

Cellular and functional MRI (CMRI) can detect and profile the temporal and spatial relationship of cells involved in graft infiltration, serving as a surrogate marker for rejection. Cells of interest (macrophages, dendritic cells, B cells) must be labeled with MRI contrast agents such as iron oxide (Fe_nO_m). Some of the most successful agents are *iron oxidenanoparticles* (Fe_2O_3 and Fe_2O_4) coated with dextran or other polysaccharide derivatives. *Superparamagnetic iron oxide (SPIO)* and *ultra-small SPIO (USPIO)* nanoparticles consist of iron core sizes of 4–5 nm and 5–8 nm, respectively. Labeling can be performed *in vitro* or *in vivo*. In the *in vivo* approach, the agents are injected and the cells naturally ingest the labeling agents by phagocytosis. One day after *in vivo* injection of USPIO in a rejecting heart, MRI can detect macrophages in the graft. The USPIO and SPIO particles are biodegradable.

Micrometer-sized particles make imaging of individual cells possible. They last longer and can be followed longitudinally. They have been effective in imaging the development of chronic rejection in rat cardiac transplants. Macrophages appear very early in chronic rejection and increase as it progresses. Many iron oxide particles are also designed to contain fluorescent tags, allowing for both MR and optical imaging. Cells that are not phagocytic, including T cells, B cells, and stem cells must be labeled *in vitro* for successful imaging *in vivo* and then injected. Polyethylene glycol-coated nanosized iron particles called ITRI-IOP that label T cells with 92–99% efficiency have been developed (Wu et al., 2010).

A two-pronged approach for assessing cellular infiltration of macrophages combined with regional functional MRI has shown even greater precision in noninvasive imaging of rejection. Tagging MRI with high-resolution strain analysis of regional wall motion can be performed. It is labor intensive, but clinically relevant correlations have been generated. Simultaneously coupling cellular infiltrates in rejection with functional abnormalities associated with rejection results in more accuracy and sensitivity (Wu et al., 2010). These novel technologies are approaching clinically feasible methods to eliminate the need for invasive biopsy monitoring of transplants grafts.

Gene therapy in transplantation

Gene therapy involves the introduction of foreign genetic material into the cell to replace, modify, or remove a defective gene or genes for the treatment of the disease. Although this technique was initially developed for the correction of genetic abnormalities caused by a single gene, such as cystic fibrosis, muscular dystrophy, and hemophilia, it has since been recognized that gene therapy can be applied in the treatment of cancer, autoimmunity, and infections as well as to disorders acquired during transplantation (Verma & Weitzman, 2005). Importantly, advances in recombinant nucleic acid technology, mapping of the human genome and a comprehensive understanding of the mechanistic basis of gene regulation have led the way in using not only DNA, but also RNA (i.e., short interfering or micro RNA), for gene regulation as a means of correcting a gene defect for the treatment of a disease. This section will only focus on the applications of DNA-based gene therapy to transplantation tolerance.

Gene delivery approaches

Gene therapy involves cloning into a DNA vector, a gene cassette that includes the gene of interest and flanking promoter and regulatory sequences required for expression (transgene), which is then introduced into target cells or tissues for expression and correction of the defect. Both germ line cells and somatic cells are potential targets for gene therapy. However, ethical constraints limit the application of gene therapy only to somatic cells for humans. Genes can be delivered into cells either *ex vivo* or *in vivo*. In the *ex vivo* approach, the gene is delivered into cells, tissues or organs of interest outside the body followed by their transplantation into a recipient for treatment purposes. The *in vivo* approach involves the direct delivery of a gene of interest into a target cell/tissue of interest in the patient.

Currently, the *ex vivo* delivery approach is the method of choice for cell-based therapies. The advantages to this approach include the following: (i) high gene transfer efficacy, (ii) the modified cells can be enriched if a selection marker is available, and (iii) transduction efficacy can be assessed before transplantation of the cells into the patient. However, genetic manipulation of the cells requires strict GMP conditions and the efficacy of transferring the gene into the cells depends upon the nature of the target cells since harvesting primary cells from various target tissues and maintaining them in culture for gene transfer may pose challenges. In this context, genetic manipulation of hematopoietic stem cells in bone marrow is highly practical and efficient because these cells can be easily obtained from patients and efficiently modified with a gene of interest using various vectors.

In vivo gene therapy, although practical, suffers from several challenges. First, the precise delivery selectively to some target cells but not others (particularly germ line cells), is challenging. However, this limitation can be overcome if the target cell-specific elements (enhancer/promoter) that regulate expression are available (transcriptional targeting). Alternatively, genes of interest can be delivered to specific cells via cell-specific receptor endocytosis or by taking advantage of tropism of viruses used as vectors for the targeted cells if such tropism exists. Second, the efficiency of gene transfer is rather low and in most cases the expression of the transferred gene is rather short lived, which necessitates multiple treatments. Continuous treatments may cause the generation of antivector immune responses, which may further limit the efficacy of gene therapy.

There are various means of delivering the gene of interest into target cells, tissues, and organs, but they can be generally divided into two basic categories: *viral and nonviral delivery methods.*

Viral vectors

Viruses serve as a convenient and efficient means of delivering foreign genetic material into cells of interest due to their exquisite ability to infect target cells and replicate within the cell to generate copious amounts of progeny. As a result, the foreign transgene integrated into the viral vector is also being produced in high copy number, which is often required for the treatment of intended diseases (Figure 15.4). Both RNA and DNA viruses have been used as vectors for gene therapy. The most common RNA viruses include retroviruses, whereas adeno and adeno-associated viruses represent the most popular DNA viruses used for gene therapy. Although the choice of viral vector is determined by the indented purpose of gene therapy, retroviruses require actively dividing cells and integration into the host genome for replication.

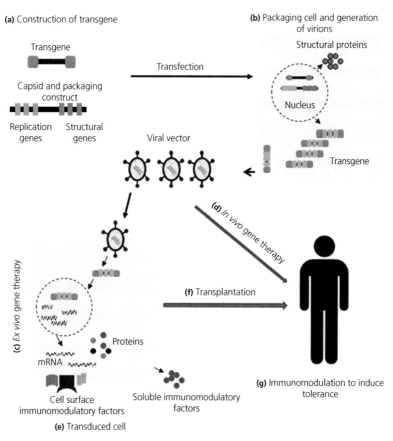

(a) Construction of transgene

Transgene

Capsid and packaging construct

Replication genes Structural genes

Transfection

(b) Packaging cell and generation of virions

Structural proteins

Nucleus

Viral vector

Transgene

(d) *In vivo gene therapy*

(c) *Ex vivo gene therapy*

Proteins

mRNA

Cell surface immunomodulatory factors

(e) Transduced cell

Soluble immunomodulatory factors

(f) Transplantation

(g) Immunomodulation to induce tolerance

Figure 15.4 Schematic diagram of *ex vivo* and *in vivo* gene therapy. The transgene of interest is cloned into an expression cassette and transfected along with a packing construct that contains both viral structural and replication genes into a packing cell line (a). Production of virions containing the transgene in packing cell line (b) is followed by their transduction into cells *ex vivo* (c) or direct administration into human (d). Transduced cells (e) are characterized for the expression of transgene and then transplanted into human for immunomodulation (f). The transgene product expressed by *ex vivo* manipulated cells or human tissues are expected to modulate the immune system for intended purposes (g).

Although integration into the host genome provides the advantage of long-term expression of the transgene, it carries the inherent risk of disrupting an essential host gene or altering the regulation of such a gene with associated undesired consequences, such as oncogenesis (Hacein-Bey-Abina et al., 2003). Viral vectors that infect nondividing cells and are stably maintained in the infected cells as extrachromosomal DNA for sustained gene expression, are preferable. The ultimate choice of the viral vector is determined by the efficacy of transducing dividing versus nondividing cells, level and duration of gene expression, need for repeated treatments, and importantly risk/benefit considerations.

Nonviral vectors

Nonviral transgene delivery presents a more practical and potentially safer alternative to viral vectors. This is primarily due to their ease of production and lack of integration into the host genome, thereby obviating the risk of insertional mutagenesis, which is a significant concern for viral vectors. Importantly, nonviral vectors lack immunogenicity and as such can be used for repeated treatments. Inasmuch as nonviral vectors do not integrate into the host genome and lack replication potential, the copy number of the transgene decreases as a function of target cell division, resulting in the lack of sustained and long-lasting expression and reduced therapeutic efficacy.

Application of gene therapy to transplantation

Gene therapy was initially developed as a treatment approach for inherited diseases caused either by the absence of certain genes or by the presence of defective genes in an autologous setting. As the gene therapy concept evolved along with our understanding of various biologic systems, its wide-spread application to the treatment of various acquired diseases was realized. This section will focus on the application of gene therapy to transplantation with particular focus on the direct manipulation of the transplant or graft recipient to promote long-term graft survival and induction of transplantation tolerance.

Cellular transplantation

Cellular transplantation serves as the most effective target for gene therapy for the induction of tolerance. Among various cellular transplants, HSC transplantation has the most potential for tolerance induction. HSC give rise to a functional immune system by differentiating into various blood and immune cells. As such, there has been a great interest to use allogeneic HSC as a means to rebuild or retune the immune system for the purpose of inducing transplantation tolerance. However, allogeneic HSC are perceived as foreign in recipients with a competent immune system, and are rejected. Therefore, the prospective graft recipients must undergo various conditioning regimens to prevent rejection and achieve engraftment. Toxicity associated with such conditioning regimens and inefficient engraftment, are some of the complications of unmanipulated allogeneic HSC transplantation. Gene therapy has the potential to overcome the complication of allogeneic HSC transplantation through the expression of various immunologic molecules that have the potential to enhance engraftment and overcome rejection.

MHC molecules serve as the most potent antigens for the rejection of allografts. Therefore, tolerance to a given allogeneic MHC molecule has the potential to overcome rejection of foreign cells, tissues, and organs matched for the same MHC molecule. Several studies tested the feasibility of using gene therapy to express allogeneic MHC molecules in syngeneic HSC and test the capacity of such genetically manipulated cells to induce tolerance to donor transplants.

Positive results from various systems have demonstrated the feasibility of this approach in rodents as well as in large animals. For example, transduction of bone marrow cells with the allogeneic H-2K^b class I MHC molecule using a retroviral vector allowed persistent expression of the transgene, and such genetically modified cells induced tolerance to donor skin grafts when used for reconstitution of conditioned syngeneic mice. Similarly, bone marrow cells transduced with allogeneic MHC class II genes were effective in inducing tolerance to transgene-matched donor kidney allografts under a transient cover of immunosuppression in miniature swine (Sonntag et al., 2001).

In addition to HSC, various other cell types such as hepatocytes, dendritic cells, mesenchymal stem cells, and endothelial cells, have been used for gene therapy-mediated transplantation tolerance. The application of genetically modified allogeneic cells expressing immunomodulatory molecules for the purpose of inducing transplantation tolerance remains to be realized in the clinic.

Solid organs

Immune responses to solid organs are more complex and have distinct characteristics than those to cellular transplants. Nonimmunologic responses precipitated by early damage to the donor organ as a result of brain death, procurement, organ preservation, surgical procedure, and reperfusion injury initiate vigorous innate immune responses that not only directly inflict damage to the graft, but also initiate and coordinate adaptive T and B cell responses that precipitate graft rejection. Adaptive immunity is controlled by using chronic immunosuppression, which has various long-term complications. Gene therapy has the potential to address various complications of solid organ transplantation by allowing the production of immunomodulatory proteins that not only have a protective effect on nonimmunologic responses, but also have the potential to induce transplantation tolerance and obviate the need for chronic immunosuppression.

Various genes encoding soluble or cell membrane immunomodulatory proteins have been used for gene therapy for solid organ transplantation in experimental settings depending on the problem and the intended treatment goal. For example, ischemic reperfusion injury has been the target of gene therapy using heme oxygenase-1. This approach prevents the graft from ischemic reperfusion injury by performing various overlapping functions, that is, reduction in free radical formation, maintenance of microcirculation, and modulation of antiinflammatory responses. Antiapoptotic genes, such as Bcl-2, BclxL, and A20, were also tested in this context to prevent ischemic reperfusion injury. Importantly, expression of these antiapoptotic genes in endothelial cells were shown not only to prevent their apoptosis in response to hypoxia and other environmental conditions, but also inhibit their activation via NF-κB, which regulates secretion of proinflammatory cytokines that perpetuate mechanisms of graft rejection (Laurence et al., 2009).

Immunomodulatory cytokines, such as IL-2, IL-4, IL-10, TGF-β, and various combinations of these cytokines were used for gene therapy to generate graft-protective responses or induction of transplantation tolerance. Genetically engineered soluble costimulatory ligands, such as CTLA4Ig, CD40Ig, and PDL1-Ig, were used to block costimulation for the induction of tolerance. Similarly, solid organs were genetically modified to express soluble donor MHC molecules to block alloantigen recognition or indoleamine 2,3 dioxygenase, an enzyme involved in T cell suppression via tryptophan catabolism (Laurence et al., 2009), to induce tolerance. Direct display of apoptosis-inducing molecules, such as FasL, on solid organs as a means of specifically eliminating alloreactive lymphocytes expressing the Fas receptor following antigen activation for the prevention of graft rejection has been tested with proof-of-feasibility data in preclinical models (Yolcu et al., 2008). However, the expression of FasL in pancreatic islets resulted in inflammation and islet necrosis, likely an unintended consequence of FasL activation of neutrophils. As well, not all cell types have an endogenous capacity to resist injury from the molecules expressed, so considerable mechanistic insight is required in selecting molecules and the cell they are delivered to.

In summary, gene therapy has great potential for the induction of transplantation tolerance. However, the realization of this potential will depend upon further improvements in delivery vehicles, sustained expression of transgenes in the target cells/tissues/organs, and the choice of transgenes with respect to their immunomodulatory capacity. Methods of gene therapy, *ex vivo* versus *in vivo*, and targets of gene therapy, cells versus tissues versus solid organs, also deserve significant consideration. Hematopoietic stem cells expressing a gene of interest present a more practical and effective approach for the induction of robust and durable tolerance by inducing not only central, but also peripheral tolerance mechanisms. Finally, the benefits of gene therapy need to be weighed against the potential risk of tumorigenesis and infections.

Taken together, tissue regeneration, nanotechnologies, gene therapy, and VCA all represent some portion of the future of transplantation. All are interrelated by the ability to provide alternative sources of tissues and organs to meet the increasing demands in the field of transplantation.

References

Brandacher G, Gorantla VS, Lee WP. Hand allotransplantation. Semin Plast Surg 2010;24: 11–17.

Cendales LC, Kanitakis J, Schneeberger S et al. The Banff 2007 working classification of skin-containing composite tissue allograft pathology. Am J Transplant 2008;8: 1396–1400.

Copelan EA. Hematopoietic stem-cell transplantation. N Engl J Med 2006;354: 1813–1826.

Dvir T, Timko BP, Kohane DS, Langer R. Nanotechnological strategies for engineering complex tissues. Nat Nanotechnol 2011;6: 13–22.

Evans MJ, Kaufman MH. Establishment in culture of pluripotential cells from mouse embryos. Nature 1981;292: 154–156.

Friedenstein AJ, Petrakova KV, Kurolesova AI, Frolova GP. Heterotopic of bone marrow. Analysis of precursor cells for osteogenic and hematopoietic tissues. Transplantation 1968;6: 230–247.

Hacein-Bey-Abina S, Von KC, Schmidt M et al. LMO2-associated clonal T cell proliferation in two patients after gene therapy for SCID-X1. Science 2003;302: 415–419.

Kanitakis J, Jullien D, Petruzzo P et al. Clinicopathologic features of graft rejection of the first human hand allograft. Transplantation 2003;76: 688–693.

Laurence JM, Allen RD, McCaughan GW et al. Gene therapy in transplantation. Transplant Rev (Orlando) 2009;23: 159–170.

Macchiarini P, Jungebluth P, Go T et al. Clinical transplantation of a tissue-engineered airway. Lancet 2008;372: 2023–2030.

Mack GS. ReNeuron and StemCells get green light for neural stem cell trials. Nat Biotechnol 2011;29: 95–97.

Ott HC, Matthiesen TS, Goh SK et al. Perfusion-decellularized matrix: using nature's platform to engineer a bioartificial heart. Nat Med 2008;14: 213–221.

Ott HC, Clippinger B, Conrad C et al. Regeneration and orthotopic transplantation of a bioartificial lung. Nat Med 2010;16: 927–933.

Petruzzo P, Dubernard JM. The International Registry on Hand and Composite Tissue allotransplantation. Clin Transpl 2011: 247–253.

Sonntag KC, Emery DW, Yasumoto A et al. Tolerance to solid organ transplants through transfer of MHC class II genes. J Clin Invest 2001;107: 65–71.

Spangrude GJ, Heimfeld S, Weissman IL. Purification and characterization of mouse hematopoietic stem cells. Science 1988;241: 58–62.

Takahashi K, Yamanaka S. Induction of pluripotent stem cells from mouse embryonic and adult fibroblast cultures by defined factors. Cell 2006;126: 663–676.

Uygun BE, Soto-Gutierrez A, Yagi H et al. Organ reengineering through development of a transplantable recellularized liver graft using decellularized liver matrix. Nat Med 2010;16: 814–820.

Verma IM, Weitzman MD. Gene therapy: twenty-first century medicine. Annu Rev Biochem 2005;74: 711–738.

Wu YL, Ye Q, Ho C. Cellular and functional imaging of cardiac transplant rejection. Curr Cardiovasc Imaging Rep 2010;4: 50–62.

Yolcu ES, Gu X, Lacelle C et al. Induction of tolerance to cardiac allografts using donor splenocytes engineered to display on their surface an exogenous fas ligand protein. J Immunol 2008;181: 931–939.

CHAPTER 16

Experimental models in discovery and translational studies

Andrew B. Adams, William H. Kitchens, and Kenneth A. Newell

Department of Surgery, Emory Transplant Center, Emory University School of Medicine, Atlanta, USA

CHAPTER OVERVIEW

- Animal models play a key role in advancing the field of transplantation.
- Small animal models provide superior insight into immunologic mechanisms, but results are often strain specific.
- Large animal models are critical for clinical translation and xenotransplantation studies.
- Experimental animal models do not perfectly predict outcomes in patients.
- Future experimental models will address outstanding needs in transplantation and better simulate the human response to transplants.

Introduction

Perhaps all aspects of modern clinical transplantation were built on a foundation of earlier experiments in animal models. This legacy traces back to the origins of transplantation in 1902, when Alexis Carrel pioneered surgical techniques allowing the successful anastomosis of blood vessels in dogs, a development enabling Ullman to perform the first successful canine renal transplants later that year. Animal models not only allowed clinicians to hurdle the technical barriers of transplantation, but they also proved vital to defining the immunologic basis of allograft rejection. For example, seminal observations by Peter Medawar using neonatal mice continue to shape current thoughts about the immunologic basis for tolerance. Additionally, nearly all immunosuppressive agents in clinical use were developed using animal models of transplantation, ranging from the demonstration by Calne and colleagues that 6-mercaptopurine (developed as azathioprine) could suppress rejection in a dog model of renal transplantation, to the

---

Transplant Immunology, First Edition. Edited by Xian Chang Li and Anthony M. Jevnikar.
© 2016 John Wiley & Sons, Ltd. Published 2016 by John Wiley & Sons, Ltd.
Companion website: www.wiley.com/go/li/transplantimmunology

most recently approved agent belatacept, which has undergone extensive testing in rodents and nonhuman primates (NHPs) prior to receiving FDA approval.

Despite the highly evolved status of organ and tissue transplantation, significant barriers persist that limit our ability to perform transplantation with optimal safety and efficacy. Animal models will undoubtedly continue to play a crucial role in overcoming these barriers. However, as transplantation science has progressed, it is evident that no animal models faithfully reproduce all features of clinical transplantation. Too often, investigators have used the most available model rather than the model best suited for a particular clinical question. In this chapter, we will first discuss the unique features of different experimental models of organ transplantation as well as how these features may make some models more suitable than others would for certain types of investigations. We will also provide examples of clinical problems in which experimental models have provided critical insights.

The need for animal models of transplantation

Technical, practical, and ethical factors limit the types of studies that can be performed in human transplant recipients. Thus, animal models remain essential for performing many basic investigations of transplant immunobiology as well as for testing new immunosuppressive strategies. However, the occasional failure of these experimental models to accurately predict clinical behavior has led many to question whether the role of these models would be diminished in the future. A prominent example where experimental transplant models failed to predict clinical results is illustrated by studies of the anti-CD154 antibodies in transplant survival. Extensive studies conducted in mice and NHPs demonstrated that anti-CD154 antibodies possessed potent immunosuppressive properties with limited adverse effects. Unexpectedly, clinical studies with anti-CD154 were halted due to thromboembolic events that were not predicted by either rodent or NHP preclinical studies. This experience aptly demonstrates that no animal model faithfully reproduces each of the key features of transplantation in humans, highlighting the importance of investigators to know the relative strengths and limitations of the different transplant models they employ in order to select the model best suited for the question of interest.

Choice of models—small animal models versus large animal models

In choosing the correct model, the first decision faced by investigators is the choice between small and large animal models. Small animal models usually employ rats or mice. Murine model systems offer numerous advantages. First, they are relatively inexpensive to purchase and house, facilitating the rapid performance of experiments with relatively large numbers of recipients. Secondly, a wide variety of inbred and congenic strains are available. Thus, it is possible to repeat experiments sequentially without the confounding changes brought about by varying degrees of genetic differences, particularly in the area of major histocompatibility complex (MHC). Furthermore, congenic markers allow the transfer of syngeneic cells, which is particularly useful for studies examining cell migration. The existence of inbred strains of mice has also facilitated the generation of genetically modified animals; these gene knockout and transgenic mice have fostered innumerable insights about the immune pathways involved in alloresponses. The vast array of antibodies, fusion proteins, and molecular reagents that are available in rodents complement these genetic approaches in rodents. These reagents can be used to identify cells *in vivo* or *in vitro*, block or enhance the function of specific pathways, or determine patterns of gene expression.

Despite these advantages, some potential limitations of small animal models must be considered in the design of experiments. First, their small size makes the transplantation of some organs technically challenging. Additionally, small animals possess a reduced number of lymphocytes relative to large animals and humans, translating into a reduced T cell repertoire diversity and a decreased T cell clone size. These two factors impact the strength and nature of alloresponses, potentially contributing to the different outcomes sometimes observed between transplants performed in humans and small animals. These differences between the T cell repertoires of mice and humans are further compounded by the standard practice of housing mice in pathogen-free environments. While this minimizes experimental variability introduced by viral infections and exposure to other pathogens, it also limits maturation of the T cell repertoire. The T cell repertoire of experimental mice is phenotypically and functionally naïve, whereas in mature humans and large animals, mature T cells comprise a significant proportion of the T cell repertoire. Others and we have shown that intentionally infecting mice prior to transplantation with a variety of viruses dramatically alters their response to a transplanted organ and can interfere with the induction of tolerance.

Another limitation of murine models is that donor-recipient strain combinations can have profound effects on the nature of the alloresponse and the outcome of transplantation. For example, in rats, some strains are known to be "low responders" that favor acceptance of transplanted organs. As well on the donor side, some strains of mice are considerably more susceptible to ischemia-reperfusion injury, which can directly alter inflammation and innate immunity that promotes alloresponses. Similarly, the host alloresponses may be dominated by Th1, Th2, or Th17 cells depending on the strain combinations chosen. A final consideration is that numerous physiologic differences exist between rodents and humans. As one example, rats are relatively resistant to calcineurin inhibitor toxicity, which must be considered in interpreting the results of studies of chronic allograft nephropathy. Combinations of these factors may result in significant differences in the outcome of transplant procedures in small animals and humans. For example, a short course of cyclosporine induces tolerance in "permissive" strains of rats and short-term blockade of costimulatory pathways such as CD28 or CD154 promotes long-term acceptance of some types of transplanted organs in mice. Neither of these therapeutic approaches is nearly as effective in humans undergoing transplantation.

Large animal models possess different advantages and limitations that largely complement those of small animal transplant models. While the relatively larger size of dogs, pigs, and NHPs increases the costs of transplantation and the complexity of caring for transplanted animals, their size is a relative advantage that has facilitated technical advances and refinements in surgical techniques necessary for successful transplantation in humans. In contrast to mice, factors that shape the current use of large animal models of transplantation include a more limited availability of genetically defined animals and a relatively meager supply of biologic agents for therapeutic use or for use as tools to dissect the alloimmune response. Additionally, almost all of these large animal models are outbred, introducing genetic variability into experiments. Selection of NHP donor-recipient pairings is particularly challenging due to the difficulty in typing macaque HLA loci and inbreeding within primate colonies, which has led to many experimental primates sharing MHC alleles. It is also true that social concerns for the welfare of large animals, particularly NHPs, have a greater impact on the design and conduct of studies as compared to small animals.

Considering these factors, large animal models are currently considered as a final pre-clinical step that is required to translate lab findings into clinical practice. No new immunosuppression drug or regimen would pass FDA scrutiny without these NHP trials. Xenotransplantation is another research field for which large animal models are uniquely suited. Due to size compatibility, transplantation of pig organs into NHP is the obvious choice for translational studies of xenotransplantation, although differences in the physiology of pig kidneys (erythropoietin species-specificity, altered phosphate handling, etc.) render them more than an immunologic challenge.

The development of belatacept illustrates the integration of small and large animal models of transplantation. Early murine transplant studies demonstrated that blockade of the CD28–CD80/CD86 pathways using a CTLA4-Ig fusion protein could dramatically prolong allograft survival. However, studies of kidney and islet transplantation demonstrated that unlike rodent models, monotherapy with CTLA4-Ig was insufficient to consistently prolong allograft survival in NHPs. This finding spurred the modification of CTLA4-Ig to increase its binding efficiency for CD80/CD86, ultimately leading to the development of belatacept, which was extensively tested in primate kidney transplant models. These large animal models laid the groundwork for subsequent successful human trials of belatacept, culminating in its FDA approval.

Choice of models—organs

Beyond choosing a small or large animal system, the choice of a specific organ to be transplanted must be well tailored to the experimental question at hand. One consideration is that experimental data clearly demonstrates a hierarchy of alloresponse strength in different transplanted organs, ranging from organs that are aggressively rejected (e.g., skin, lungs, and intestine) to those that may occasionally demonstrate even spontaneous tolerance (e.g., liver and kidney allografts). Although poorly explained, these organ-specific differences likely reflect variations in immunogenicity, vulnerability to injury, and ability to regenerate. These factors should be considered when selecting an experimental model. For example, the mouse model of kidney transplantation may not be well suited for studies of acute rejection, as, in some strain combinations (B6 to Balb/c), fully allogeneic kidney transplants can survive long-term in the absence of immunosuppression. The high rate of spontaneous acceptance needs to be factored into studies, often necessitating larger study numbers and longer observation times. Similarly, use of the mouse lung transplant model for studies of chronic injury and rejection are made more difficult by the intense immune response that results in early acute rejection.

All experimental transplant models require careful assessment of graft status, and the technique employed to accomplish this is fundamentally impacted by the choice of a model organ. Murine skin grafts, one of the simplest models, require only visual assessment of the graft. Technical considerations in other murine models (e.g., cardiac and intestine transplant) require grafts to be placed heterotopically without the removal of the primary organ. As such, the survival of the recipient is not dependent on the transplanted organ, rendering determination of graft function more difficult as it is limited to inspection (palpation of intra-abdominal heart grafts and visualization of the stoma for intestine grafts) and the review of histologic changes. The former is subjective and imprecise while the latter requires euthanizing experimental recipients, increasing the time and cost of experiments if graft function at multiple time-points is required. Other models such as kidney and islet transplantation can be performed in recipients who have undergone removal of the native organs (kidneys) or chemical ablation (islets). These models offer the advantage that graft status can be assessed by recipient survival as well as direct functional measurements (creatinine or blood glucose) in addition to histology. Kidney transplantation into fully nephrectomized recipient mice is technically very challenging. However, transplantation into recipients leaving a life supporting native kidney in place may subtly alter lymphocyte traffic and other responses that may alter results. Again, careful controls and recognizing the limitations imposed by all animal models is essential to transplant research.

Small animal transplant models (see Table 16.1)

Skin transplantation

Skin grafting has been widely used as a model of transplantation including its use in Peter Medawar's seminal studies of transplantation tolerance. Skin grafts are relatively quick and do not require the microsurgical skills necessary for other murine transplant models. Furthermore, skin is highly immunogenic and thus provides a stringent model, well suited for screening studies of new approaches to immunosuppression and mechanistic studies of the alloimmune response. Skin grafts are also ideal models for studies of tolerance, as the ability

Table 16.1 Small animal models of transplantation.

Organ/tissue	Species	Immunologic fate	Outcome measure	Common uses
Skin	Mouse	Acutely rejected (M, R)	Graft survival	Immunosuppression
				Mechanisms of rejection
				Tolerance
Heart	Mouse/rat	Acutely rejected (M, R)	Graft survival—contraction	Immunosuppression
			Histology	Mechanisms of rejection
				Tolerance
Kidney	Mouse/rat	Chronic rejection (M)	Recipient survival	Ischemia/reperfusion injury
		Acute rejection (R)	Function (Cr)	Immunosuppression
			Histology	Protective immunity
				Effect of brain death on graft
Intestine	Mouse/rat	Acutely rejected (M, R)	Histology (heterotopic)	Immunosuppression
			Recipient survival (orthotopic)	Mechanisms of rejection
				Ischemia/reperfusion injury
Liver	Mouse/rat	Spontaneously accepted (M)	Recipient survival	Ischemia/reperfusion injury
			Function (liver enzymes)	
		Acutely rejected (R)	Histology	

Continued

Table 16.1 Continued

Hepatocytes	Mouse	Acutely rejected	Graft function (hA1AT)	Immunosuppression Mechanism of rejection
Pancreas	Mouse	Acutely rejected	Graft/recipient survival	Rarely used
Islets	Mouse	Acutely rejected	Graft/recipient survival	Immunosuppression Mechanisms of rejection
Trachea	Mouse	Acutely rejected	Histology	Model of chronic rejection
Lung	Mouse/rat	Acutely rejected	Histology	Immunosuppression Mechanisms of rejection Interplay auto and lloimmunity Interplay viral and lloimmunity
Limb/CTA	Mouse/rat	Acutely rejected	Graft survival	Immunosuppression Mechanisms of rejection Tolerance

to easily apply a second third-party skin graft can confirm the donor-specific nature of unresponsiveness to the primary allograft. Unlike clinically transplanted organs, skin grafts are not primarily vascularized following transplantation. Whether this has an impact on the immune response is uncertain.

Heart transplantation

Heterotopic transplantation of hearts into the abdominal cavity of recipients is perhaps the most widely used experimental model of vascularized organ transplantation (Figure 16.1). Compared to other vascularized transplant models, it requires simpler microsurgical techniques. Allograft function can be serially assessed by palpation of the transplanted heart through the abdominal wall, as well as by histologic evaluation at the time of recipient sacrifice. The potential bias that comes with palpation alone in survival analyses makes observations by blinded scoring essential. As well, aortic pulsation may be transmitted to the transplanted heart to make interpretation more difficult. Similar to clinical

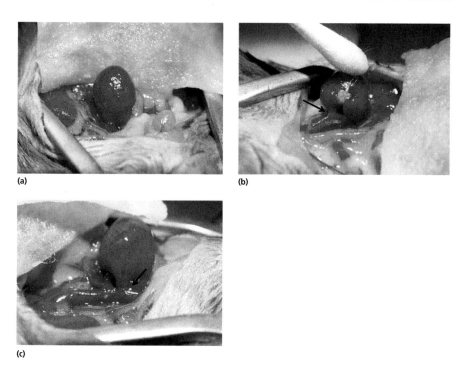

Figure 16.1 Mouse heterotopic heart transplant. (a) Mouse heart allograft, placed heterotopically in the abdomen of recipient mouse. (b) Black arrow indicates donor aorta (Ao) to recipient aorta (Ao) anastomosis. (c) Black arrow denotes donor pulmonary artery (PA) to recipient inferior vena cava (IVC).

transplants, heterotopic cardiac allografts can develop cardiac allograft vasculopathy that is evident on histology, making this a good model of chronic allograft rejection. Additionally, this model can be used in tolerance studies, as a second heart can be transplanted in a cervical location to assess tolerance to a primary intra-abdominal allograft. Again, while heart transplant has many advantages, the disadvantages of this technique include the subjectivity of allograft palpation, as well as the fact it is not a life-sustaining organ, which may alter the immunologic response.

Kidney transplantation

Kidney transplantation in small animals has been used to investigate ischemia/reperfusion injury, the impact of viral pathogens such as polyoma virus on the immune response, and the interplay between injury mediated by nephrotoxic agents and immune-mediated injury. Kidney transplantation in rats has been used with great success to examine the effects of brain death on organ injury. A major advantage of this model is the relative ease of performing bilateral native nephrectomies. Monitoring serum creatinine in this setting provides a simple, inexpensive and clinically applicable method for serially assessing graft function.

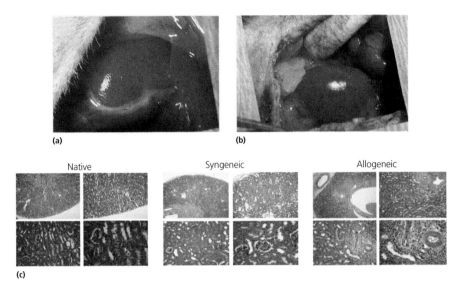

(a)   (b)

Native   Syngeneic   Allogeneic

(c)

Figure 16.2 **Mouse kidney transplant**. (a) Native kidney, (b) transplant kidney, and (c) histology of native, syngeneic, and rejecting allogeneic kidney transplant.

Partially offsetting this advantage is the technical difficulty of kidney transplantation in small animals and the relatively high technical failure rate related primarily to complications associated with the ureteral anastomosis. As mentioned earlier, in some strain combinations of mice, transplanted kidneys are not acutely rejected but undergo a chronic, immunologically mediated injury perhaps making this model better suited for studies of chronic injury as opposed to acute immune-mediated rejection (Figure 16.2).

Intestinal transplantation

As in kidney transplantation, intestinal transplantation in rodents, particularly mice, is technically challenging, limiting its widespread use as a transplant model. Although successful orthotopic intestinal transplantation in mice has been reported, heterotopic positioning of the graft is the more commonly used method (Figure 16.3). In this setting recipient nutrition and survival are independent of the transplanted graft. Graft assessment is largely dependent on histologic evaluation. Inspection of the stoma or quantification of the absorption of nutrients instilled via the stoma (i.e., maltose that is broken down to glucose by enzymes in the brush border of the intestine) has been used to gain more crude estimates of the graft status.

Lung and trachea transplantation

Similar to intestinal transplants, murine lung allografts are characterized by both major interactions with the external environment and the presence of secondary and tertiary lymphoid organs within the graft. These features make the lung

Stoma   Graft   Histology

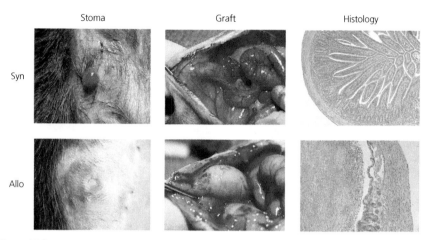

Syn

Allo

Figure 16.3 Mouse intestine transplant. Syngeneic and rejecting allogeneic mouse intestine transplant.

transplant model (as well as the intestinal transplant model) well suited for studies of cell migration and studies examining the interplay of infections and alloimmunity. Rodent models of lung transplantation also provided important insights into the interplay between alloimmunity and autoimmunity to antigens exposed by ischemic, infectious, and alloimmune-mediated injury. In contrast to whole lung transplant, tracheal transplant (usually heterotopic) has been widely employed as a model of chronic rejection, as it manifests many of the histologic findings of obliterative bronchiolitis. However, these models also have significant limitations including the fact that the grafts are not primarily vascularized; they are large airways being used to mimic a process that affects predominantly small airways, and they do not contain the same lymphoid structures as transplanted lungs.

Islet and pancreas transplantation

Although there are reports of whole organ pancreas transplantation being performed in rats and mice, these models are rarely used due to their technical difficulty. In contrast, rodent models of islet transplantation have been widely employed to investigate the immune response to allogeneic islets, nonimmune factors affecting islet engraftment, and the effect of the site of implantation on islet function. Islets may be implanted either under the kidney capsule or injected intra-portally into the liver, similar to the approach used clinically.

Liver and hepatocyte transplantation

Orthotopic liver transplantation is technically feasible in both rats and mice, although in most mouse models the graft does not receive arterial blood flow (Figure 16.4). In most strain combinations, mice accept fully allogeneic livers indefinitely even in the absence of immunosuppression, clearly limiting the utility of this model for investigating alloimmunity. In contrast to whole organ

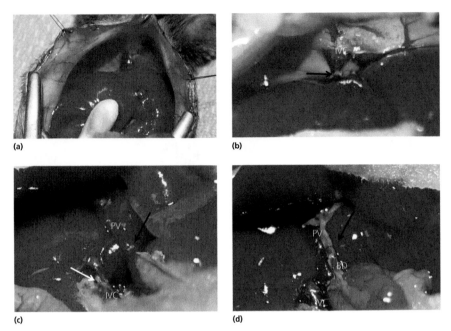

Figure 16.4 Mouse liver transplant. (a) Mouse liver allograft placed orthotopically in the abdomen of recipient mouse. (b) Suprahepatic inferior vena cava (IVC) anastomosis denoted by black arrow. (c) Infrahepatic inferior vena cava (IVC) anastomosis denoted by white arrow and portal vein (PV) anastomosis by black arrow. (d) Bile duct (BD) anastomosis with stent denoted by black arrow.

liver allografts, mice reject allogeneic hepatocytes (injected into the recipient spleen) in all strain combinations tested. Assessment of graft survival has been facilitated by the use of hepatocytes from transgenic donors that express human α-1 anti-trypsin (hA1AT). In this model decreases in serum levels of hA1AT reflect rejection.

Large animal transplant models

Three species predominate experimental use in large animal transplant models: dog, pig, and nonhuman primate. Each of these model organisms closely approximate the general physiology and basic anatomy of humans. The histology and timing of unmodified rejection is essentially equal to that seen in humans and the putative mechanisms of rejection involve similar networks of T cells.

Dogs were the most prevalently used species in early transplantation research, based mostly on their historical role in surgical training. Many of the technical issues related to vascular anastomoses were perfected in the canine model. Indeed, the first successful use of immunosuppressant (6-MP and azathioprine) was tested in the canine renal transplant model by Calne and colleagues. More recently, the use of dogs in experimental research has declined due in large part to social pressures to avoid the use of domesticated animals.

The porcine model has several advantages over both dog and nonhuman primates. First, there is little social pressure countering porcine research as society generally accepts their use for human consumption. In addition, techniques to produce genetically manipulated knockout and transgenic pigs have been developed. While early experiments in transplantation exclusively used outbred pigs, more recently David Sachs and colleagues have developed well-characterized inbred pigs homozygous for certain swine leukocyte antigen (SLA) loci. Pig organs have also become the primary source for experimental xenotransplantation. Porcine organs are ideal for xenotransplants as they have similar organ size to nonhuman primate recipients; the production of α-1,3-galactosyltransferase gene knockout pigs as well as pigs transgenic for various complement regulatory factors including human decay accelerating factor (CD55) or membrane cofactor protein (CD46) also facilitates the use of pig organs in xenotransplant experiments.

Nonhuman primates have become the principal model for pre-clinical studies in recent years. The burgeoning number of therapeutic monoclonal antibodies or fusion proteins has highlighted the importance of nonhuman primate experimental subjects, as many of these biologics have a high degree of human specificity, which preclude testing in other large animal models. Although some baboons have been used in xenotransplant studies, in general, macaques (cynomologous and rhesus) are the predominant nonhuman primate species currently employed in transplantation as they exhibit sufficient homology to humans, are small-sized, and relatively available for use. Ethical and legislative prohibitions prevent the use of chimpanzees in invasive transplant studies.

Kidney transplantation

Kidney transplantation is relatively commonly being performed in large animal models; particularly in nonhuman primates and pigs (Figure 16.5). In general, the transplanted kidney is life sustaining as most researchers perform bilateral native nephrectomies so that the monitoring of serum chemistries accurately reflects allograft function. In addition to the ease with which one can measure allograft function, access to histologic specimens via percutaneous needle biopsy is also feasible. Adequate donor tissue can be sampled serially and evaluated without the need for a major intervention. The model can be technically challenging and often requires microsurgical techniques limiting its use to those with surgical expertise. Technical complications include arterial or venous thrombosis, urine leak and ureteral stricture.

Islet and pancreas transplantation

With the resurgence of clinical islet transplantation, there has been an accompanying increase in the use of large animal models of islet transplantation. The most common models tend to use either nonhuman primates or dogs as recipients.

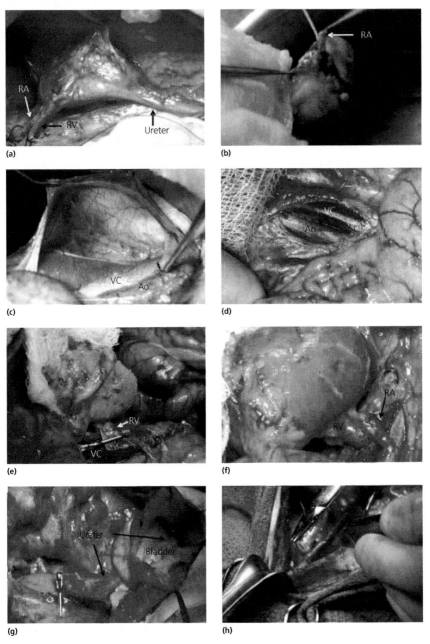

Figure 16.5 Nonhuman primate kidney transplant. (a) Donor kidney isolated on a pedicle consisting of the renal vein (RV), renal artery (RA) and ureter. (b) The donor kidney is excised and flushed with UW preservation solution. (c) A retroperitoneal pocket lateral to the vena cava (VC) is raised. (d) The recipient's VC and aorta (Ao) are prepared for anastomosis. (e) The venous anastomosis has been completed and the donor RV clamped to permit restoration of flow through the VC. (f) The completed vascular anastomoses consisting of end to side donor RV to VC and donor RA to aorta. (g) The bladder has been incised and the donor ureter passed through the retroperitoneal pocket and through the posterior wall of the bladder. (h) The bladder is closed in two layers.

Pigs (wild-type or genetically modified, e.g., Gal ko) are primarily used as donors for xenogeneic studies. The induction of diabetes in the recipient animal is usually accomplished chemically with beta cell toxins such as streptozotocin, but can also be achieved surgically via total pancreatectomy. In addition, there have been occasional reports using spontaneously diabetic animals as recipients. One advantage of the islet model is the diminished requirements for microsurgical techniques when compared to other large animal models. The donor islets can be transferred by intra-portal injection or by placement beneath the capsule of the liver, spleen or kidney. The latter technique provides a distinct advantage for serial examination of the islet allograft via percutaneous biopsy. Immunologically the islet model is probably somewhat less strenuous when compared to the other organ models, but it still provides a robust enough immune response that unmodified rejection occurs within days. The source of donor islets, particularly for xenogeneic studies, includes unmodified adult islets, cultured neonatal islet clusters and islets from genetically manipulated donors. Allograft function is generally assessed with serum glucose measurements, interval glucose tolerance testing, and measurement of c-peptide. While whole organ pancreas transplantation has been performed and reported in large animal models, as an experimental model it has been limited.

Heart transplantation

While one of the most famous cases of xenotransplantation involved the use of a baboon heart into a newborn human infant, "Baby Fae," the application of xenogeneic transplantation has remained challenging and elusive. Orthotopic cardiac transplantation in large animal models, mainly nonhuman primates and dogs, was used extensively in the development of surgical techniques for clinical cardiac transplantation, but is now rarely used. Instead, most researchers employ the heterotopic heart model using various species including dogs, nonhuman primates, and pigs. The final location of the donated organ can be in the neck or the abdomen. As in small animal models, function is generally assessed by palpation, and EKG monitoring although left ventricular pressure monitoring by telemetry via implantable detectors has also been used. The transplanted heart is not life sustaining nor load dependent and some argue as such, it does not accurately recapitulate the clinical scenario. One additional disadvantage of this model is the need for open cardiac biopsy to obtain allograft tissue for histology although theoretically endomyocardial biopsies could be performed as in humans.

Intestinal transplantation

Intestinal transplantation testing in animals was instrumental in the development of the surgical techniques that are now employed. However, small bowel transplantation today as an experimental model is much less common and reports in literature are sporadic. Dogs and pigs continue to be used as recipients more often than nonhuman primates. In addition to models of isolated intestinal transplantation, models of combined liver-intestine or multivisceral transplantation have been reported, which provide insights into the immunologic "protection" afforded to intestinal allografts by liver transplants.

Use of experimental models to address key challenges

Ischemia-reperfusion injury (IRI)
Some of the first uses of animal models of organ transplantation involved the search for better means of preserving organs. Syngeneic rodent transplant models played a critical role in the development of the University of Wisconsin (UW) organ preservation solution. Rodent models continue to play an important role in the field of organ preservation by allowing the assessment of how supplements added to preservative solutions can prolong organ storage times. Again, the caveat is the significant strain variation in responses to ischemia (i.e., B6 being more susceptible than Balb/c).

Acute rejection
Animal models have been widely used to define the mechanisms of acute rejection and guide the development of therapeutic agents. These models have provided definitive evidence of the central role of T cells in acute rejection. Indeed, rejection is often abrogated when murine transplant recipients are treated with T cell-depleting monoclonal antibodies (such as anti-CD3, anti-CD4 or anti-CD8) or when immunodeficient mice (SCID, RAG$^{-/-}$, or TCR-knockout) are used as recipients. Rodent models of transplantation have also been used to define the contributions of key costimulatory pathways, cytokines, chemokines, and cytolytic effector molecules to the process of acute rejection. Rodent models of transplantation were critical in demonstrating that disruption of costimulatory pathways (including CD28, OX40L, 4-1BB, CD154, CD70, and ICOS), chemokine signaling pathways (including CCR5, CCR7, CXCL9, CXCL10, and CXCR3) and cytokines (including IFNγ, IL-5, IL-10, and IL-12) alters the development of acute rejection of heart or kidney transplantation. Conversely, the critical role of FoxP3$^+$ regulatory T cells (Tregs) in preventing allograft rejection was also documented in a series of antibody-depletion and adoptive transfer experiments using murine models of transplantation.

Chronic rejection
Chronic allograft rejection is a dominant factor limiting the lifespan of transplanted organs. Rodent transplant models are ideal for studying chronic rejection, as this process is dramatically accelerated in many small animal transplant systems compared to human transplants. The most widely used model to study chronic renal injury is the transplantation of a minor MHC mismatch kidney from a Fischer 334 rat into a Lewis rat. When a short course of cyclosporine is added, this regimen reliably reproduces progressive and chronic injury,

although in this model injury results from both the alloimmune response and cyclosporine toxicity. While the ready availability of genetically manipulated mice and mouse monoclonal antibodies makes the use of mice in experimental studies of chronic injury appealing, use of mice in studies of chronic kidney allograft injury have been limited by both the technical challenges of this model and concerns about whether murine renal transplants accurately recapitulate alloresponses in human renal allografts (since many of these mouse kidney transplants are spontaneously accepted). Other experimental models of chronic alloresponses include heterotopic tracheal transplants in mice (which develop a bronchiolitis obliterans-like lesion). Limitations of this model are that it uses a large airway to model a small airway disease process, it is not primarily vascularized, and there is no interplay between environmental antigens and the trachea, unlike in clinical lung transplant. To address these concerns, rat and, subsequently, mouse models of orthotopic lung transplantation have been developed. These were employed to explore the impact of autoimmunity on antigens such as collagen type V on alloresponses, as well as the role of viral-induced epithelial injury on the development of bronchiolitis obliterans.

Animal models of cardiac allograft vasculopathy (CAV) are also commonly used to study chronic rejection. Although rat models of CAV (usually LEW-to-F344) have been described, most of these systems have used mouse strain combinations in which acute injury is minimized by limiting MHC disparity. Examples include MHC class II (bm12-to-B6) and MHC class I (bm1-to-B6) mismatched strain combinations. Despite many similarities in the histologic appearance of allograft injury between human CAV and injury patterns in these rodent models, concern has been voiced that these models represent injury mediated by blunted acute effector mechanisms rather than distinct mechanisms responsible for chronic injury in humans.

Composite tissue allotransplantation (CTA)

Rodent, large animal, and NHP models have been developed to investigate the immunologic response, functional recovery, and technical feasibility of CTA. The most widely used CTA model for the study of tolerance induction is that of limb transplantation. Experimental models of limb transplantation, as well as face transplantation, have been developed in rodents, swine, and NHPs. While tolerance-inducing regimens, usually comprising transient immunosuppression together with a source of donor bone marrow, have been effective in some rodent models, these regimens have been largely ineffective in promoting tolerance in large animal and NHP CTA models.

Tolerance

Experimental animal models of transplant tolerance have provided both key mechanistic insights and unrealized clinical expectations. Experimental models of transplantation have definitively demonstrated roles for deletion, regulation or suppression, anergy potentially leading to apoptosis, and ignorance in the induction and/or maintenance of tolerance. Three experimental approaches have been devised that attempt to exploit the natural process of thymic deletion (central tolerance) in a clinically applicable design. The first is the intrathymic administration of donor antigen in combination with depletion of peripheral lymphocytes. This strategy effectively induces tolerance to islet or heart allografts in rats and mice, but it is ineffective in NHP, perhaps due to the decline in thymic function with age. A different approach that also exploits central deletion is transplantation of a thymokidney in MHC mismatch pigs. When combined with a short course of cyclosporine and depletion of peripheral T cells, thymokidneys that were created by placing fragments of minced donor thymus under the renal capsule experienced long-term survival in the absence of immunosuppression.

A third strategy using central deletion as a means of promoting tolerance is to create a state of hematopoetic "mixed chimerism." Studies by David Sachs and colleagues found that nonmyeloablative conditioning of recipients could be coupled with a transplant of donor bone marrow cells to create this mixed chimerism, in which there is persistence of hematopoetic cells of both donor and recipient origin. Establishment of mixed chimerism in recipients promoted indefinite acceptance of allografts from donors of the same strain, even once immunosuppression is fully weaned. Mixed chimerism has been extended to murine, porcine, NHP and now human transplant recipients. However, unlike mouse models of transplantation where long-term survival of allografts is associated with persistence of high levels of mixed hematopoietic chimerism following the cessation of immunosuppression, in NHPs chimerism is transient even in those with long-term survival of allografts. This suggests that different mechanisms may be responsible for tolerance in rodent and NHP transplant recipients.

In addition to central mechanisms, peripheral mechanisms of tolerance exist that deal with autoreactive T cells that escape the thymus. Peripheral mechanisms of tolerance include anergy and peripheral deletion and regulation. Animal experimental models have demonstrated that these peripheral mechanisms of tolerance can be exploited through either blockade of costimulatory pathways necessary for alloreactive T cell activation or through adoptive transfer of *ex vivo* expanded Tregs, both of which have been successful strategies for tolerance induction in a variety of murine transplant models.

Unfortunately, current animal models of transplantation have significant limitations that prevent the direct extrapolation of their results to clinical transplantation. Of note, strategies such as the intrathymic administration of donor antigen or transient blockade of important costimulatory pathways have failed to promote tolerance in NHPs and humans as was routinely observed in rodents. Expanding regulatory cells has proven an effective means of generating tolerance to allografts in rodents, but to date has not been successfully exploited in NHPs or humans. Although mixed chimerism induction has allowed human transplant recipients to be weaned off immunosuppression in small clinical trials, even this approach seems to confer less robust tolerance in NHPs and humans than in rodents. Several factors contribute to the increased difficulty of tolerance induction in these large animal models, specifically the greater representation of memory T cells in NHPs and humans, the greater diversity of T cell repertoire in these large animal transplant models and the fact that (unlike experimental transplants), donors for human clinical transplants are usually brain dead and have a highly inflammatory milieu. Assuming that a future goal of experimental animal models of transplantation is to more accurately predict the outcome of tolerance-promoting strategies in human transplant recipients, investigators will need to modify the existing models to address some or all of these factors.

Summary and future directions

Animal models have played, and will almost certainly continue to play a critical role in identifying barriers to successful transplantation and evolving new strategies to increase the success of clinical transplantation. However, it is also readily apparent that animal models often fail to accurately reproduce key features of the response of humans to transplanted organs. As the field of transplantation moves forward, it will be necessary to identify those features responsible for the discrepant outcome of transplantation in animal models and humans. The following three examples highlight the areas in which refinement of models would increase their utility as preclinical tools.

Models of B cell mediated injury and "humoral" immunity

The role of B cells and alloantibodies in transplantation is being increasingly recognized as a cause of both early and late allograft injury. Currently, most interventions to avoid or treat antibody-mediated rejection (such as treatment with IVIG or proteosome inhibitors) are tested in human transplant recipients rather than experimental animal systems. In fact, there is a paucity of animal models of hyper-acute rejection mediated by alloantibodies. In many rodent models, transfer of memory B cells or even the direct transfer of alloantibody (in the form of serum from immunized mice or monoclonal antibodies targeting donor MHC molecules) fails to provoke acute antibody-mediated rejection. This may be due to the relatively low titer of alloantibodies in wild-type mice. These studies are also crippled by the absence of effective B-cell depleting antibodies in mice, similar to rituximab (anti-CD20) in humans. The development of animal transplant models that more closely reflect the important role of B cells and alloantibodies in transplantation would provide an important tool for developing strategies to protect allografts from antibody-mediated injury.

MHC typing in NHP

Despite the critical role that NHP studies play in bridging basic and clinical research, there has been a stunning lack of knowledge regarding the degree of relatedness and MHC-matching amongst transplant pairs. While rodent, canine, and to some extent porcine (SLA-defined miniature swine) models have detailed data regarding MHC disparity and genetics, experimental NHP transplant studies typically rely on mixed lymphocyte cultures and rudimentary MHC typing assays to determine relatedness between donor and recipient pairs. This lack of detailed knowledge has contributed to the variability seen when results from new therapies are compared between investigators or when successful outcomes in the monkey have not accurately predicted outcomes in humans.

Nonhuman primate immunogenetics (particularly macaque immunogenetics) are quite complex. Although macaque MHC shares significant sequence homology with human HLA, the rhesus MHC region is significantly larger than its human counterpart mostly due to gene duplication and expansion in the mamu B alleles. While humans express six different class I alleles from their two chromosomes (two each of HLA-A, B, and C), a heterozygous rhesus theoretically may express 8 mamu-A alleles and up to 28 mamu B alleles. Until recently, sophisticated typing techniques to reliably determine an individual animal's MHC type, thereby providing an accurate map of disparity between donor and recipient pairings, have been unavailable. Developments of microsatellite typing techniques and pyrosequencing breakthroughs have allowed much more accurate determination of MHC disparity between NHP transplant pairings. These new techniques have permitted directed breeding strategies where defined MHC haplotype matching can be achieved. A sample pedigree and inheritance map is shown in Figure 16.6a. Not surprisingly the level of MHC disparity significantly impacts outcomes. The degree of MHC disparity and its impact on the alloresponse is highlighted in Figure 16.6b and c. The vigor of alloresponses is enormously impacted by the degree of MHC matching between donors and recipients, as shown in a rhesus renal transplant model using different donor-recipient pairings. Adoption of better techniques to define MHC-matching in large animal transplant models will allow for a more accurate representation of MHC disparity in future NHP studies. This information may allow for models that more reliably predict outcomes when therapies are translated to patients.

Humanized mice

An "ideal" experimental model would accurately recapitulate human immune responses while offering the benefits of a rodent transplant system (e.g., low costs, easy scalability, and access to abundant monoclonal antibodies). Efforts to develop such a model have culminated in the production of so-called "humanized mice." These mice are generated by reconstituting NOD-*scid* IL2r γ^{null} or NOD-Rag1^{null} IL2r γ^{null} (which lack the IL-2 receptor gamma chain and have resulting profound defects in T, B, NK cell and dendritic cell function) with

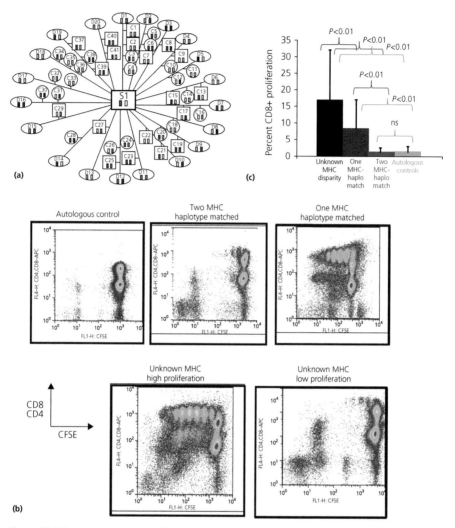

Figure 16.6 Impact of Improved NHP MHC typing. (a) Pedigree and inheritance map for one macaque sire (S1), his mating pairs and his offspring. (b and c) CFSE mixed lymphocyte reaction analysis reveals increasing alloproliferation (loss of CFSE fluorescence) with increasing MHC disparity.

human peripheral blood cells, G-CSF-mobilized human stem cells, umbilical cord blood, or fetal liver cells. These human cells expand in their murine host, preserving the unique diversity of the human T cell repertoire. These humanized mice have been used successfully to model alloresponses in skin and islet transplants, confirm the tolerogenic effects of *ex vivo* expanded Tregs, and study human autoimmune diseases.

However, this model is not without disadvantages. First, the recipients are prone to develop human antimouse graft-versus-host disease (GVHD), usually around 30 days post-bone marrow transplant. This model therefore is of limited use in the study of chronic rejection. Additionally, some critical growth factors for immune cell function display some degree of species specificity. For example, mouse BLyS cannot support human B cell survival, potentially altering B cell and humoral rejection responses.

The development of these humanized mice epitomizes the critical role played by animal transplant models in transplantation research. Both basic transplant immunology and highly translatable clinical studies fundamentally employ animal models to test hypotheses. Success in these studies is largely dictated by proper selection of both the animal system (large vs. small animal) and the correct organ type to transplant. A comprehensive knowledge of the relative advantages and disadvantages of these different systems is paramount to ensure successful studies as well as clinical translations.

Further reading

D Bedi, Animal models of chronic allograft injury: contributions and limitations to understanding the mechanism of long-term graft dysfunction. Transplantation 2010;90:935.

P Boros, Organ transplantation in rodents: novel applications of long-established methods. Transplant Immunol 2007;18:44

K. Brown, What have we learned from experimental renal transplantation?. Nephron Exp Nephrol 2010;115: e9.

L Cornell, Kidney Transplantation: Mechanisms of rejection and acceptance. Annu Rev Pathol Mech Dis 2008;3:189.

B Ekser, Overcoming the barriers to xenotransplantation: prospects for the future. Expert Rev Clin Immunol 2010;6:219.

L Kean, Transplant tolerance in non-human primates: progress, current challenges and unmet needs. Am J Transplant 2006;6:884.

C Kingsley, Transplantation tolerance: lessions from expt rodent models. Transpl Int 2007;20:828.

E Kuo, Animal models for bronchiolitis obliterans syndrome following human lung transplantation. Immunol Res 2005;33:69.

X.C Li, The significance of non–T-cell pathways in graft rejection: implications for transplant tolerance. Transplantation 2010;90:1043.

Long E, Wood KJ, Regulatory T cells in transplantation: transferring mouse studies to the clinic. Transplantation 2009;88(9):1050–1066.

K.A Newell, Experimental models of small bowel transplantation. Curr Opin Organ Transplant 2003;8:209.

R Pierson, Current status of xenotransplantation and prospects for clinical application. Xenotransplantation 2009;16:263.

M Sato, Translational research: animal models of obliterative bronchiolitis after lung transplantation. Am J Transplant 2009;9:1981.

M Siemionow, Advances in the development of expt CTA models. Transpl Int 2010;23:2.

M Sykes, Hematopoietic cell txpl for tolerance induction: animal models to clinical trials. Transplantation 2009;87:309.

M Thomsen, Reconstitution of a human immune system in immunodeficient mice: models of human alloreaction in vivo. Tissue Antigens 2005;66:73.

J Wehner, Immunological challenges of cardiac transplantation: the need for better animal models to answer current clinical questions. J Clin Immunol 2009;29:722.

Y Zhai, Liver ischemia and reperfusion injury: new insights into mechanisms of innate-adaptive immune-mediated tissue inflammation. Am J Transplant 2011;11:1563.

B Zhang, Mouse models with human immunity and their application in biomedical research. J Cell Mol Med 2009;13:1043.

Index

Page numbers in *italics* refer to illustrations; those in **bold** refer to tables

Transplant Immunology, First Edition. Edited by Xian Chang Li and Anthony M. Jevnikar.
© 2016 John Wiley & Sons, Ltd. Published 2016 by John Wiley & Sons, Ltd.
Copyright ® American Society of Transplantation 2016.
Companion website: www.wiley.com/go/li/transplantimmunology